Contents

Letter to Student 2
Letter to Parent/Guardian 3

Chapter One: What Is the SSAT? 4–6
What Is the Purpose of the SSAT? 4
How Is the SSAT Designed? 4
The SSAT Is Reliable 4
The SSAT Is a Norm-Referenced Test 4–5
The SSAT Is a Standardized Test 5
Should I Guess on the SSAT? 5
SSAT Practice Online 6

Chapter Two: About the Middle Level SSAT 7–60
The Sections of the Middle Level Test 7–9
Test Overview 9
The Writing Sample 10–11
The Quantitative Section 12–13
    Sample Questions: Quantitative 14–39
The Reading Comprehension Section 40–43
    Sample Questions: Reading Comprehension 44–46
The Verbal Section: Synonyms 47–48
    Prefixes, Suffixes, and Roots 49–52
    Sample Questions: Synonyms 53
The Verbal Section: Analogies 54–56
    Sample Questions: Analogies 57–58
Summing It Up 59

Chapter Three: Scores 61–66
What Your Scores Mean 61
Formula Scoring 61
The Score Report 62–64
Supporting the Test Taker 65

Chapter Four: The Character Skills Snapshot 67–72
What Is the Character Skills Snapshot? 67
How Was the Snapshot Designed? 67
What Does the Snapshot Measure? 68
The Sections of the Snapshot 69
How Is the Snapshot Administered? 69
Is the Snapshot Reliable? 69
The Snapshot Is a Norm-Referenced Assessment 70
Strategies for Taking the Snapshot 70
Sample Questions 71–72

Middle Level Practice Tests 73–214
Trying Out the Middle Level SSAT 74–76
Practice Test I 77–112
Practice Test II 113–144
Practice Test III 145–178
Practice Test IV 179–214

Evaluating Your Middle Level SSAT 215–230
How Did You Do? 216
Scoring the Practice Tests 216
Computing Your Raw Score 217
Answer Keys 218–229
Equating Raw Scores to Scaled Scores 230

Dear Student,

The private schools you'll find in books and on television may be interesting, but the real world of private schools is even more amazing. You're reading this guide because you think that a private school might be right for you, and you're ready for one of the first steps—taking the SSAT.

This book will introduce you to the SSAT, the test format, and what to expect on test day. It contains practice tests that resemble the one you'll be taking, plus preparation tips to help you do your best on the SSAT and the Character Skills Snapshot.

The Official Study Guide for the SSAT gives you:

- The definition of an admission test
- Descriptions of the test sections
- Test-taking strategies
- An introduction to the Character Skills Snapshot
- Plenty of sample questions to practice
- Full-length practice tests
- Information about how to interpret scores
- Registration and test day checklists

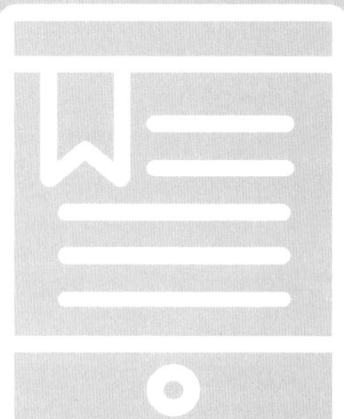

What won't you find here? Shortcuts, tricks, or gimmicks. This is the only book that contains sample questions and practice tests written by the SSAT assessment developers and the test-taking strategies to help you to do your best. There are some valuable hints that can help you stay on track and maximize your time. But when it comes down to it, getting familiar with the test format and scoring, studying specific content types covered on the test, and solving practice questions is the best way to prepare for the SSAT. In addition to this guide, we offer an online practice program (see page 6) that provides even more sample questions, subject quizzes, and practice tests.

The path ahead will be exciting, and you'll probably learn a lot about yourself on the way. We wish you the best as you prepare for this journey, which will help you apply to a school that can change your life.

The SSAT Assessment and Research Team

Dear Parent/Guardian,

Congratulations on your decision to explore a private school education for your child! For more than 50 years, the SSAT has been the gold standard in admission testing for the world's best private schools. We know that the process of taking the SSAT can be fraught with concern and distress, but it needn't be. The SSAT is one important step on the road to a private school education—one that should be taken seriously but should not cause undue anxiety.

The results of admission testing, while integral to an application, are just one of many factors considered by admission officers when determining if your child and their school make a great match. The degree of emphasis placed on scores depends on the school and on other information, such as transcripts and teacher recommendations. For the vast majority of schools, students with a wide range of SSAT scores are admitted.

Here are a few questions that admission officers contemplate when reviewing an applicant's scores:

- Are the scores consistent with the student's academic record?
- Do the scores highlight areas of academic strength or weakness?
- How do these scores compare with those of other students in the applicant pool?
- How do these scores compare with students who have enrolled over the last few years?

As a parent, you have a central role to play in helping your child to succeed in the school application process by reminding them to keep the SSAT in perspective. Schools are most interested in finding out who your child is.

There are a multitude of sources, both on- and offline, that promise to prepare your child for the SSAT and increase their test score. This guide was created by our assessment development team to support your child's preparation efforts with legitimate information, test-taking strategies, and practice tests. We encourage you to use this guide as your official source for SSAT preparation and the Character Skills Snapshot information. On page 65, we share tips to help you support your student during this important preparation for taking the SSAT.

Finally, we urge you to use the ssat.org website not only to register your child for the test but also to access information about the private school application process, search for schools that are the right fit for your child and your family, and take advantage of our online practice program.

We hope *The Official Study Guide for the Middle Level SSAT* will help to make your family's experience of testing and applying to private school a successful and enjoyable one.

Good luck!

Heather Hoerle

Heather Hoerle, Executive Director & CEO, The Enrollment Management Association

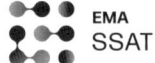

Chapter One: What Is the SSAT?

What Is the Purpose of the SSAT?

The SSAT is designed for students who are seeking entrance to private schools worldwide. The purpose of the SSAT is to measure the verbal, quantitative, and reading skills students develop over time—skills that are needed for successful performance in private schools. The SSAT provides private school admission professionals with meaningful information about the possible academic success of potential students at their institutions, regardless of background or experience.

The SSAT is not an achievement test, although knowledge of a certain amount of mathematical content is necessary to do well on the quantitative sections of the test. Your most recent classroom math test, for example, was probably an achievement test: Your teacher designed it to evaluate how much you know about what was covered in class. The SSAT, on the other hand, is designed to measure the overall verbal, quantitative, and reading skills you have acquired, instead of focusing on your mastery of specific course materials.

SSAT tests are not designed to measure other characteristics, such as initiative, resilience, or teamwork, that may contribute to your success in school. As a complement to the SSAT's assessment of cognitive skills, we also offer the Character Skills Snapshot, which was designed expressly to measure character skills valued by private schools. To learn more about the Snapshot, visit ssat.org/snapshot.

How Is the SSAT Designed?

The SSAT measures three constructs: verbal, quantitative, and reading skills that students develop over time, both in and out of school. It emphasizes critical thinking and problem-solving skills that are essential for academic success.

The overall difficulty level of the SSAT is built to be at 50%–60%. This means that on average, 50%–60% of the test takers can answer the questions correctly. The distribution of question difficulties is set so that the test will effectively differentiate among test takers, who vary in their level of abilities.

To develop the SSAT, The Enrollment Management Association convenes content committees composed of content experts and independent school teachers. The committees write and review items, and reach consensus regarding the appropriateness of the questions. Questions judged to be acceptable after the committee review are then pretested and analyzed. Questions that are statistically sound are selected and assembled into test forms.

The SSAT Is Reliable

The SSAT is a highly reliable test. A test is said to have a high reliability if it produces similar results under consistent conditions. Reliability coefficients range between 0.00 (no reliability) and 1.00 (perfect reliability). On the SSAT, the scaled-score reliability is higher than 0.90 for both the verbal and quantitative sections, and is approaching 0.90 for the reading section.

The SSAT Is a Norm-Referenced Test

A norm-referenced test interprets an individual tester's score relative to the distribution of scores for a comparison group, referred to as the *norm group*. The SSAT norm groups consist of all the test takers (same grade) who have taken the test for the first time on one of the Standard SSAT administrations in the United States and Canada typically within the past three years.

The SSAT reports percentile ranks, which are referenced to the performance of the norm group. For example, if you are in the sixth grade, and your percentile rank on the March 2019 verbal section is 90%, it means that verbal scores for 90% of all the other sixth-grade students (who have taken the test for one of the SSAT administrations in the United States and Canada, typically using the most recent three years of data) fall below your scaled score. The score report also provides this information for your grade. The same scaled score on the SSAT may have a slightly different percentile rank from year to year, and the SSAT percentile ranks should not be compared to those of other standardized tests because each test is taken by a different group of students.

In contrast, a criterion-referenced test interprets a test-taker's performance without reference to the performance of other test takers. For example, your percent correct from a classroom math test would be 90% if you answered 90% of the questions correctly. Your score is not referenced to the performance of anyone else in your class.

It is important to remember that the SSAT norm group is highly competitive. You are being compared to all the other students (same grade) who are taking this test for admission into private schools. Most important to remember is that the SSAT is just one piece of information considered by schools when making admission decisions, and for the vast majority of schools, students with a wide range of SSAT scores are admitted.

The SSAT Is a Standardized Test

The SSAT is scored in a consistent (or standard) manner. It adheres to standard administration processes and practices, based on the testing mode. The reported (or scaled) scores are comparable and can be used interchangeably, regardless of which test form was taken. A scaled score of 500 on the June 2018 Middle Level verbal section, for example, has the same meaning as the scaled score of 500 from the December 2016 Middle Level verbal section, although the forms are different. This score interchangeability is achieved through a statistical procedure referred to as *score equating*. Score equating is used to adjust for minor form difficulty differences, so that the resulting scores can be compared directly.

Standard also refers to the way in which tests are developed and administered. A standard process for writing, testing, and analyzing questions—before they ever appear on a live test—is used. Further, The Enrollment Management Association provides precise instructions to be followed by qualified and experienced test administrators from the moment students are admitted to the test center until the time of dismissal. Any deviations from the uniform testing conditions are reported in writing by the test administrator to The Enrollment Management Association. Of course, a student may apply for testing accommodations, but the processes and procedures for the test's administration remain the same.

Should I Guess on the SSAT?

The answer is: It depends. You must first understand how the test is scored.

When your test is scored, you will receive one point for each correct answer. One quarter of a point is deducted for each incorrect answer. You will not receive or lose points for questions that are not answered. If you guess, try guessing only when you can eliminate at least one (but optimally more than one) answer choice.

A few things to keep in mind:

Keep moving. Do not waste time on a question that is hard for you. If you cannot answer it, make a note of it, skip over it, and move on. If you have time left in the section, go back to it then.

Take care with each question. You receive one point for each correct answer, no matter how hard or easy the questions are. Approach all questions with equal consideration; don't risk losing points to careless errors on seemingly easy questions.

Check your answer sheet. If taking the test on paper, mark your answers in the correct row on the answer sheet. Be especially careful if you skip questions.

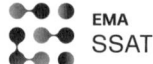
EMA
SSAT

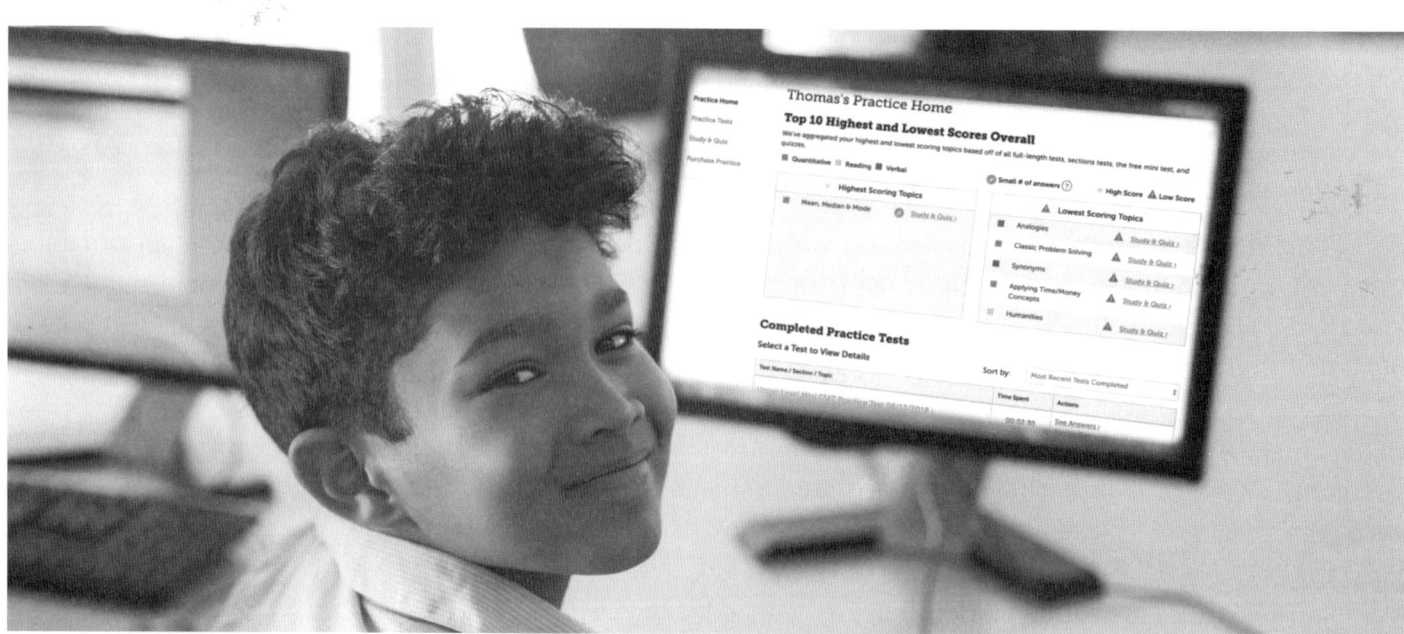

SSAT Practice Online

A perfect complement to this study guide, our online practice program is another official source for SSAT practice. SSAT Practice Online helps you prepare by providing practice questions similar to those appearing on the SSAT, and identification of exactly which topics you should focus on before you test. Other key features include: section tests that target quantitative, reading, or verbal practice; SSAT topic quizzes with tips on how to answer each question; and study tools. Visit ssat.org/practice or access the program via your SSAT account.

ssat.org/practice

Students who use a fee waiver for the SSAT registration are also provided free access to the online practice program for both the Middle and Upper Level SSAT, as well as free access to the Admission Academy, a resource to help families navigate the K–12 private school admission process.

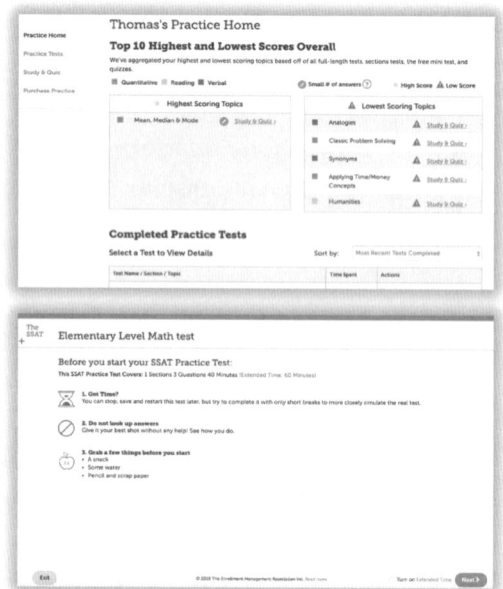
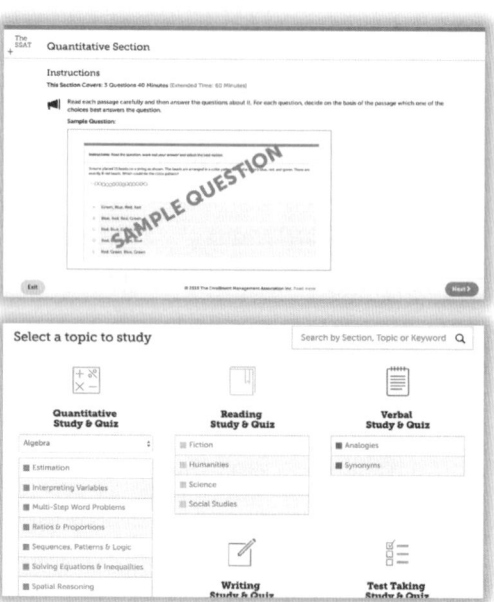

Chapter Two: About the Middle Level SSAT

The SSAT is a multiple-choice test that consists of verbal, quantitative (math), and reading comprehension sections. The Middle Level SSAT is for students in grades 5–7 and provides admission officers with an idea of your academic ability and "fit" in their schools. The best way to ensure that you perform as well as you possibly can on the SSAT is to familiarize yourself with the test. Understanding the format of the test and reviewing practice questions will make your test-taking experience easier. You'll feel more comfortable with the test and be able to anticipate the types of questions you'll encounter.

This chapter will introduce you to the kinds of questions you'll see on the Middle Level SSAT and the best ways to approach them. The sample questions that accompany each section will give you some practice before you tackle the practice tests that appear later in the book. In this chapter, we will also provide test-taking strategies that you should know when you take the Middle Level SSAT. The bonus of these test-taking strategies is that they may also help you perform better on the tests you take in school!

The Middle Level Test Consists of FIVE Sections:

1. Writing Sample

Number of questions: You will have a choice between two prompts.

What it measures: Your ability to think creatively, organize your ideas, and write clearly

Scored section: No, but it is provided to the schools you have selected to receive your score reports.

Time allotted: 25 minutes

Topics covered: Students are given a choice between two prompts: one prompt is a creative story-starter, and the other is a personal essay question. You choose one of them and write either a story or an essay.

> The best way to make sure you perform as well as you can on the SSAT is to become familiar with the test.

2. Quantitative (Math) Section

Number of questions: 50, divided into two parts

What it measures: Your ability to solve quantitative problems

Scored section: Yes

Time allotted: 30 minutes for the first 25 problems, and 30 minutes for the final 25 problems

Topics covered: These problems test quantitative reasoning based on the following topics:

Number Concepts and Operations
- Decimals: Place Value and Computations
- Fractions: Concepts and Computations
- Integers: Computations and the Order of Operations
- Arithmetic Word Problems
- Number Sense/Number Theory
- Ratio, Rate, Proportions, and Converting Units
- Percent
- Estimation
- Sequences and Patterns

Continued on next page

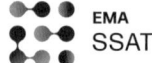

2. Quantitative (Math) Section *(continued)*

Geometry
- Length, Perimeter, Area
- Radius, Diameter, Circumference
- Surface Area and Volume
- Angle Relationships
- Visual/Spatial Reasoning

Algebra
- Simple Linear Equations and Inequalities
- Algebra Word Problems
- Simplification and Evaluation of Algebraic Expressions

Data Analysis
- Graphs and Tables
- Mean, Median, Mode, Range
- Probability
- Counting

3. Reading Comprehension Section

Number of questions: 40

What it measures: Your ability to understand and interpret what you read

Scored section: Yes

Time allotted: 40 minutes

Topics covered: There are 7–8 reading passages, each 150–350 words in length. Passages are either literary or expository. Literary passages are drawn from works of fiction or poetry. Expository passages examine topics in the fields of science, social science, history, or the humanities.

Literary passages:
- Fiction
- Poetry

Expository passages:
- Science
- Social Science
- History
- Humanities (art, music, etc.)

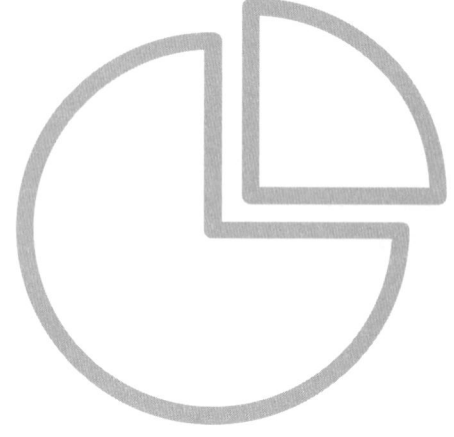
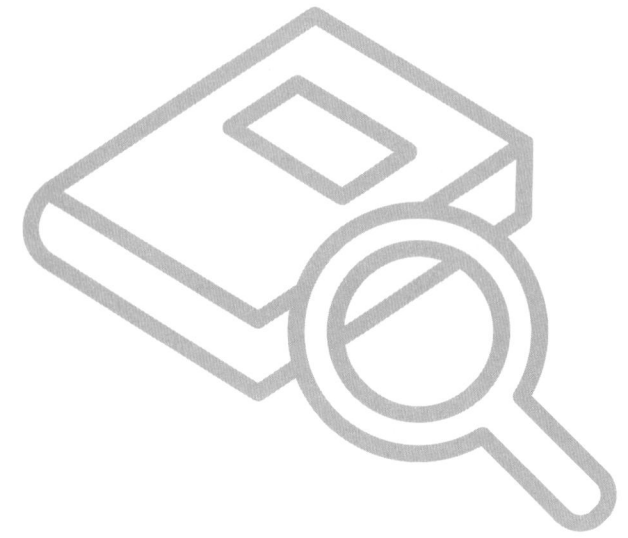

4. Verbal Section

Number of questions: 60 (30 synonyms and 30 analogies)

What it measures: Your ability to understand the meanings of words and to recognize relationships between words with different meanings

Scored section: Yes

Time allotted: 30 minutes

Topics covered: These questions ask you to identify words that have similar meanings (synonyms) and identify word pairs that have similar relationships (analogies). The words tested are nouns, adjectives, or verbs.

5. Experimental Section

Number of questions: 16

What it measures: Verbal, reading comprehension, and quantitative skills

Scored section: No

Time allotted: 15 minutes

Topics covered: Six verbal, five reading, and five quantitative questions

Testing accommodation students requiring 1.5x time are not required to complete the experimental section.

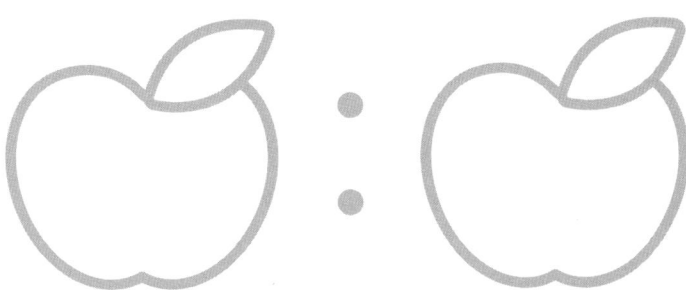

Test Overview

Section	Number of Questions	Time Allotted to Administer Each Section
Writing Sample	1	25 minutes
Break		10 minutes
Section 1 (Quantitative)	25	30 minutes
Section 2 (Reading)	40	40 minutes
Break		10 minutes
Section 3 (Verbal)	60	30 minutes
Section 4 (Quantitative)	25	30 minutes
Section 5 (Experimental)	16	15 minutes
Totals	**167[1]**	**3 hours, 10 minutes**

[1]*Of the 167 items including the writing sample, 150 questions are scored.*

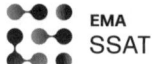

1. The Writing Sample

At the beginning of the test, you will be asked to write a story or an essay in 25 minutes. You'll have a choice between two prompts. You may choose either (A) a creative story-starter or (B) a personal essay question.

What Are the Directions for the Writing Sample Section of the Test?

Schools would like to get to know you better through a story you tell or an essay you write. If you choose to write a story, use the sentence presented in A to begin. Make sure that your story has a beginning, middle, and end. If you choose to write a personal essay, base your essay on the topic presented in B. Please fill in the circle next to your choice.

How Are the Writing Prompts Presented?

EXAMPLE:	(A) All I wanted was a glass of water. *or* (B) What is your favorite game to play? Describe the game and tell why you like it.

Just the Facts
The Writing Sample

Number of questions: You will have a choice between a creative story-starter and a personal essay question.

What this measures: Your ability to organize your ideas and write clearly.

Scored: No, but it is delivered to the schools you have selected to receive your score reports.

Time allotted: 25 minutes

Tips for Getting Your Writing Sample Started

Read the prompts carefully. Take a few minutes to think about them and choose the one you prefer. Then, organize your thoughts before you begin writing (scrap paper for organizing your thoughts will be provided when you test). Be sure that you use a pencil, that your handwriting is legible, and that you stay within the lines and margins. Remember to be yourself and let your ideas flow or your imagination soar!

Remember: Your writing sample will not be scored. Schools use it to get to know you better through your writing.

If you want to change what you have written, erase or neatly cross out the words you want to eliminate and add the new words so they are legible. Two line-ruled pages will be provided. Don't feel as if you have to fill both pages—just do your best to provide a well-written story or essay.

Practice Writing Samples

This book includes practice writing sample prompts, which can be found at the beginning of the practice tests. Each sample includes directions, two prompts, and an answer sheet similar to the one you'll receive during the actual test.

Writing Sample Test-Taking Strategies

1. While creativity is encouraged, remember that the admission officers in the schools to which you are applying will be reading your writing sample. Be sure that your story or essay is one that you would not hesitate to turn in for a school assignment.

2. Read both prompts. Take a couple of minutes to think about what you're going to write. You can use your scrap paper to organize your thoughts.

3. Choose a working title for your story or essay. The Middle Level SSAT doesn't require a title, but a working title will help to keep you on track.

4. If you choose to write a story, make sure it has a beginning, a middle, and an end. Get involved in your story. Give details, describe emotions, and have fun.

5. If you choose to write a personal essay, be sure to provide interesting details to illustrate your thoughts and feelings.

6. If there's time, check your writing for spelling, punctuation, and grammatical errors.

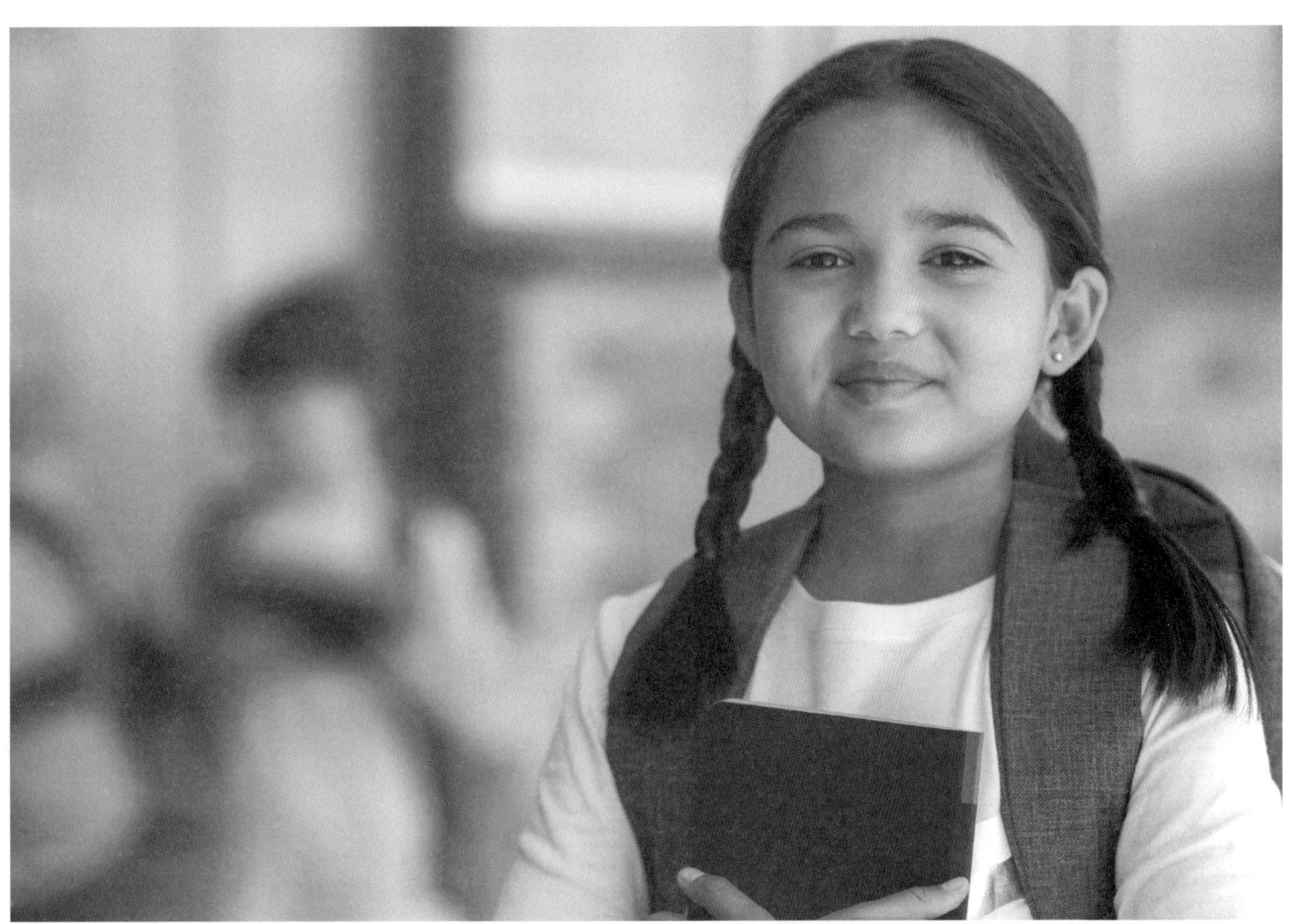

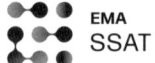

2. The Quantitative Section

The quantitative (math) section of the Middle Level SSAT measures your knowledge of number concepts and operations, geometry, algebra, and data analysis. The words used in SSAT problems refer to mathematical operations with which you are already familiar.

What Are the Directions for the Quantitative Section on the Test?

Following each problem in this section, there are five suggested answers. Work each problem in your head, in the blank space at the right of the page if taking the test on paper, or on scrap paper if taking the test on the computer. Then, look at the five suggested answers and decide which one is best.

How Are the Quantitative Problems Presented?

> **Just the Facts**
> The Quantitative Section
>
> **Number of questions:**
> 50, divided into two parts
>
> **What this measures:**
> Your ability to solve problems involving number concepts and operations, geometry, algebra, and data analysis
>
> **Scored session:** Yes
>
> **Time allotted:**
> 30 minutes for the first 25 problems and 30 minutes for the final 25 problems

Many of the problems that appear in the quantitative section of the Middle Level SSAT are structured in mathematical terms that directly state the operation you need to perform to determine the best answer choice.

EXAMPLE:	$13, 25, 37, \ldots.$ In the sequence above, 13 is the first number. Each number after the first is 12 more than the preceding number. What is the 10th number in the sequence? (A) 35 (B) 49 (C) 72 (D) 121 (E) 133 **The correct answer is (D).**

Other questions are structured as word problems. A word problem often does not specifically state the mathematical operation or operations that you will need to perform in order to determine the answer. In these problems, your task is to carefully consider how the question is worded and the way the information is presented to determine what operations you will need to perform.

EXAMPLE:	Kathy and Donna ran a 3-mile race. Kathy ran the first 2 miles at a speed of 6 miles per hour and walked the last mile at a speed of 4 miles per hour. Donna ran the first mile at a speed of 10 miles per hour and walked the last 2 miles at a speed of 3 miles per hour. Which of the following statements is true about the timing of the race for Kathy and Donna? (A) Kathy finished the race 3 minutes ahead of Donna. (B) Kathy finished the race 4.5 minutes ahead of Donna. (C) Kathy finished the race 11 minutes ahead of Donna. (D) Donna and Kathy finished the race at the same time. (E) Donna finished the race 4 minutes ahead of Kathy. **The correct answer is (C).**

Quantitative Test-Taking Strategies

1. Read the problem carefully.

2. Pace yourself. Try not to spend too much time on one problem.

3. Be sure to use the "Use This Space for Figuring" area of your test book to do the scratch work. If taking the computer-based test at a Prometric test center, you will receive a white board. If taking the SSAT at Home, you may use scrap paper.

4. Always check to see if you have answered the question asked in the problem. Circling what's being asked can be helpful, so you don't mistakenly choose the wrong answer.

5. Watch for units of measure. Be sure you know and understand in which unit of measure the answer is supposed to be given.

6. Draw pictures. If you find that a problem is complicated, you can draw a graph, diagram—anything that will allow you to understand what the problem is asking.

7. Remember to mark your answers on the answer sheet if taking the test on paper! If your problem is solved in the test book but not marked on the answer sheet, it will not be counted.

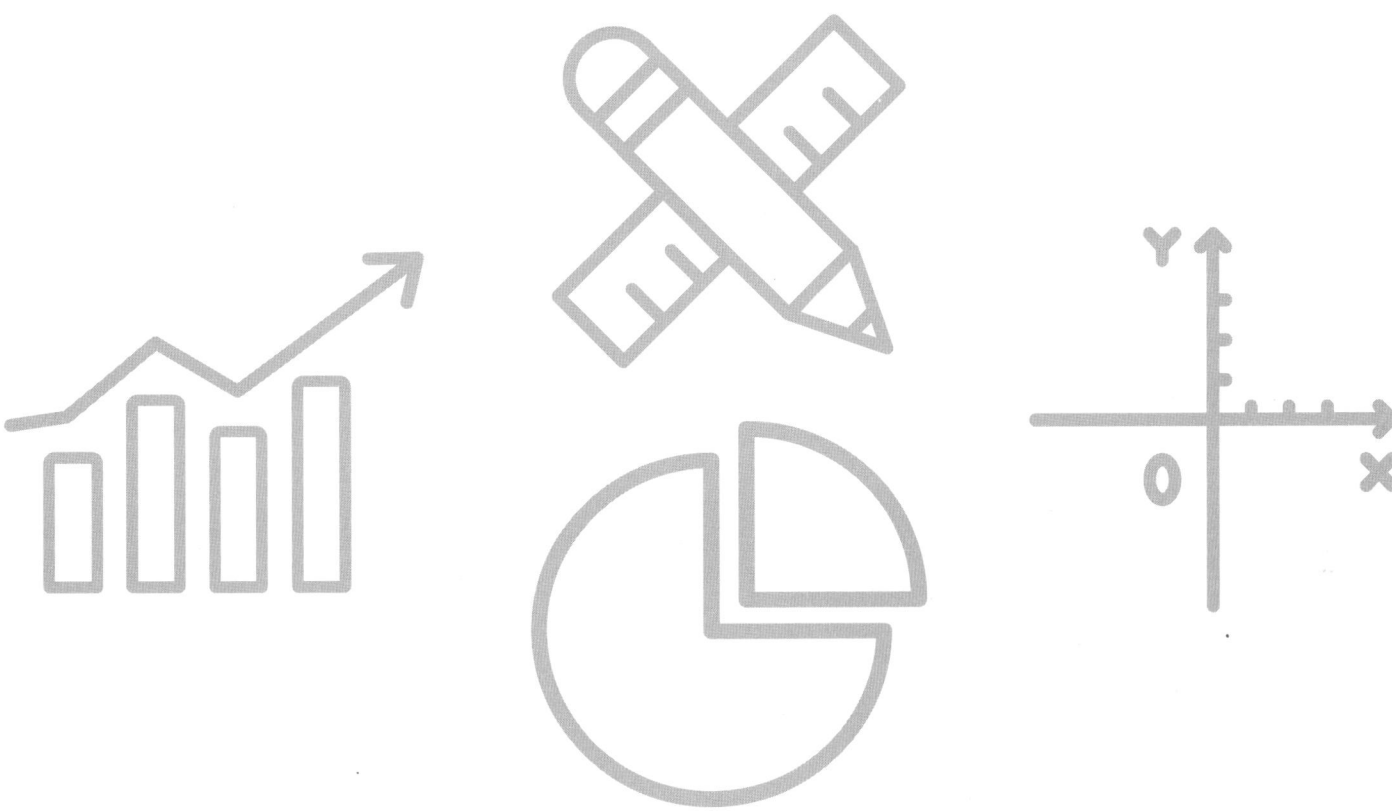

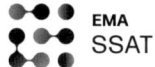

Sample Questions: Quantitative

On the following pages, you will find sample questions from these topics: Number Concepts and Operations, Geometry, Algebra, and Data Analysis. Each topic may also include a brief overview of related content.

Section I: Number Concepts and Operations

In this section, you will find 26 sample questions and related overviews of mathematics concepts in Number Concepts and Operations. The answers to these 26 questions are located at the end of this section.

Decimals: Place Value and Computations

> A **decimal point**, which is placed after a whole number, separates the whole-number part of a number from its fractional part. Nonzero digits to the left of the decimal point indicate values greater than one. Digits to the right of the decimal point indicate values less than one.
>
> For example:
> Thirty-five and six-tenths is 35.6 written as a decimal number.
> 426.98 has 4 hundred**s**, 2 ten**s**, 6 ones, 9 ten**ths**, and 8 hundred**ths**.
>
> $426.98 = 400 + 20 + 6 + \frac{9}{10} + \frac{8}{100}$

1. Which of the following decimals is greatest?
   - (A) 1.065
   - (B) 1.654
   - (C) 1.645
   - (D) 1.456
   - (E) 1.045

2. Calculate: 1.1 + 20.3 + 4.97
   - (A) 7.11
   - (B) 8.10
   - (C) 25.47
   - (D) 26.37
   - (E) 71.1

3. What is the value of 2.1 × 1.5 ?
   - (A) 315
   - (B) 31.5
   - (C) 3.15
   - (D) 0.315
   - (E) 0.0315

Fractions: Concepts and Computations

A **fraction** has a numerator and a denominator. The numerator is above the fraction bar, and the denominator is below the fraction bar. The numerator is divided by the denominator.

For example: $\frac{1}{2}$ ↔ numerator
↔ denominator

When fractions have the same numerator but different denominators, the one with the larger denominator is smaller.

For example: $\frac{1}{8} < \frac{1}{4}$

4. The figure shown is divided into 6 triangles of equal size. The shaded region represents what fraction of the figure?

    (A) $\frac{1}{4}$

    (B) $\frac{1}{3}$

    (C) $\frac{1}{2}$

    (D) $\frac{2}{3}$

    (E) $\frac{5}{6}$

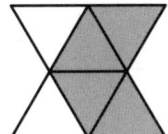

5. Compute: $\frac{3}{2} + \frac{2}{5} - \frac{1}{4}$

    (A) $\frac{1}{5}$

    (B) $\frac{4}{11}$

    (C) $\frac{27}{20}$

    (D) $\frac{4}{3}$

    (E) $\frac{33}{20}$

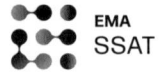

6. What is the value of $\frac{5}{3} \div \frac{3}{2}$?

    (A) $\frac{1}{10}$
    (B) $\frac{9}{10}$
    (C) $\frac{10}{9}$
    (D) $\frac{5}{2}$
    (E) 10

$$\frac{5}{3} \div \frac{3}{2} = \frac{5}{3} \times \frac{2}{3} = \frac{10}{9}$$

Integers: Computations and the Order of Operations

Integers are the whole numbers and their opposites: …, −2, −1, 0, 1, 2, …

The whole numbers are **positive** integers, and their opposites are **negative** integers. The number 0 is neither positive nor negative.

The **order of operations** is the method for simplifying an expression with multiple operations. The order is as follows:

1) Perform operations inside grouping symbols.

2) From left to right, find the value of powers.

3) From left to right, multiply and divide.

4) From left to right, add and subtract.

7. Compute: $8 \times (-4) \times (-3)$ BEDMAS
    (A) −32 32×3
    (B) −27 $= 96$
    (C) 27
    (D) 32
    (E) 96

8. Simplify: $6 + (-1)^2 \times (8 + 2)$
    (A) 15 $6 + ^{-1} \times 10 =$
    (B) 16 $6 + -10$
    (C) 50
    (D) 60
    (E) 70

Arithmetic Word Problems

Arithmetic word problems have real-life settings and can be solved using one or more steps. Some may require you to add, subtract, multiply, or divide the numbers in the problem. Others may require different problem-solving strategies like working backwards, drawing a picture, guessing and testing, or making a pattern.

9. Yesterday Jaaron ran 5.1 kilometers. Today he ran 2.01 kilometers. How many more kilometers did he run yesterday than today?
    (A) 3.11
    (B) 3.09
    (C) 2.09
    (D) 1.50
    (E) 1.40

10. Karen has $\frac{1}{3}$ of a pie and Mara has $\frac{1}{4}$ of the pie. What is the total fraction of the pie that Karen and Mara have?
    (A) $\frac{1}{6}$
    (B) $\frac{1}{2}$
    (C) $\frac{7}{12}$
    (D) $\frac{5}{6}$
    (E) $\frac{4}{3}$

11. A bookstore receives a shipment of 120 books. Of the books, $\frac{1}{3}$ are hardcover, and the rest are paperback. Of the paperback books, $\frac{3}{4}$ are fiction. How many paperback fiction books are in the shipment?
    (A) 20
    (B) 30
    (C) 60
    (D) 80
    (E) 90

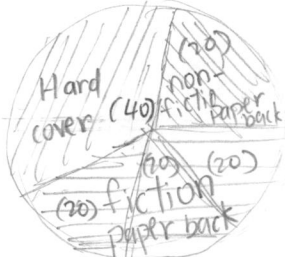

12. An elevator in a building is currently on floor 21. After the elevator goes up 8 floors, down 5 floors, then up 4 floors, on which floor will the elevator be located?
    (A) 9
    (B) 14
    (C) 20
    (D) 28
    (E) 30

    21+8−5+4=
    29−5+4=
    24+4=28

Number Sense / Number Theory

A **factor** of a number n is any integer that divides exactly into the number n. The number n is **divisible** by each of its factors. A **prime number** p is any integer with exactly <u>two</u> factors: 1 and p. An **even number** is an integer with the digit 0, 2, 4, 6, or 8 in the ones place. An **odd number** is an integer with the digit 1, 3, 5, 7, or 9 in the ones place.

13. Which of the following is divisible by 15?
    (A) 159 ✗
    (B) 225 ✓
    (C) 415
    (D) 560
    (E) 663 ✗

14. Which of the following is the least common multiple of 18, 24, and 60?
    (A) 6
    (B) 72
    (C) 120
    (D) 360
    (E) 720

15. How many prime numbers are between 30 and 60?
    (A) Seven
    (B) Eight
    (C) Nine
    (D) Ten
    (E) Eleven

    2, 3, 5, 7, 11, 13, 17, 19 ...
    31, 37, 41, 43, 47, 53, 57

16. If k is an odd number, which of the following is an even number?
    (A) k + 2
    (B) k – 10
    (C) 3k + 1
    (D) 4k – 1
    (E) k(k + 4)

17. Which of the following is NOT a factor of 60 × 33?
    (A) 12
    (B) 20
    (C) 36
    (D) 40
    (E) 55

Ratio, Rate, Proportion, and Converting Units

> A **ratio** compares one quantity with another quantity by division. When two ratios are equal, they form a **proportion**. A ratio that compares quantities with different units of measure (for example, miles per hour) is called a **rate**. A ratio can be expressed in several ways.
>
> For example, the ratio 5 to 10 can also be expressed as $\frac{5}{10}$ or 5:10.

18. A school reports a student-to-teacher ratio of 6:1. How many students does the school have, if there are 45 teachers in the school?
    (A) 285
    (B) 270
    (C) 225
    (D) 151
    (E) 51

19. A train traveled 100 miles from City W to City X in 2 hours. The train then traveled 120 miles from City X to City Y in 80 minutes. What was the average speed, in miles per hour, at which the train traveled from City W to City Y?
    (A) 53
    (B) 66
    (C) 70
    (D) 73
    (E) 80

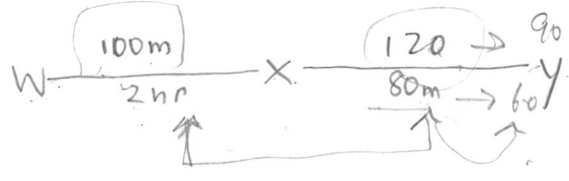

20. A length of 100 meters is closest to which of the following lengths, in inches? (1 inch is approximately equal to 2.5 centimeters.)

   (A) 40
   (B) 250
   (C) 400
   (D) 2,500
   (E) 4,000

Percent

Percent (%) is a ratio that compares a number to 100 by division.

For example, $\frac{40}{100}$ = 40%. The number 3 is 75% of 4 because $\frac{3}{4} = \frac{75}{100}$ = 75%.

21. Two friends went out to lunch and split the cost equally. The meal's cost was $20.40. Tax is an additional 5% on the meal's cost. The friends decide to leave 20% of the meal's cost (not including tax) for a tip. How much will each friend spend on the meal?

   (A) $10.33
   (B) $12.64
   (C) $12.75
   (D) $21.42
   (E) $25.50

22. After changing the number 20 by a certain percent, the result is 50. Which of the following represents this percent change?

   (A) A decrease of 40%
   (B) An increase of 30%
   (C) An increase of 60%
   (D) An increase of 150%
   (E) An increase of 250%

Estimation

> Estimation problems can be presented in either a real-life or an abstract setting. When solving an estimation problem, round the numbers as close to the given number as possible. It may be to your advantage to look at the answer choices first before you begin to round numbers.

23. Of the following, which is closest to 110.2 × 39.998 ?

    (A) 8,000
    (B) 4,400
    (C) 4,000
    (D) 3,300
    (E) 3,000

24. Each morning from Monday through Friday, Mr. Ruiz travels 19.8 miles to work. After work, he travels 10.1 miles to a local gym. Then he travels home a distance of 9.9 miles. Of the following, which is closest to the total number of miles Mr. Ruiz travels Monday through Friday?

    (A) 100
    (B) 150
    (C) 200
    (D) 250
    (E) 300

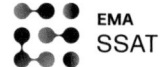

Sequences and Patterns

For sequence problems, the pattern for generating the sequence will be stated. You may be asked to find a number or a figure in the patterns, or be given a number in the sequence and asked which term it is.

25. The first number in a sequence is 2, and the second number in the sequence is 5. Each number after the second is the product of the two preceding numbers. What is the sum of the first four numbers of the sequence?

    (A) 12
    (B) 50
    (C) 67
    (D) 500
    (E) 840

26. The first three figures in a geometric pattern are shown. The area of the first figure is 1. The area of each figure after the first is half the area of the preceding figure. What is the area of the 6th figure?

    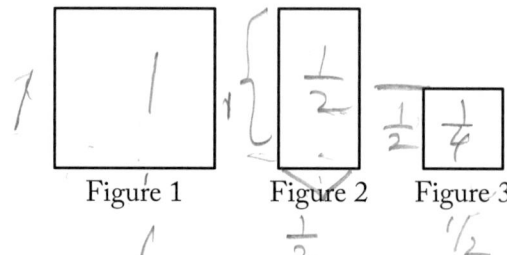
    Figure 1   Figure 2   Figure 3

    (A) $\frac{1}{32}$

    (B) $\frac{1}{16}$

    (C) $\frac{1}{10}$

    (D) $\frac{1}{8}$

    (E) $\frac{1}{6}$

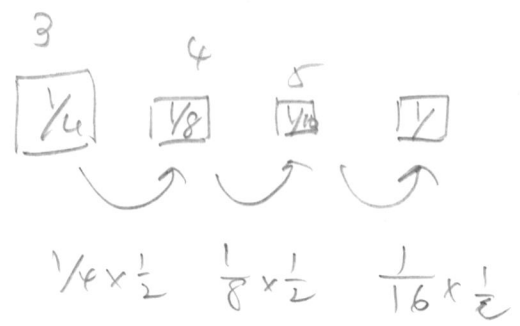

Answer Key
Section I: Number Concepts and Operations

1. **Answer (B) 1.654**

2. **Answer (D) 26.37**

      1.1
     20.3
   + 4.97
   ────
    26.37

3. **Answer (C) 3.15**
   Multiply without decimals: $21 \times 15 = 315$
   2.1 has 1 decimal place.
   1.5 has 1 decimal place.
   so, 2.1×1.5 has two decimal places:
   $315 \rightarrow 3.15$

4. **Answer (D) $\frac{2}{3}$**
   $\frac{4}{6} = \frac{2}{3}$

5. **Answer (E) $\frac{33}{20}$**
   The least common multiple of 2, 4, and 5 is 20.
   $\frac{3}{2} = \frac{30}{20}; \frac{2}{5} = \frac{8}{20}; \frac{1}{4} = \frac{5}{20}$
   $\frac{30}{20} + \frac{8}{20} - \frac{5}{20} = \frac{33}{20}$

6. **Answer (C) $\frac{10}{9}$**
   $\frac{5}{3} \div \frac{3}{2} = \frac{5}{3} \times \frac{2}{3} = \frac{10}{9}$

7. **Answer (E) 96**
   $8 \times -4 = -32; -32 \times -3 = 96$

8. **Answer (B) 16**
   $6 + (-1)^2 \times (8 + 2)$
   $6 + 1 \times 10 = 6 + 10 = 16$

9. **Answer (B) 3.09**

     5.10
   − 2.01
   ────
     3.09

10. **Answer (C) $\frac{7}{12}$**
    The lowest common denominator is
    $\frac{1}{3} \times \frac{4}{4} = \frac{4}{12}; \frac{3}{4} \times \frac{3}{3} = \frac{3}{12}$ *(correction: $\frac{2}{3} = \frac{8}{12}$... as shown: $\frac{1}{3} = \frac{4}{12}; \frac{1}{4} = \frac{3}{12}$)*
    $\frac{4}{12} + \frac{3}{12} = \frac{7}{12}$

11. **Answer (C) 60**
    There are $\frac{2}{3} \times 120 = 80$ paperback books.
    Of those, $\frac{3}{4} \times 80 = 60$ are fiction.

12. **Answer (D) 28**
    $21 + 8 - 5 + 4 = 29 - 5 + 4 = 24 + 4 = 28$

13. **Answer (B) 225**
    Numbers that are divisible by 15 are divisible by 3 and by 5. Only 225, 415, and 560 are divisible by 5. Of these three numbers, only 225 is also divisible by 3.
    So 225 is divisible by 15.

14. **Answer (D) 360**
    $18 = 2 \times 3 \times 3$
    $24 = 2 \times 2 \times 2 \times 3$
    $60 = 2 \times 2 \times 3 \times 5$
    So, the LCM of 18, 24, and 60 is
    $(2 \times 2 \times 2) \times (3 \times 3) \times 5 = 8 \times 9 \times 5 = 360$.

Answer Key
Section I: Number Concepts and Operations (continued)

15. **Answer (A) Seven**

    There are seven prime numbers between 30 and 60. They are 31, 37, 41, 43, 47, 53, and 59.

16. **Answer (C) $3k + 1$**

    Odd times odd gives an odd number, so $3k$ is odd. Odd plus odd gives an even number, so $3k + 1$ is even.

17. **Answer (D) 40**

    $60 \times 33 = (2 \times 2 \times 3 \times 5) \times (3 \times 11)$
    $= 2 \times 2 \times 3 \times 3 \times 5 \times 11$

    Of the choices, $40 = 2 \times 2 \times 2 \times 5$, which has one more 2 in its prime factorization than 60×33, so 40 is not a factor of 60×33.

18. **Answer (B) 270**

    $\dfrac{\text{students}}{\text{teachers}} = \dfrac{6}{1} = \dfrac{x}{45}$

    $6(45) = 1(x)$
    $270 = x$

19. **Answer (B) 66**

    Average speed $= \dfrac{\text{total distance}}{\text{total time}}$

    2 hours = 120 minutes
    120 minutes + 80 minutes = 200 minutes
    200 minutes $= \dfrac{200}{60}$ hours $= \dfrac{10}{3}$ hours

    $\dfrac{100 \text{ mi} + 120 \text{ mi}}{\frac{10}{3} \text{ hr}} = \dfrac{220 \text{ mi}}{\frac{10}{3} \text{ hr}}$

    $= 220 \times \dfrac{3}{10}$

    = 66 miles per hour

20. **Answer (E) 4,000**

    1 meter = 100 centimeters
    100 m = 10,000 cm

    $\dfrac{10{,}000 \text{ cm}}{x \text{ in}} = \dfrac{2.5 \text{ cm}}{1 \text{ in}}$

    $x = \dfrac{10{,}000}{2.5} = \dfrac{10{,}000}{25} = 4{,}000$

21. **Answer (C) $12.75**

    Tip: $0.2 \times \$20.40 = \$4.08$
    Tax: $0.05 \times \$20.40 = \$1.02$
    Total: $\$20.40 + \$5.10 = \$25.50$
    Cost per friend: $\$25.50 \div 2 = \$12.75$

22. **Answer (D) An increase of 150%**

    The number 20 increases 30 units to 50, which is represented by a percent increase of

    $\dfrac{30}{20} = \dfrac{150}{100} = 150\%$

23. **Answer (B) 4,400**

    110.2×39.998 is approximately $110 \times 40 = 4{,}400$.

24. **Answer (C) 200**

    $19.8 \approx 20$ miles; 10.1 miles ≈ 10 miles; 9.9 miles ≈ 10 miles; $20 + 10 + 10 = 40$ and $40 \times 5 = 200$

25. **Answer (C) 67**

    The first four numbers of the sequence are 2, 5, 10, 50. The sum is $2 + 5 + 10 + 50 = 67$.

26. **Answer (A) $\dfrac{1}{32}$**

    Following the pattern, the first 6 figures have areas $1, \dfrac{1}{2}, \dfrac{1}{4}, \dfrac{1}{8}, \dfrac{1}{16}, \dfrac{1}{32}$. So, the area of the 6th figure is $\dfrac{1}{32}$.

Section II: Geometry

For this section, you will find 10 sample questions and related overviews of mathematics concepts in Geometry. Geometric figures such as polygons, circles, or solids may appear in these questions. The answers to these 10 sample questions are located at the end of this section.

Length, Perimeter, and Area

Perimeter is the distance around a two-dimensional figure.
Area is the number of square units inside a two-dimensional figure.

For example:
In the square shown,
Perimeter = 4(5) = 20 units
Area = 5(5) = 25 square units

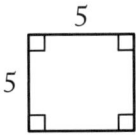

27. What is the perimeter of the triangle shown?

    (A) 21.9 cm
    (B) 19.4 cm
    (C) 18.3 cm
    (D) 15.8 cm
    (E) 12.2 cm

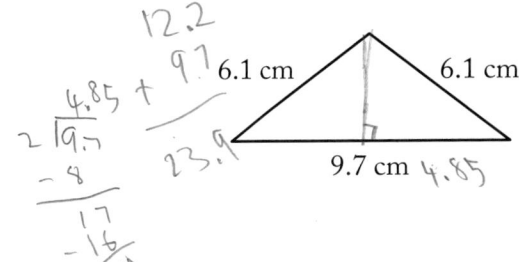

28. A diagram of a field is shown. What is the area of the field, in square feet?

    (A) 37,000
    (B) 30,000
    (C) 15,000
    (D) 700
    (E) 500

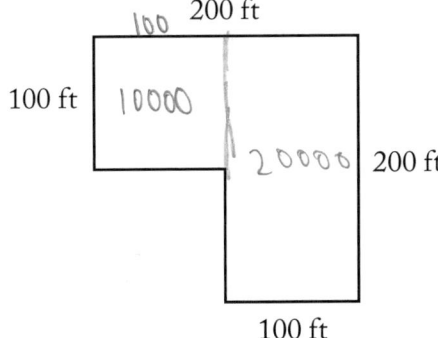

Radius, Diameter, and Circumference

The **radius** of a circle is a line segment with one endpoint at the center of the circle and the other endpoint on the circle. The **diameter** of a circle is a line segment that passes through the center of the circle and has endpoints on the circle. The **circumference** of a circle is the distance around the circle.

The radius r, diameter d, circumference C, and area A of a circle are all related by the formulas shown in the box.

$$d = 2r \quad C = 2\pi r$$
$$A = \pi r^2 \quad C = \pi d$$
$$\pi \approx 3.14 \text{ units}$$

For example, in the circle shown with center C, line segments $\overline{AC}, \overline{BC},$ and $\overline{CD}$ are each a radius of the circle. Line segment $\overline{BD}$ is a diameter of the circle. If $BC = 10$, then $r = 10$, $d = 20$, $C = 20\pi$, and $A = 100\pi$.

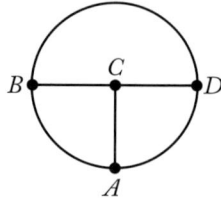

29. The figure shown represents the wheel on a model with center S. If the wheel has made 5 complete revolutions, and $RT = 11$cm, then, of the following, which is the best estimate for the distance traveled by the wheel?

    (A) 55 cm
    (B) 110 cm
    (C) 165 cm
    (D) 220 cm
    (E) 330 cm

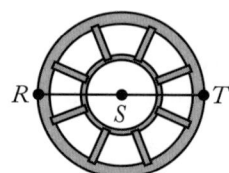

30. For the circle shown with center Q, if $PQ = 4$ inches, which of the following is the area, in square inches, of the circle?

    (A) 2π
    (B) 4π
    (C) 8π
    (D) 10π
    (E) 16π

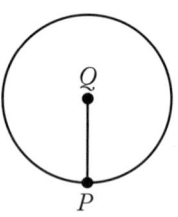

Surface Area and Volume

Surface area is the total area of the surfaces of a three-dimensional figure.
Volume is the number of cubic units inside a three-dimensional figure.

For example: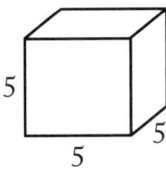

In the cube shown,

Surface area = 6(5)(5) = 150 square units

Volume = 5(5)(5) = 125 cubic units

---

31. For an art project, Tomas will paint the rectangular solid shown. He will paint the two shaded faces yellow and the remaining 4 faces blue. If RU = 3 meters, UT = 2 meters, and ST = 1 meter, what is the ratio of the areas, in square meters, of the faces painted yellow to the faces painted blue?

    (A) 1 to 1
    (B) 1 to 3
    (C) 2 to 1
    (D) 3 to 5
    (E) 6 to 5

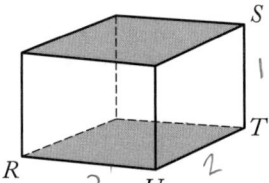

32. A case of 8 boxes is packed as shown. Each box is a cube with sides of 2 meters. What is the volume of the case, in cubic meters?

    (A) 192
    (B) 128
    (C) 96
    (D) 64
    (E) 48

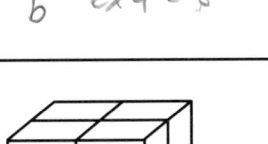

Angle Relationships

> An **angle** consists of two segments, or two rays, that have the same endpoint. Angles are measured in degrees (°). The sum of the angles along a straight line is 180°. The sum of the internal angles of a triangle is also 180°. A square or rectangle has four 90° angles. The sum of the angles around the center of a circle is 360°.

33. In the figure, lines k and m intersect at a point with a line segment as shown. What is the value of y?

    (A) 30
    (B) 60
    (C) 75
    (D) 120
    (E) 150

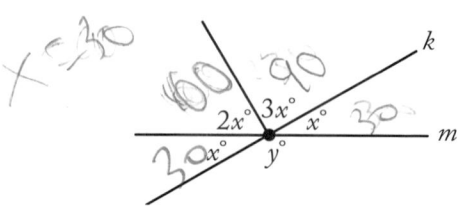

34. The figure shows an isosceles triangle with the base side extended. What is the value of $x + y$?

    (A) 105
    (B) 140
    (C) 145
    (D) 180
    (E) 210

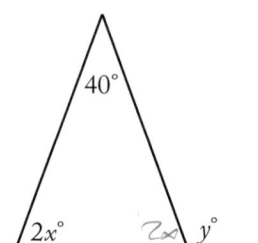

35. The figure shows two parallel lines intersected by a transversal line. What is the value of k?

    (A) 20
    (B) 30
    (C) 40
    (D) 50
    (E) 60

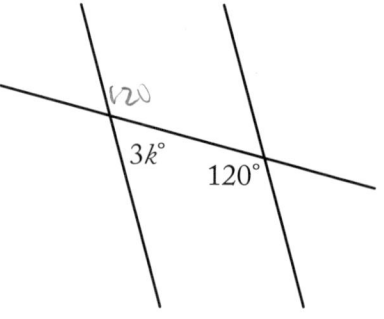

Visual/Spatial Reasoning

Problems that test Visual/Spatial Reasoning are all different. Examples of some types of problems that may be tested include visualizing different faces of a cube as the cube is turned, or rotating a figure about a point.

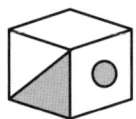 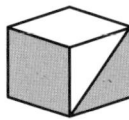 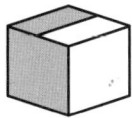

36. The figure above shows three views of a cube. Each face of the cube is different. Which of the following could be another view of the cube?

(A)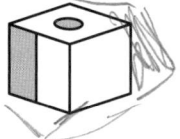

(B)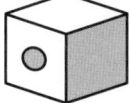

(C)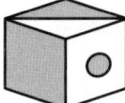

(D)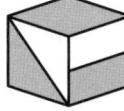

(E)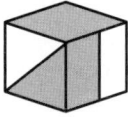

Answer Key
Section II: Geometry

27. Answer (A) 21.9 cm
6.1 cm + 6.1 cm + 9.7 cm = 21.9 cm

28. Answer (B) 30,000
The figure can be broken into 2 figures: one square with side lengths 100 feet by 100 feet, and one rectangle with side lengths 200 feet by 100 feet. $A = (100 \times 100) + (200 \times 100) = 10{,}000 + 20{,}000 = 30{,}000$.

29. Answer (C) 165
$C = \pi d \approx 3 \times 11 = 33$ cm
So 5 revolutions is $5 \times 33 = 165$ cm.

30. Answer (E) 16π
$A = \pi r^2 \rightarrow A = \pi(4)^2 = 16\pi$

31. Answer (E) 6 to 5
Area of yellow is $6m^2 + 6m^2 = 12m^2$.
Area of blue is
$3m^2 + 2m^2 + 3m^2 + 2m^2 = 10m^2$.
So the ratio of the areas is 12 to 10 or 6 to 5.

32. Answer (D) 64
Each box has volume $2m \times 2m \times 2m = 8$ m^3. There are 8 boxes. So the volume is
8×8 m$^3 = 64$ m^3.

33. Answer (E) 150
$3x + x + 2x = 180$
$6x = 180$
$x = 30$
$x + y = 180 \rightarrow 30 + y = 180 \rightarrow y = 150$

34. Answer (C) 145
Because the triangle is isosceles, $2x = 70$, so $x = 35$.
$y = 180 - 70 = 110$
so $x + y = 35 + 110 = 145$.

35. Answer (A) 20
The angles shown are supplementary angles, so
$120 + 3k = 180 \rightarrow 3k = 60 \rightarrow k = 20$.

36. Answer (A)
Based on the given information, only choice A can be a view of the cube. The other four answer choices lead to contradictions in the three views that were given.

Section III: Algebra

For this section, you will find 6 sample questions and related overviews of mathematics concepts in Algebra. The answers to these 6 sample questions are located at the end of this section.

Simple Linear Equations and Inequalities

Algebra is a form of mathematics that uses variables, expressions, equations, and inequalities to represent situations and to solve problems. A **variable** is a letter, like x, which represents a number or quantity. The following are examples of expressions, equations, and inequalities.

Expressions : $2 + x$ and $3y^2$

Equations : $4b - 10 = 2$ and $2(a + 6) = 20$

Inequalities : $\frac{c}{3} \geq 6$ and $2r < 20$

$$10 + 2x = x + 1$$

37. What is the solution to the equation above?

  (A) 10

  (B) $\frac{11}{3}$

  (C) 3

  (D) $\frac{1}{3}$

  (E) -9

$$2 + 4x > 30$$

38. For the inequality above, what is the least possible integer value of x ?

  (A) 6
  (B) 7
  (C) 8
  (D) 9
  (E) 10

Algebra Word Problems

An algebra word problem can be presented in either a real-life or an abstract setting. Some word problems will require you to set up and solve an equation or inequality to arrive at the final answer. Other word problems will require you to translate words into an expression, equation, or inequality, which will be the final answer.

39. If 4 less than half a number n is 16, what is the value of n?
    (A) 12
    (B) 20
    (C) 24
    (D) 32
    (E) 40

40. Maria has x dollars and Alex has 5 dollars more than Maria. If Alex gives Maria 6 dollars, how many dollars will Alex have left?
    (A) $x - 1$
    (B) $x + 1$
    (C) $5x + 1$
    (D) $6x + 1$
    (E) $6x - 1$

Simplification and Evaluation of Algebraic Expressions

Some algebra problems on the test may involve simplifying algebraic expressions by combining like terms, or by substituting values into expressions.

$$\frac{4a - 3b + c}{-(8a + 3b + 2c)}$$

41. Which of the following is equivalent to the expression above?
    (A) $-4a - c$
    (B) $-4a + 3c$
    (C) $4a - 6b - c$
    (D) $-4a - 6b - c$
    (E) $-4a - 6b + 3c$

42. If $x = 5$ and $y = -2$, what is the value of $2(x - y)^2$?
    (A) 196
    (B) 98
    (C) 81
    (D) 28
    (E) 18

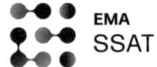

Answer Key
Section III: Algebra

37. **Answer (E)** -9

$$10 + 2x = x + 1$$
$$10 + x = 1$$
$$x = -9$$

38. **Answer (C)** 8

$$2 + 4x > 30$$
$$4x > 28$$
$$x > 7$$

So $x = 8$ is the least possible integer value of x.

39. **Answer (E)** 40

4 less than half n is 16 is the same as

$$\frac{1}{2}n - 4 = 16$$
$$\frac{1}{2}n = 20$$
$$n = 40$$

40. **Answer (A)** $x - 1$

$$x + 5 - 6 \rightarrow x - 1$$

41. **Answer (D)** $-4a - 6b - c$

$$\begin{array}{r} 4a - 3b + c \\ -(8a + 3b + 2c) \\ \hline \end{array}$$

$$\begin{array}{r} 4a - 3b + c \\ -\ 8a - 3b - 2c \\ \hline -4a - 6b - c \end{array}$$

42. **Answer (B)** 98

$$2(x - y)^2 \rightarrow 2(5 - (-2))^2$$
$$= 2(7)^2 = 2(49) = 98$$

Section IV: Data Analysis

For this section, you will find 8 sample questions and related overviews of mathematics concepts in Data Analysis. The answers to these 8 sample questions are located at the end of this section.

Graphs and Tables

Graphs are used to present numerical information in visual form. A **bar graph** uses bars to make comparisons between parts of the data. A **line graph** uses line segments to show changes in the data over time. A **circle graph** uses a divided circle to compare parts of the data to the whole data set. A **dot plot** uses dots to display the number of each value in a data set. Examples of each are shown below.

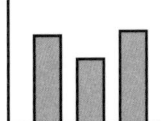
Bar Graph

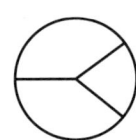
Line Graph

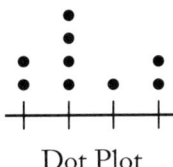
Circle Graph

Dot Plot

43. The circle graph shows the percent of a day that Maurice spends on different activities on Wednesday. On Saturday, Maurice plans on spending twice as much time on chores and sports as he does on Wednesday. Which of the following is the best estimate of the number of hours he will spend on chores and sports on Saturday?

    (A) 4.3
    (B) 8.2
    (C) 12.5
    (D) 14.2
    (E) 15.8

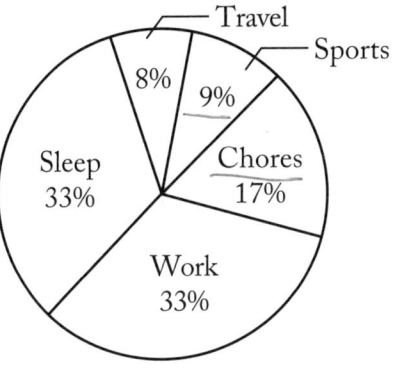

Maurice's Wednesday

44. The bar graph shows the number of students in the Oldtown Middle School concert choir by grade. The music director predicts that next year the number of 8th graders in the concert choir will decrease by 10%. How many 8th graders will be in the concert choir next year?

    (A) 10
    (B) 18
    (C) 20
    (D) 25
    (E) 27

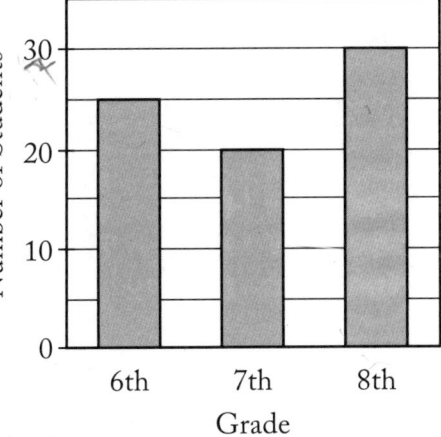

Oldtown Middle School Concert Choir

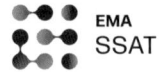

Mean, Median, Mode, Range

> For a list of values:
> - The **mean** is the sum of the values divided by the number of values;
> - The **median** is the middle value, when the list is placed in either increasing or decreasing order;
> - The **mode** is the value in the list that occurs the most; and
> - The **range** results from subtracting the least value from the greatest value in the list.

6, 15, 3, 15, 11, 0, 20

45. What is the mean of the list above?

(A) 10
(B) 11
(C) 14
(D) 15
(E) 20

44, m, 11, 78, 93, 29, 72

46. If m is the median for the list of seven numbers above, what is the greatest possible value of m?

(A) 71
(B) 72
(C) 78
(D) 82
(E) 93

96°, 87°, 100°, 91°, 87°, 98°, 99°

47. The daily high temperatures, in degrees Fahrenheit, for seven days in Cactus Town are shown above. What is the mode of the high temperatures, in degrees Fahrenheit?

(A) 96°
(B) 94°
(C) 91°
(D) 87°
(E) 13°

48. There are five integers in a list. The maximum value is 18 and the range is 11. The mode is half as large as the maximum value. If the list has one mode, what is the least possible sum of the numbers in the list?

(A) 51
(B) 53
(C) 56
(D) 58
(E) 60

Probability

Probability is the measure of the likelihood that an event will occur. The probability of an event is a number between 0 and 1. The closer a probability is to 0, the less likely an event will occur. The closer a probability is to 1, the more likely an event will occur. The probability of an event, P, is calculated by the ratio:

$$P = \frac{\text{number of specific outcomes}}{\text{total number of outcomes}}$$

49. In Jad's closet, he has 5 striped shirts, 2 white shirts, 6 blue shirts, and 7 yellow shirts. If he selects a shirt at random from the closet, what is the probability of selecting a striped shirt or a yellow shirt?

(A) $\frac{1}{4}$
(B) $\frac{7}{20}$
(C) $\frac{2}{5}$
(D) $\frac{3}{5}$
(E) $\frac{3}{4}$

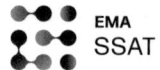

Counting

Counting problems on the test may involve determining the number of paths to get from one point to another or determining the number of combinations that are possible in certain situations.

Red	Orange	Yellow	Green
Apple	Cantaloupe	Banana	Apple
Grape	Peach	Mango	Grape
Raspberry			Kiwi
Strawberry			Melon

50. A store makes centerpieces using different fruits. For each centerpiece, customers select one fruit from each of the columns in the table shown. How many different centerpieces are possible?

    (A) 6
    (B) 12
    (C) 32
    (D) 48
    (E) 64

Answer Key
Section IV: Data Analysis

43. **Answer (C) 12.5**
    Twice as much time on chores and sports is $2 \times (9\% + 17\%)$ or 52%, so $(0.52)(24) = 12.48 \approx 12.5$.

44. **Answer (E) 27**
    $30 \times 0.1 = 3$
    $30 - 3 = 27$

45. **Answer (A) 10**
    $$\frac{6 + 15 + 3 + 15 + 11 + 0 + 20}{7} = \frac{70}{7} = 10$$

46. **Answer (B) 72**
    The median m is the middle number of the ordered list. The six numbers in increasing order are 11, 29, 44, 72, 78, and 93, so $44 \leq m \leq 72$, and so the greatest value of m is 72.

47. **Answer (D) 87°**
    The mode is the most common value in the list, or 87°.

48. **Answer (A) 51**
    The maximum is 18, so the mode is 9, and the minimum is $18 - 11 = 7$. So the list with the least possible sum is 7, 8, 9, 9, 18. So the sum is $7 + 8 + 9 + 9 + 18 = 51$.

49. **Answer (D) $\frac{3}{5}$**
    $$P = \frac{\text{number of striped and yellow shirts}}{\text{total number of shirts}}$$
    $$= \frac{5 + 7}{5 + 2 + 6 + 7} = \frac{12}{20} = \frac{3}{5}$$

50. **Answer (E) 64**
    $4 \times 2 \times 2 \times 4 = 8 \times 8 = 64$

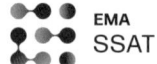

3. The Reading Comprehension Section

The reading comprehension section presents several reading passages, each followed by a series of questions designed to measure how well you understand what you have read. The questions ask not only about the ideas presented in the passage but also about the ways in which the author expresses those ideas. Passages are of two kinds: literary and expository. Literary passages are excerpts from works of fiction or poetry. They generally tell part of a story or develop a certain theme. Expository passages explore topics related to the humanities (art, music, etc.), history, science (biology, astronomy, technology, etc.), or social science (psychology, anthropology, etc.).

> **Just the Facts**
> Reading Comprehension
>
> **Number of questions:**
> 40
>
> **What it measures:**
> Your ability to understand and interpret what you read
>
> **Scored section:**
> Yes
>
> **Time allotted:**
> 40 minutes

What Are the Directions for the Reading Comprehension Section on the Test?

Read each passage carefully and then answer the questions about it. For each question, decide on the basis of the passage which one of the choices best answers the question.

What Types of Questions Are Presented in the Reading Comprehension Section?

There are five basic question types in the reading comprehension section. Examples of each question type are provided below:

1. Basic information

Understanding what is directly stated in the passage

Examples:
- According to the passage, the elephant's diet consists mainly of...
- In the second stanza, the poet indicates that she is...
- According to the passage, what accounts for the enduring popularity of Bach's music?
- What is the main idea of the passage?
- In the final paragraph, the author argues for...

2. Inference

Understanding what is implied but not directly stated in the passage

Examples:
- It can be inferred from the passage that the "old cabin" (line 8) was...
- The author's description of his childhood suggests that he...
- The author assumes that her readers are...
- The "grave concerns" mentioned in line 6 were most likely...
- The description of the "office" (line 10) implies that it was...

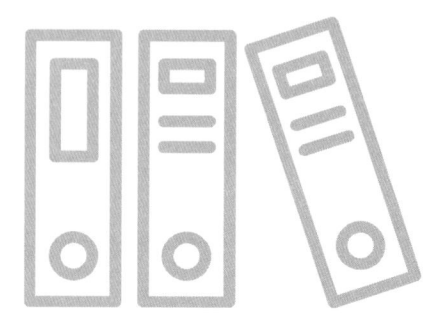

3. Language
Interpreting the author's use of specific words and phrases
Examples:
- As used in line 16, the word "fair" most nearly means…
- In line 7, the expression "safety net" refers to…
- In line 10, the pronoun "they" refers to…
- To describe the effects of the storm, the author makes use of which literary device?
- In the third stanza, the poet develops a metaphor drawn from the realm of…
- Throughout the poem, the "candle" serves as a symbol of…
- The rhyme scheme of the poem's last stanza is…

4. Purpose
Understanding the author's writing strategy: how the writing is structured and why it is structured that way
Examples:
- The main purpose of the final paragraph is to…
- The author mentions "fairy tales" (line 1) in order to…
- The narrator repeats the word "paper" (lines 6–7) in order to…
- Why is the detective's sentence left unfinished in line 17?
- The list in the third paragraph serves to…
- The examples cited in the second paragraph are intended to…
- How does the third paragraph relate to the second paragraph?

5. Tone
Recognizing the tone, mood, or style of the passage or the attitude of the author, speaker, or character
Examples:
- In the second paragraph, the author adopts a tone of…
- In the second stanza, the poet sounds a note of…
- In the first paragraph, the narrator creates an atmosphere of…
- The style of the passage is best described as…
- As indicated in the quotation (lines 9–10), Lawry's attitude toward modern art is one of…

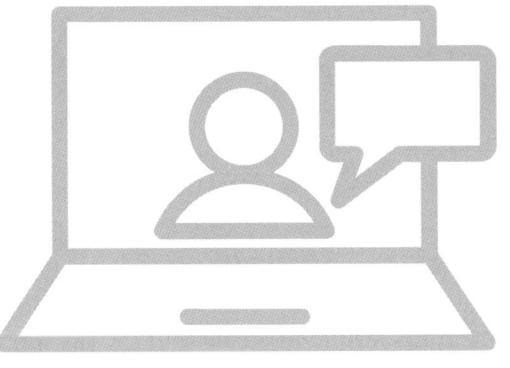

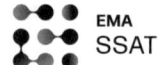

How Are the Reading Comprehension Questions Presented?

The SSAT presents each passage (or poem) with a corresponding group of three to eight questions. The directions instruct you to read each passage and answer the questions about it.

> Little Jim was, for the time, Engine Number 36 and he was making the run between Syracuse and Rochester. He was fourteen minutes behind time, and the throttle was wide open. As a result, when he swung around the curve at the flower bed, a wheel of his cart destroyed a tulip. Number 36 slowed down at once and looked guiltily at his father, who was mowing the lawn. The doctor had his back to the accident,
> Line 5 and he continued to pace slowly to and fro, pushing the mower.
> Jim dropped the handle of the cart. He looked at his father and at the broken flower. Finally, he went to the tulip and tried to stand it up, but it would only hang limply from his hand. Jim could not repair it. He looked again toward his father.

1. It can be inferred from the passage that the main cause of Jim's accident was
   (A) excessive speed
   (B) mechanical failure
   (C) lack of visibility
   (D) poor road conditions
   (E) miscommunication

   The correct answer is (A). The words "the throttle was wide open" (line 2) imply that Jim was traveling at top speed, and the words "As a result" (line 2) indicate that this was the reason that the wheel of his cart accidentally "destroyed a tulip" (line 3).

2. It can be inferred from the passage that Jim's father was a
   (A) farmer
   (B) doctor
   (C) gardener
   (D) train engineer
   (E) business executive

   The correct answer is (B). In line 4 the narrator indicates that Jim's father "was mowing the lawn" and in the next sentence (lines 4–5) refers to the person "pushing the mower" as "The doctor," so it may reasonably be inferred that Jim's father was a doctor.

3. After the accident, Jim was apparently most concerned about
   (A) getting to his destination
   (B) the damage to his cart
   (C) his father's reaction
   (D) preventing future collisions
   (E) the injuries he had sustained

   The correct answer is (C). The narrator indicates that immediately after the accident Jim "looked guiltily at his father" (lines 3–4) and then "looked at his father and at the broken flower" (line 6) and then "looked again toward his father" (line 8). The fact that Jim looked repeatedly at his father suggests that he was worried about what his father's reaction would be.

How Do You Answer the Reading Comprehension Questions?

As you read, determine the main idea. Identify the important details that move the narrative along or create a mood or tone. In expository passage, identify the details that support the writer's argument or illustrate the ideas being presented. The first sentence of each paragraph will give you a general sense of the topic. Identify the topic of each paragraph and underline or make note of key facts. Try to figure out the writer's intention, or purpose of the passage. Notice the writer's attitude, tone, and general style.

> These habits can help you understand what you read, whether you are taking the SSAT, preparing for a history test, or getting ready to write an essay for your English class.

Reading Comprehension Test-Taking Strategies

1. Take time to read and understand the first sentence of each paragraph. This will provide you with a general sense of the topic.

2. Scan the answer choices, since they are generally short and provide excellent clues. If an answer choice refers you to a specific line in the passage, underline or make note of that line for reference.

3. Read each passage carefully. Follow the author's reasoning. Notice attitude, tone, and general style.

4. Pay attention to words such as always, never, every, and none. They may play an important role in the answer.

5. Identify the topic of each paragraph, key facts, and the author's purpose for writing. Underline or make note of the key facts for quick reference.

6. Read all answer choices carefully before you choose. When you find an answer choice that fails to satisfy the requirements of the question and statement, cross it out.

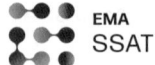

Sample Questions: Reading Comprehension

Directions: Read each passage carefully and then answer the questions about it. For each question, decide on the basis of the passage which one of the choices best answers the question.

> It is often said that what separates man from beast is the ability to think logically. This is not true. A deer passing through the forest scents the ground and detects a certain odor. A sequence of ideas is generated in the mind of the deer. Nothing in the deer's experience has ever produced that odor except a wolf, and so the deer infers that wolves have passed that way.
>
> Line 5 But it is a part of the deer's scientific knowledge, based on previous experience, that wolves are dangerous beasts. So, combining direct observation in the present with the application of a general principle based on past experience, the deer reaches the very logical conclusion that it would be wise to turn around and run in another direction. All this implies an understanding and use of scientific principles. And, strange as it may seem to speak of a deer possessing scientific
>
> 10 knowledge, yet there is really no absurdity in the statement. The deer does possess scientific knowledge that differs in degree only, not in kind, from the knowledge of a physicist. Nor is the animal less scientific in the application of that knowledge than is the man. The animal that could not make accurate scientific observations of its surroundings and deduce accurate scientific conclusions from them would soon pay the penalty for its lack of logic.

1. The author's primary purpose in the passage is to
   (A) expose common errors of logic
   (B) compare two different methods
   (C) propose a new observational technique
   (D) challenge a widely held belief
   (E) differentiate two species of animal

2. The "direct observation" (line 6) made by the deer involved
   (A) seeing
   (B) hearing
   (C) smelling
   (D) tasting
   (E) touching

3. As it is used in line 9, the word "as" most nearly means
   (A) though
   (B) when
   (C) like
   (D) that
   (E) since

4. The "penalty" (line 14) that the deer would have to pay for a lack of logic would most likely be
   (A) getting lost in the forest
   (B) being attacked by wolves
   (C) failing to attract a mate
   (D) going without food
   (E) losing its habitat

>   Seven daughters had Lord Archibald,
>   All children of one mother.
>   I could not say in one short day
>   What love they bore each other.
> *Line 5* A garland of seven lilies wrought—
>   Seven sisters that together dwell!
>   But he—bold knight as ever fought—
>   Their father—took of them no thought,
>   He loved the wars so well.

5. In lines 3–4, the speaker suggest that the sisters' love was

    (A) insincere
    (B) well hidden
    (C) indescribably strong
    (D) tragically short-lived
    (E) potentially destructive

6. As it is used in line 4, the word "bore" most nearly means

    (A) make weary
    (B) drill into
    (C) gave birth
    (D) felt toward
    (E) put up with

7. Line 5 provides an example of which literary device?

    (A) simile
    (B) metaphor
    (C) alliteration
    (D) onomatopoeia
    (E) hyperbole

8. The passage suggests that, as a father, Lord Archibald was

    (A) stern
    (B) proud
    (C) protective
    (D) considerate
    (E) neglectful

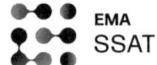

Answer Key: Reading Comprehension

1. **(D)** In the first sentence the author refers to a widely held ("often said") belief that animals do not think logically. In the second sentence the author challenges this belief, declaring it to be false. In the rest of the passage the author presents an extended argument showing why the belief is false.

2. **(C)** The author presents a scenario in which a deer "scents the ground and detects" the odor of a wolf (lines 2–3). This is the only direct observation that the deer makes, and it involves only the sense of smell.

3. **(A)** Of the five answer choices, "though" is the only word that makes sense when substituted for "as" in the passage: "And, strange though it may seem to speak of a deer possessing scientific knowledge, yet there is really no absurdity in the statement."

4. **(B)** The author is making the general point that animals would not be able to survive if they did not use logic. In the case of the deer, this means that if the deer did not logically conclude that the smell of the wolf implied danger, the deer would not take action to avoid the danger and would probably fall prey to the wolves, thus paying a penalty for its lack of logic.

5. **(C)** The words "I could not say in one short day" indicate that the sisters' love was so tremendous that the speaker would be unable to adequately describe it even if he had all day to do so.

6. **(D)** Of the five answer choices, "felt toward" is the only expression that makes sense when substituted for "bore" in the passage: "I could not say in one short day what love they felt toward each other."

7. **(B)** A metaphor is an expression that likens one thing to another by saying or implying that the one thing is the other. In line 5, the poet likens Lord Archibald's seven daughters to a flowery wreath by calling them "A garland of seven lilies wrought."

8. **(E)** The words "he…their father…took of them no thought" (lines 7–8) indicate that Lord Archibald did not think about and thus neglected his daughters.

4. The Verbal Section

The verbal section of the Middle Level SSAT presents two types of questions: **synonyms** and **analogies**. The synonym questions primarily test the strength of your vocabulary. The analogy questions test not only your knowledge of individual words but also your ability to recognize logical relationships between pairs of words.

Synonyms

Synonyms are words that have the same or nearly the same meaning as another word. For example, *fortunate* is a synonym for *lucky*; *hoist* is a synonym for *raise*; and *melody* is a synonym for *tune*. Synonym questions on the SSAT ask you to choose a word that has a meaning similar to that of a given word.

What Are the Directions for the Synonym Section on the Test?

Each of the following questions consists of one word followed by five words or phrases. You are to select the one word or phrase whose meaning is closest to that of the word in capital letters.

How Are the Synonym Questions Presented?

Synonym questions present a single word in capital letters followed by five answer choices in lowercase letters.

EXAMPLE:	1. PREMONITION: (A) opening (B) firmness (C) discovery (D) conspiracy (E) forewarning The correct answer is (E), forewarning.

> **Just the Facts**
> The Verbal Section
>
> **Number of questions:**
> 60 (30 synonyms and 30 analogies)
>
> **What it measures:**
> Your ability to understand the meanings of words and to recognize relationships between words with different meanings
>
> **Scored section:**
> Yes
>
> **Time allotted:**
> 30 minutes

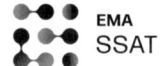

How Do You Answer Synonym Questions?

There is only one correct response, so make sure you consider all of the choices carefully. Don't just pick the first word that seems approximately right. If you're having difficulty deciding between two word choices, try making up a short sentence using the capitalized word and then ask yourself which choice would be the best substitute for the capitalized word in that sentence.

How Can You Build Your Vocabulary?

The best way to prepare is to read as much as you can to build your vocabulary. If you encounter an unfamiliar word in your reading, make sure you look it up in a dictionary (either online or in print). Keep track of the word and its meaning on an index card, notepad, or in notes on your smartphone. Keeping track of new words or words that are unfamiliar to you will help you build a tremendous vocabulary.

Another way to prepare is to learn the meaning of the word parts that make up many English words. These word parts consist of **prefixes, suffixes,** and **roots**. If you encounter an unfamiliar word, you could take apart the word and think about the parts.

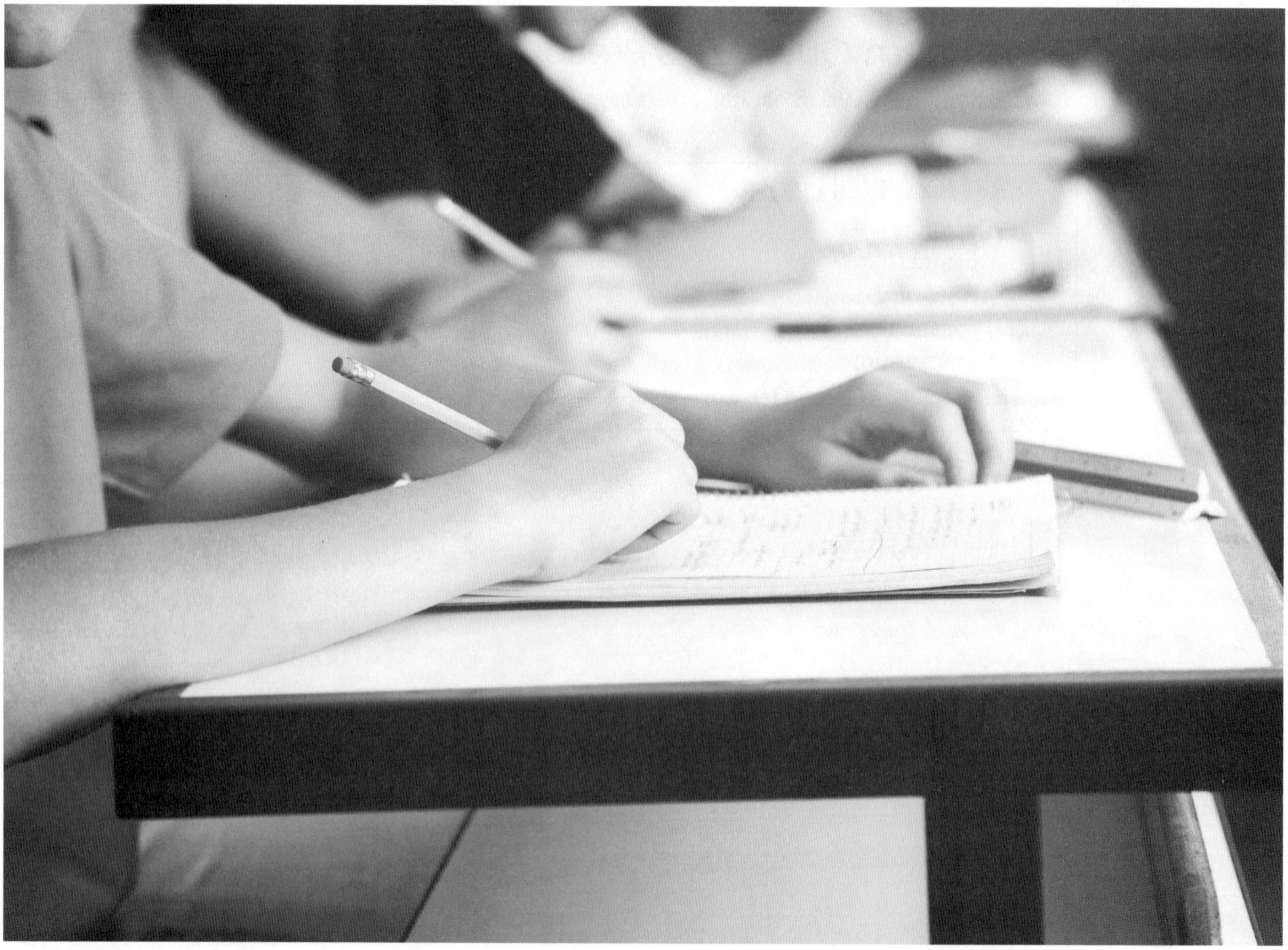

> The greater your vocabulary, the greater your chance of getting the correct answer.

Prefixes

Prefix	Meaning	Example
a-, an-	not, without	anonymous, amoral
ab-	from	abnormal
ad-	to, toward	advance, adhere
ante-	before	antebellum
anti-	against, opposite	antibacterial, antithesis
auto-	self	autobiography, automobile
bi-	two	bicycle, binary
circu(m)-	around	circumference, circulate
de-	away from	derail, defend
dia-	through, across	diagonal
dis-	away from, not	disappear, disloyal
en-	put in, into	encircle, enlist
ex-	out of	exit, exhale
extra-	outside of, beyond	extraordinary
hyper-	over, more	hyperactive, hyperbole
in-, ill-, im-	not	inanimate, illicit, impossible
in-, ill-, im-	in, into	insert, illuminate, impose
inter-	between	interact
intra-	within	intrastate
macro-	large	macroeconomics
mal-	bad, wrong	malady, malpractice
micro-	small	microscope
mono-	one	monopoly, monotonous
multi-	many	multicolor, multiply
non-	without, not	nonsense
peri-	around	perimeter, periscope
post-	after	postscript
pre-, pro-	before, forward	preview, prologue
semi- (also hemi-)	half	semicircle, hemisphere
sub-	under	subway, submarine
syn-, sym-	same	synonym, sympathy
trans-	across	transport, transit
tri-	three	triangle, triple
un-	not	unkind
uni-	one, together	unity, unique

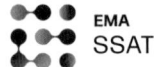

Suffixes

Suffix	Meaning	Example
-able (-ible)	able to be	habitable, edible
-acy	state or quality	privacy, literacy
-al	relating to, belonging to	theatrical
-an (-ian)	relating to, belonging to	equestrian
-ance, -ence	state or quality	brilliance, patience
-ant	a person	informant, participant
-arian	a person	librarian, vegetarian
-cide	act of killing	genocide
-cracy	rule, government, power	aristocracy
-dom	state or quality	wisdom, freedom
-dox	belief	orthodox
-en	make a certain way	sharpen, sadden
-er, -or	person doing something	lover, actor
-ese	relating to a place	Japanese
-esque	in the style of/like	arabesque, grotesque
-fy	make a certain way	beautify, terrify, magnify
-ful	full of	graceful
-gam/-gamy	marriage, union	monogamous
-gon/-gonic	angle	decagon, trigonometry
-hood	state, condition, or quality	parenthood
-ile	relating to, capable of	juvenile, mobile
-ious, -ous	characterized by	contagious, studious
-ish	having the quality of	childish
-ism	doctrine, belief	socialism
-ist	person doing or advocating	dramatist, communist
-ity, -ty	quality of	ferocity
-ive	having a tendency	talkative, divisive
-ize	make a certain way	prioritize, advertize
-log(ue)	word, speech	analogy, dialogue
-ment	condition or action	ailment, assessment
-ness	state or quality	happiness, kindness
-phile	one who loves	bibliophile
-phobia	abnormal fear of	acrophobia
-ship	quality or position of	craftsmanship, dictatorship
-sion, -tion	action or condition	destruction, tension

Word Roots G = Greek   L = Latin

Root	Meaning	Example
ann, enn (L)	year	anniversary, perennial
anthrop (G)	man	anthropomorphism
ast(er) (G)	star	astrology, asterisk
audi (L)	hear	audible, audience
auto (G)	self	autobiography
bene (L)	good	beneficial
bio (G)	life	biography, biology
chron (G)	time	chronology, chronicle
civ (L)	citizen	civilization, civilian
cred (L)	believe	credential, incredible
dem(o) (G)	people	democracy, epidemic
dict (L)	say	predict, dictator
duc (L)	lead, make	conduct, reduce
gen (G & L)	give birth	genesis, generation
geo (G)	earth	geometry
graph (G)	write	autograph, graphic
jur, jus (L)	law	juror, justice, injure
log, logue (G)	thought, word	logical, prologue
luc (L)	light	lucid, translucent
man(u) (L)	hand	manual, manufacture
mand (L)	order	command, mandate
min (L)	small	minimal, diminish
mis, mit (L)	send	missile, transmit
nov (L)	new	novel, innovate
omni (L)	all	omnivore, omniscient
pan (G)	all	panorama, panacea
pater, patr (G & L)	father	paternal, patriarchy
path (G)	feel	sympathy
phil (G)	love	philosophy, philanthropist
phon (G)	sound	phonetic, telephone
photo (G)	light	photosynthesis
poli (G)	city	political, metropolis
port (L)	carry	deport, report
scrib, script (L)	write	prescribe, inscription
sens, sent (L)	feel	sentiment, resent
sol (L)	sun	solar, parasol

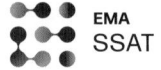

Word Roots   G = Greek   L = Latin

Root	Meaning	Example
tele (G)	far off	television
terr (L)	earth	terrestrial, inter
tract (L)	drag, draw	detract, traction
vac (L)	empty	evacuation, vacant
vid, vis (L)	see	invisible, video
vit (L)	life	vitality, vitamin
zo (G)	life	zoology

Sample Questions: Synonyms

Directions: Each of the following questions consists of a word followed by five words or phrases. You are to select the one word or phrase whose meaning is closest to the word in capital letters.

1. POISE:
   (A) creativity
   (B) respect
   (C) sympathy
   (D) composure
   (E) secrecy

2. BRANDISH:
   (A) shout
   (B) wave
   (C) emerge
   (D) struggle
   (E) label

3. RADIANT:
   (A) youthful
   (B) successful
   (C) impressive
   (D) glowing
   (E) peaceful

4. VERSATILE:
   (A) vigilant
   (B) adaptable
   (C) friendly
   (D) poetic
   (E) wise

5. WAFT:
   (A) jut
   (B) dive
   (C) drift
   (D) paddle
   (E) explore

6. SWAGGER:
   (A) fall
   (B) strut
   (C) guzzle
   (D) mumble
   (E) bet

7. SCURRY:
   (A) rush
   (B) bluff
   (C) topple
   (D) scribble
   (E) disperse

8. EGREGIOUS:
   (A) sociable
   (B) pitiful
   (C) flagrant
   (D) contemplative
   (E) communicable

Answer Key: Synonyms

1. (D) composure
2. (B) wave
3. (D) glowing
4. (B) adaptable
5. (C) drift
6. (B) strut
7. (A) rush
8. (C) flagrant

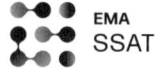

Verbal Analogies

An **analogy**, very generally, is a statement saying that one thing is similar to another thing. A simple example would be "Life is like a roller-coaster ride." The analogy questions in the verbal section of the SSAT ask you to compose a special kind of analogy, called a verbal analogy because it has to do with the meanings of words. A verbal analogy is a statement saying that the relationship between one pair of words is similar to the relationship between another pair of words. For example, the verbal analogy "Swim is to water as fly is to air" says that the verb "swim" is related to the noun "water" in the same way that the verb "fly" is related to the noun "air." To swim is to move through water, just as to fly is to move through the air.

> The analogy portion of the SSAT asks you to identify the answer that best matches the relationship between two words.

What Are the Directions for the Verbal Analogies Section on the Test?

The following questions ask you to find relationships between words. For each question, select the answer choice that best completes the meaning of the sentence.

What Are the Things to Remember When Doing Analogies?

Parts of Speech

The parts of speech in the first word pair must match the parts of speech in the second word pair. If, for example, the words in the first pair are noun/adjective, then the words in the second pair must also be noun/adjective.

Word Order

If the first pair of words expresses a particular relationship, the second pair must express the same relationship in the same order.

Exactness

Sometimes two or more of the given choices would make sense. When this happens, choose the answer that most exactly fits the relationship between the words in the stem of the question.

How Are Verbal Analogies Presented?

The SSAT analogy questions present a **stem** followed by five **options**. The stem is an incomplete sentence, and each option offers a different way of finishing the sentence. The stem has the form **A is to B as**, (with **A** and **B** representing the first word pair), and the options have the form **C is to D** (with **C** and **D** representing the second word pair). When the stem and an option are put together, the result is a sentence of the form **A is to B as C is to D**.

EXAMPLE:	1. Loud is to hear as (A) sad is to cry (B) bright is to see (C) rude is to speak (D) angry is to feel (E) bland is to taste **The correct answer is (B).**

What Are Verbal Analogy Relationships?

Below are examples of some of the most common types of analogical relationships that you will find on the SSAT. This list is not complete; there are other types of verbal relationships not represented here.

1. **Antonyms**: X is the opposite of Y.
   EXAMPLE: Success is to failure as joy is to sadness.

2. **Degree:** To be X is to be extremely Y.
   EXAMPLE: Furious is to angry as enormous is to large.

3. **Type:** An X is a kind of Y.
   EXAMPLE: Sonnet is to poem as elm is to tree.

4. **Specific Type:** An X is a [gender] Y.
   EXAMPLE: Father is to parent as brother is to sibling.

5. **Specific Manner:** To X is to Y quickly.
   EXAMPLE: Glance is to look as jot is to write.

6. **Part:** An X is part of a Y.
   EXAMPLE: Chapter is to book as singer is to chorus.

7. **Specific Part:** An X is the outer part of a Y.
   EXAMPLE: Shell is to egg as rind is to orange.

8. **Specific Part:** An X is a unit of Y.
   EXAMPLE: Blade is to grass as grain is to sand.

9. **Associated Characteristic:** An X is Y.
   EXAMPLE: Liar is to dishonest as genius is to intelligent.

10. **Associated Characteristic:** Someone who Xes is Y.
    EXAMPLE: Attack is to aggressive as donate is to generous.

11. **Associated Characteristic:** Something X pertains to a Y.
    EXAMPLE: Solar is to sun as nautical is to ship.

12. **Associated Action:** An X Ys.
    EXAMPLE: Fugitive is to flee as arbiter is to decide.

13. **Associated Action:** Something that is X is easily Yed.
    EXAMPLE: Obvious is to see as weak is to overpower.

14. **Negative Association:** Someone who is X is NOT Ying.
    EXAMPLE: Awake is to sleep as silent is to talk.

15. **Negative Association:** Someone who is X lacks Y.
    EXAMPLE: Foolish is to wisdom as dauntless is to fear.

16. **Negative Association:** Something that is X cannot Y.
    EXAMPLE: Numb is to feel as immobile is to move.

17. **Associated Tool:** An X typically uses a Y.
    EXAMPLE: Farmer is to plow as navigator is to compass.

18. **Associated Material:** An X typically works with Y.
    EXAMPLE: Carpenter is to wood as tailor is to fabric.

19. **Associated Location:** An X is kept in a Y.
    EXAMPLE: Book is to library as artwork is to museum.

20. **Associated Location:** One Xes in a Y.
    EXAMPLE: Prosecute is to courtroom as compete is to arena.

21. **Purpose:** An X is used to Y.
    EXAMPLE: Pen is to write as shovel is to dig.

22. **Specific Purpose:** An X is used to measure Y.
    EXAMPLE: Yardstick is to length as scale is to weight.

23. **Purpose:** An X provides Y.
    EXAMPLE: Shield is to protection as blanket is to warmth.

24. **Specific Purpose:** An X protects a Y.
    EXAMPLE: Helmet is to head as glove is to hand.

25. **Product:** An X produces Y.
    EXAMPLE: Cow is to milk as bee is to honey.

26. **Result:** Something that Xes increases in Y.
    EXAMPLE: Expand is to size as accelerate is to speed.

27. **Result:** One becomes an X by Ying.
    EXAMPLE: Student is to enroll as soldier is to enlist.

28. **Result:** What has Xed is Y.
    EXAMPLE: Perish is to dead as depart is to absent.

29. **Result:** Something X elicits Y.
    EXAMPLE: Humorous is to laughter as pathetic is to pity.

30. **Expression:** An X expresses Y.
    EXAMPLE: Smile is to pleasure as sneer is to contempt.

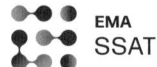

How Do You Solve Verbal Analogy Questions?

A useful strategy for solving analogies is to use a **bridge sentence**. A bridge sentence is a sentence that defines the relationship between two words using the letters **X** and **Y** in place of the words themselves. For instance, the bridge sentence **An X is not Y** defines the relationship between the words **coward** and **brave**.

When those words are substituted for **X** and **Y**, the result is a true sentence: "A coward is not brave." Of course, there are other word pairs that fit the same bridge sentence—for example, **fool** and **wise**. What this tells you is that the relationship between **coward** and **brave** is the same as the relationship between **fool** and **wise**. The two word pairs are analogous.

> Be careful of the order of the words when you're determining the corresponding relationships.

When answering an analogy question, the first thing to do is figure out the relationship between the two main words in the stem and then try to represent that relationship in a bridge sentence. So, for instance, if the main words in the stem are **tulip** and **flower**, you'll probably recognize that a tulip is a kind of flower, and so you'll then formulate the bridge sentence **An X is a kind of Y**. Now that you have your bridge sentence, you can try out each of the word pairs in the options and see which pair fits the bridge sentence. For instance, if **stick** and **stone** are the words in one of the options, then you substitute these words for **X** and **Y** in the bridge sentence to produce the sentence "A stick is a kind of stone." But this sentence is obviously not true, and that tells you that the option with **stick** and **stone** is not the correct answer choice. If another option contains the words **apple** and **fruit**, then you substitute these words for **X** and **Y** to get the sentence "An apple is a kind of fruit." Since this sentence is true, the option that produced it must be the correct answer. You've solved the analogy!

Try this strategy out on the sample questions that follow.

Verbal Test-Taking Strategies

1. The best way to improve your vocabulary is to read, read, and read some more.
2. Take note of unfamiliar words and look up their meanings.
3. Review the words you don't know.
4. Practice your vocabulary by taking the practice tests in this book. If you missed any of the verbal questions, read the questions and answers again, so you'll understand why you answered those questions incorrectly. Look them up and write them down.

Sample Questions: Analogies

Directions: The following questions ask you to find relationships between words. For each question, select the answer choice that best completes the meaning of the sentence.

1. Shore is to island as
   (A) arc is to circle
   (B) membrane is to cell
   (C) orbit is to satellite
   (D) element is to compound
   (E) scale is to note

2. Tether is to restrain as
   (A) pen is to erase
   (B) freezer is to shiver
   (C) book is to write
   (D) bracket is to support
   (E) loaf is to slice

3. Knoll is to mountain as
   (A) leaf is to tree
   (B) grass is to meadow
   (C) pond is to lake
   (D) valley is to plateau
   (E) ocean is to wave

4. Grimace is to pain as
   (A) nod is to agreement
   (B) cheer is to victory
   (C) scowl is to frown
   (D) laugh is to joke
   (E) clench is to fist

5. Chaos is to orderly as
   (A) bravery is to confident
   (B) weather is to climatic
   (C) music is to soothing
   (D) danger is to safe
   (E) evidence is to persuasive

6. Clamorous is to quiet as
   (A) acrid is to bitter
   (B) dull is to smooth
   (C) savory is to delicious
   (D) tepid is to bland
   (E) brilliant is to dim

7. Zeal is to enthusiasm as
   (A) delight is to sorrow
   (B) patience is to irritation
   (C) terror is to speechlessness
   (D) curiosity is to openness
   (E) bliss is to happiness

8. Chassis is to car as
   (A) frame is to house
   (B) trunk is to tire
   (C) address is to mailbox
   (D) intersection is to traffic
   (E) furniture is to room

9. Bewilder is to confusion as
   (A) surprise is to boredom
   (B) befriend is to discord
   (C) reprimand is to pride
   (D) threaten is to fear
   (E) accuse is to suspicion

10. Resist is to passive as
    (A) stretch is to flexible
    (B) hurry is to careless
    (C) grumble is to satisfied
    (D) investigate is to energetic
    (E) empathize is to tolerant

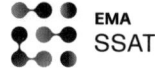

Answer Key: Analogies

1. **(B) membrane is to cell**
   An X forms the outer boundary of a Y.

2. **(D) bracket is to support**
   The purpose of an X is to Y something.

3. **(C) pond is to lake**
   X is a small geographic feature, and Y is a larger one.

4. **(A) nod is to agreement**
   To X is an indication of Y.

5. **(D) danger is to safe**
   X is a state in which things are not Y.

6. **(E) brilliant is to dim**
   Being X is the opposite of being Y.

7. **(E) bliss is to happiness**
   X is intense Y.

8. **(A) frame is to house**
   An X is the underlying structure of a Y.

9. **(D) threaten is to fear**
   To X someone causes that person to feel Y.

10. **(C) grumble is to satisfied**
    One who Xes is not Y.

Summing It Up

Here are a few things to keep in mind when you take the Middle Level SSAT:

- Make sure that you understand the directions before you start to work on any section. If there is anything that you do not understand, read the directions again.

- You don't need to answer every question on the test to score well. Some of the questions will be very easy and others will be difficult. Most students find that they do not know the answer to every question in every section. By working as quickly as you can without rushing, you should be able to read and think about every question.

- If you are not sure of an answer to a question, make note of it and move on. Make sure you also skip that question. If taking the test on paper, skip filling in that question's answer bubble on your answer sheet. If you have time remaining in that section, you can come back to questions you have not answered.

- If taking the test on paper, you may make as many marks on the test booklet as you need to. Just be sure to mark your answers on the answer sheet!

- Answers written in the test book will not count toward your score. Space is provided in the book for scratch work in the quantitative sections. Check often to make sure that you are marking your answer in the correct row on the answer sheet.

- If you decide to change an answer, be sure to erase your first mark on the answer sheet completely. If taking the SSAT at Home or computer-based SSAT, make sure you change your answer before completing the section.

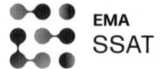

THIS PAGE INTENTIONALLY LEFT BLANK.

Chapter Three: Scores

What Your Scores Mean

If you're like most people, you'll quickly scan the score report trying to find **the** magic number that will tell you whether the scores are "good." With an admission test like the SSAT, this is not an easy thing to do. First, remember that the purpose of an admission test is to offer a common measure of academic ability that can be used to compare all applicants. In the case of the SSAT, the testing population is a relatively homogeneous one—students applying to college-preparatory private schools. Given this, it is important to keep in mind that your scores are being compared only to students in this academically elite group.

As described in Chapter 1, admission tests differ from other tests such as classroom and achievement tests in significant ways. Achievement and classroom tests assess a specific body of knowledge that was covered. If all students perform well, the teacher and school system have fulfilled their objective. If all students performed well on an admission test, it would lose its value in helping differentiate between and among candidates.

Formula Scoring

The SSAT uses a method of scoring known in the testing industry as "formula scoring." Students earn one point for every correct answer, receive no points for omitted questions, and lose $\frac{1}{4}$ point for each incorrect answer. This is different from "right scoring," which computes the total score by counting the number of correct answers, with no penalty for incorrect answers. Formula scoring is used to eliminate the test taker's gain from random guessing.

This is why we suggest that you omit questions for which you cannot make an educated guess. Since most students have not encountered this kind of test before, it is an important concept to understand and experience prior to taking the SSAT. SSAT score reports provide detailed information by section on the number of questions right, wrong, and not answered to aid families and schools in understanding your test-taking strategies and scores.

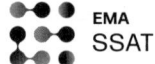

The Score Report

It cannot be said often enough: *admission test scores are only one piece of the application*. The degree of emphasis placed on scores in a school's admission process depends on that school and on other information, such as transcripts, applicants' statements, and teacher recommendations.

The descriptions indicated by the letters below correspond to the lettered sections on the sample score report on page 63.

Ⓐ About You

Parents and students should review this section carefully. Is the student's name spelled correctly? Is the date of birth listed correctly? And—very important—when registering the student, was his/her current grade listed? The student's current grade is used to determine which test form he/she will take and dictates the comparison or norm groups. If the grade to which the student is applying is used for registration, he/she may get the wrong form and his/her SSAT scaled score will be compared with students a year (or grade) older. If any of this information is incorrect, contact The Enrollment Management Association immediately.

Ⓑ About the Test You Took

Again, parents and students should review this information for accuracy. For Test Level, the student will have taken the Middle Level SSAT since he/she is applying to grades 6–8. The Upper Level SSAT is for students in grades 8–11 who are applying to grades 9–12. There is a different score scale for each of these levels.

Ⓒ About Your Scores

SSAT scores are listed by section so you can understand the student's performance on each of the three scored sections: verbal, quantitative/math, and reading comprehension. A total score (a sum of the three sections) is also reported. For the Middle Level SSAT, the lowest number on the scale (440) is the lowest possible score a student can earn, and the highest number (710) is the highest possible score a student can earn.

Scores are first calculated by awarding one point for each correct answer and subtracting one quarter of one point for each incorrect answer. These scores are called raw scores. Raw scores can vary from one edition of the test to another due to differences in difficulty among different editions. A statistical procedure called *score equating* is used to adjust for these differences. After equating, the reported scores or scaled scores (e.g., the scores on the 440–710 scale for the Middle Level test) can be compared to each other across forms.

Score Range

Even after equating adjustments are made, no single test score provides a perfectly accurate estimate of proficiency. Many factors can affect a student's score. We provide a scaled-score range to suggest where a student's scores might fall if taking a different version of the test. Assuming the student's ability remains the same, there is a high likelihood that the scores would fall within the range indicated.

Continued on page 64

The Official Study Guide for the Middle Level SSAT

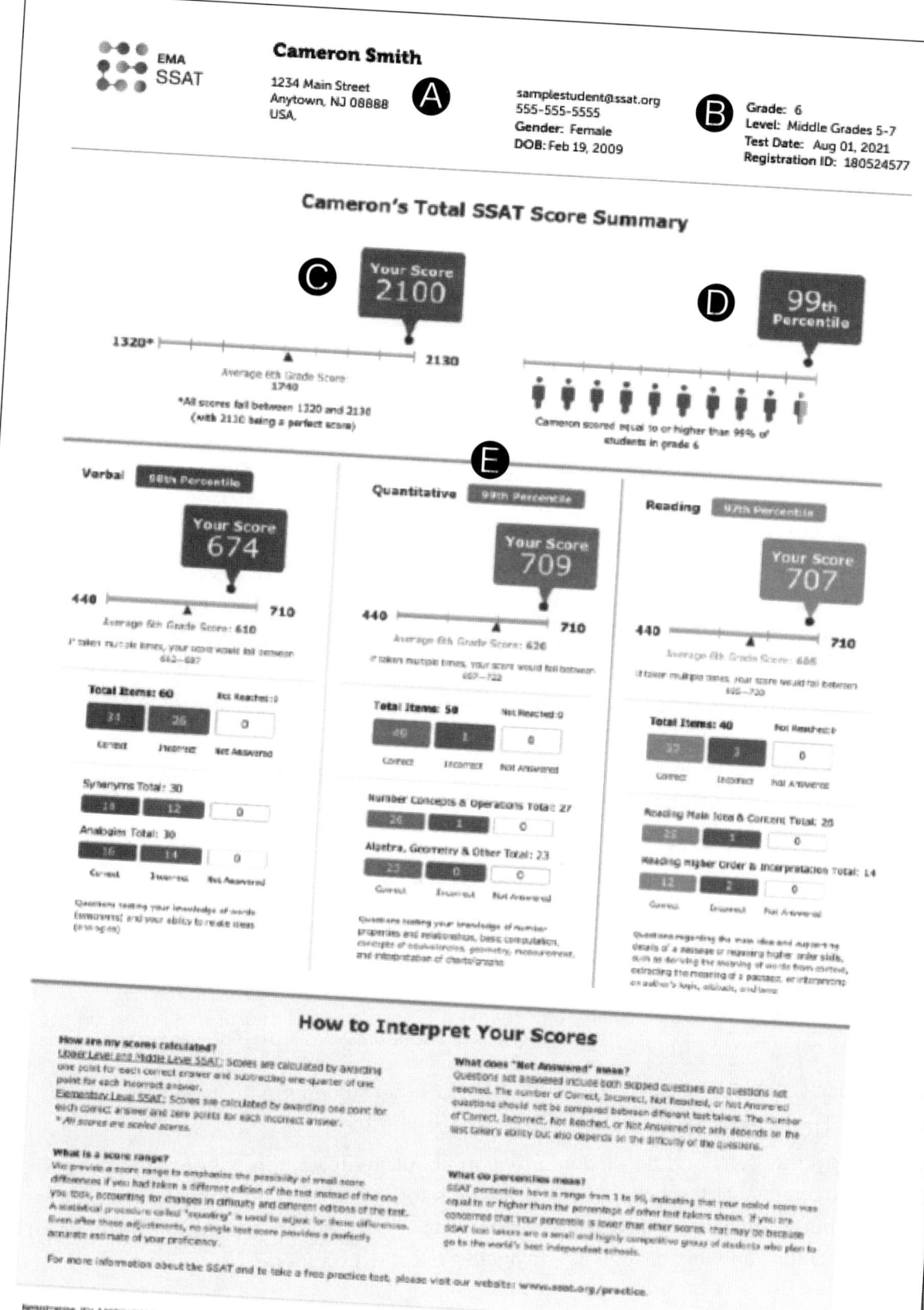

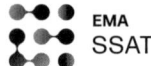

D SSAT Score Information

Beginning with the 2021–2022 academic year, SSAT provides reference information based on one norm group. The norm group, such as all students in grade 6, contains all test takers in the same grade level who have taken one of the Standard SSAT administrations in the United States and Canada typically within the past three years. If a test taker completed the SSAT in previous years, a second norm group, such as female students in grade 6, would have been displayed, indicating test takers of the same grade level and gender who have taken one of the Standard administrations in the United States and Canada within the past three years. The difference between the two norm groups is that the total norm group contains both male and female test takers, whereas the second norm group is gender specific. You will only see the grade-specific norm group going forward. You will also see the average scaled score attained by the group.

SSAT Percentile

The SSAT reports percentile ranks. The percentile rank is the percentage of students in the norm group whose scores fall below your scaled score. For example, if a seventh-grade student's verbal scaled score is 680 and the percentile rank is 72 on the verbal section in the total group, 72% of all seventh-grade students in the norm group had a verbal score lower than 680.

Many parents express concern that their student's SSAT percentiles are lower than those they have earned on other tests. Please remember that SSAT test takers are members of a small and highly competitive group of students who plan to attend some of the world's best schools. Do not be discouraged by what seems to be a lower score than the student usually attains on standardized testing.

> It is important to remember that SSAT test takers are members of a small and highly competitive group of students who plan to attend some of the world's best private schools. Being in the middle of this group is still impressive!

International and Flex test scores are not included in the comparison norm group. However, international testers' scaled scores are compared to the domestic/Standard/first-time test-taker norm group described above.

SSAT Average Score

SSAT average scores provide additional context information for your SSAT scaled score on each of the three scored sections (verbal, quantitative/math, and reading). These average scores are based on the same norm group used to provide the SSAT percentiles.

The SSAT average score is the average performance of all other students in the total norm group.

E Test Question Breakdown

This section provides useful and detailed information about the test's content and the student's test-taking strategies. Look carefully at the ratio of wrong answers to unanswered questions. If the student had many wrong answers but omitted few or no questions, meaning that they were guessing quite a bit instead of skipping questions they couldn't answer, that could have an adverse effect on scores.

Supporting the Test Taker

Here are a few simple things you can do to help your student perform as well as possible on the SSAT.

Practice! Practice! Practice! Help your student structure time to take the practice tests in the next chapter. Act as the proctor—administer the timed practice tests while approximating testing conditions as closely as possible.

Review and encourage! Review any incorrect answers. Which sections or types of questions proved most difficult? Focus, encourage, and help your student sharpen those skills. Examine your student's guessing strategy. Try to determine the cause of the errors so that your student can develop a strategy for avoiding similar mistakes on the actual test.

Some common pitfalls:
- Accidentally marking the wrong circle on the answer sheet when the student knows the correct answer
- Making simple arithmetic mistakes

Double-checking answers and not rushing can help with this.

Extra help! If taking the practice tests reveals that your student lacks a particular skill that is necessary for success, seeking extra help for your student may be useful. If you would rather self-direct this process, consider signing up for SSAT Practice Online. With diagnostic tools, progress indicators, and study tools, it provides a full year of help and feedback.

Perspective is everything! Keep the importance of the SSAT in perspective and help your student do the same. The SSAT is an important and valuable part of the application package and students should prepare for it. But remember that the SSAT is just *one* part of the entire package. Schools will weigh your student's test scores along with other information.

Retaking the test? Scheduling options are available at ssat.org should your student want to retake the SSAT. In general, the lower the initial scores, the more likely the scores will increase the second time.

Rest up and eat well! Make sure your student gets enough sleep on the days leading up to the test and that he or she eats a healthy breakfast on the day it is administered.

Be prepared for the unexpected! If your student panics, freezes, or gets sick during the administration of the SSAT, she or he has the option to leave the test. It's important for you to know that if your child does leave the test, the results will be canceled. It's your responsibility, however, to alert The Enrollment Management Association immediately so that the scores are voided and not sent to schools. Please note that your fee for the canceled test will not be refunded, but for a service charge, you may reschedule for a new test date.

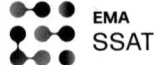

THIS PAGE INTENTIONALLY LEFT BLANK.

Chapter Four: The Character Skills Snapshot

What Is the Character Skills Snapshot?

The Character Skills Snapshot is an online assessment tool designed for students in grades 5 to 11 who are seeking entrance to private schools for grades 6 to 12. The purpose of the Snapshot is to measure essential character skills deemed important by private schools. The Snapshot is considered one new and important piece of the student admissions process, but it should not be used independently of other pieces of information to make admissions decisions.

What Is the Purpose of the Snapshot?

We know that schools care about students and how they grow—not just in cognitive skills such as writing and math, but also growing into good citizens with initiative, resilience, and social awareness—those skills that carry them forward into a successful adult life.

While character education is a hallmark of a private school education and is a salient piece of every school's mission, gaining insight into an applying student's current character skill development has been largely a matter of intuition and an investigative screening of the application. While many schools assess character in some way (e.g., via student interviews or teacher recommendations), reliance on unstandardized or inconsistent methods to assess character skills can introduce bias and subjectivity into the admissions process. This highlights the need for a standardized and empirically supported approach.

The Snapshot is meant to provide a snapshot in time of a student's character skills—it is not a fixed, absolute measure. It provides a way for schools to get to know a student better and an opportunity for them to enumerate the ways in which their communities can enrich and develop a student's developing skills.

How Was the Snapshot Designed?

The development of the Snapshot was research- and data-driven. Over the last six years, The Enrollment Management Association has put considerable time and resources toward developing the Snapshot. Spearheaded by the recommendation of the Think Tank on the Future of Assessment, EMA worked with 56 private schools and Educational Testing Service to conceptualize, build, pilot, and launch the Character Skills Snapshot. The Snapshot, a revolutionary new tool for the admissions process, enables member schools to include a standardized measure of character into their admissions process.

Prior to launching the Snapshot, multiple pretesting and field trials were conducted with more than 12,000 students completing the assessment. Additionally, user testing was conducted with parents to gain feedback on the design and content elements of the results reports, as well as the assessment itself.

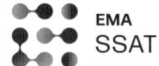

What Does the Snapshot Measure?

The Snapshot measures seven character skills.

Character Skill	Definition	Example Preferences
Initiative	This skill describes the student's inclination to work on assignments in a timely manner and emphasizes the point at which a student chooses to start work rather than when the student finishes work.	Starts working on assignments early Does not do things at the last minute
Intellectual Engagement	This skill focuses on the student's enjoyment of and willingness to pursue learning opportunities, regardless of how much difficulty they might present.	Enjoys challenging assignments and tasks Likes to learn more about topics of interest
Open-Mindedness	This skill describes the student's willingness to try new things.	Is open to trying new and unfamiliar approaches Does not avoid trying new activities, experiences, music and/or food
Resilience	This skill highlights the student's ability to adjust to unexpected situations and changing circumstances.	Readily adapts when plans change Is comfortable in stressful situations
Self-Control	This skill focuses on the student's ability to monitor and control his or her thoughts and actions, and what he or she says to others.	Thinks carefully about what he or she says Thinks things through before making a decision
Social Awareness	This skill describes a student's ability to recognize the appropriate ways to interact with others.	Adapts behavior based on the particular context Attempts to resolve conflicts and act appropriately
Teamwork	This skill highlights the student's ability to engage in supportive behaviors and emphasizes empathetic qualities that enable productive collaboration with others.	Attempts to comfort friends when they are upset Tries to resolve conflicts between people in a group

The Character Skills Snapshot Consists of TWO Sections

The first section has 20–30 forced-choice questions, depending on the form. A forced-choice question presents three short statements and asks you to select the response that is MOST like you and the response that is LEAST like you. One option will always be left blank. (See Sample Questions at the end of this chapter.)

The second section has 10 situational judgment scenarios. You are asked to read each scenario then read the four corresponding responses. You are asked to rate the appropriateness of each response using a scale of 1 (not appropriate) to 4 (very appropriate). You can use the same ratings for each response. For example, if you think each response is very appropriate, you can use a rating of 4 for each option.

How Is the Snapshot Administered?

The Snapshot is administered online. After parents consent for their student(s) to take the Snapshot and respond to an integrity statement, the student can then log into their Student Access Portal and begin the Snapshot.

The tool is untimed, but usually takes about 30 minutes to complete.

Is the Snapshot Reliable?

Yes, the Snapshot is reliable. Reliability is a measure of consistency. Think of it this way: If you weigh yourself every day for a week and the scale registers the same weight, you can say that the scale is reliable. In statistics, reliability is measured on a scale from 0–1: "0" means no reliability at all and "1" means perfect reliability, which is rarely achieved in reality. Depending on the purpose of the test, the desired range of reliability can vary. For a noncognitive assessment like the Snapshot, a reliability of 0.7 or higher is preferable. The Snapshot has achieved this target reliability.

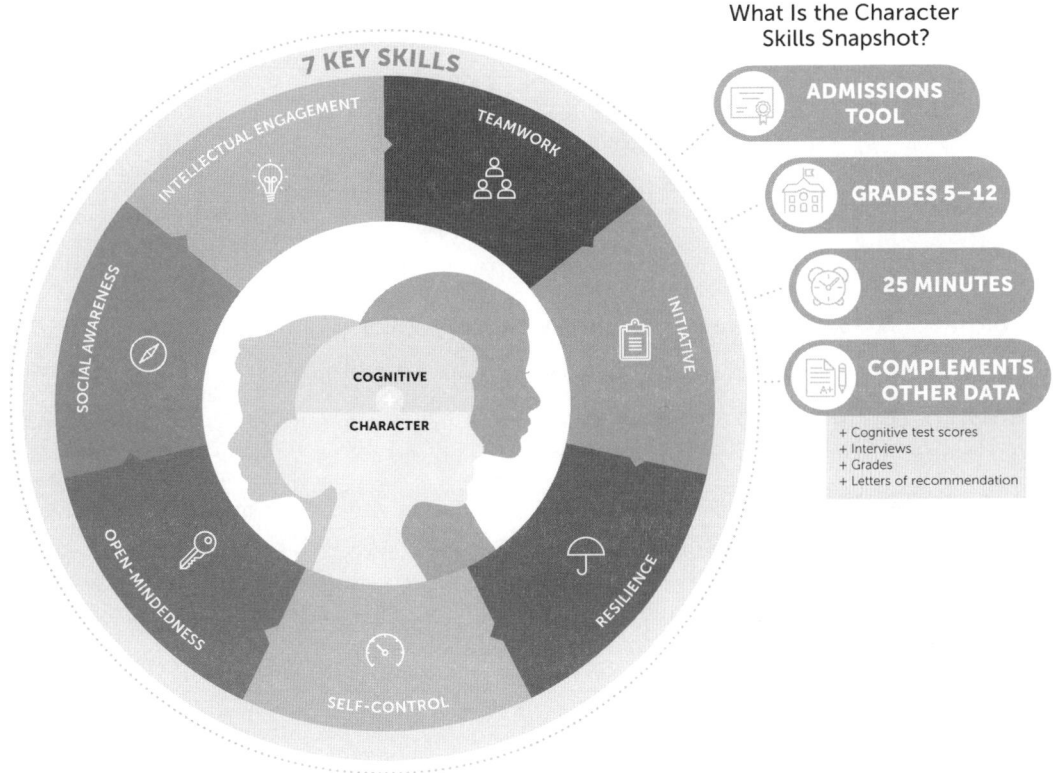

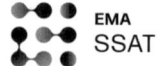
EMA
SSAT

The Snapshot Is a Norm-Referenced Assessment

A norm-referenced assessment interprets an individual's results compared to the results distribution of a comparison group, referred to as the norm group. The Snapshot norm groups are based on a group of approximately 5,000 students who took the Snapshot during a given academic year. There are two norm groups for the Snapshot, determined by grade band. The middle-level norm group consists of all students in grades 5–7 applying to grades 6–8. The upper-level norm group consists of all students in grades 8–11 applying to grades 9–12.

The Snapshot reports results for each of the seven skills in three performance categories: Emerging, Developing, and Demonstrating.

Emerging	**Developing**	**Demonstrating**
The student's result fell into the lowest 25% (0–25th percentile) of scores in the comparison sample.	The student's result fell into the middle 50% (above 25th and below 75th percentile) of scores in the comparison sample.	The student's results fell in the upper 25% (at or above 75th percentile) of scores in the comparison sample.
The student is starting to show signs of this skill. Note that emerging does not imply a student does not have any of this skill.	The student displays the skill but is continuing to develop it.	The student displays a clear understanding and use of this skill. Note that demonstrating a skill does not imply that a student has mastered the skill. There is still room to grow.

Strategies for Taking the Snapshot

Relax. The Snapshot provides you with an opportunity to share more about yourself and your preferences as they relate to the seven character skills with schools. Remember, it is only one piece of the application.

Answer honestly. Remember this is the way you see yourself—not how your parents, your friends, your teacher, or your coach would describe you.

Select the choice that is MOST like you or the choice that is LEAST like you. You are sometimes going to have to make a difficult choice. You may see multiple options that are all like you or not like you at all.

Consider your answers carefully. The assessment will not allow you to go back and change your answers. Once a selection is made, it is final.

Do not misrepresent yourself. Trying to answer questions in such a way as to make yourself look good on any one skill may have an adverse effect on some of the other skills. Don't overthink your answers, just be yourself!

Sample Questions
Forced-Choice

Select the statement that describes you most accurately and the statement that describes you least accurately. There will always be one statement in each set of three that will not be dragged into the "most" and "least" boxes.

| I say the first thing that comes to my mind. | I get bored when trying to solve difficult problems. | I avoid being emotionally involved in other people's problems. |

Most like me: I avoid being emotionally involved in other people's problems.

Least like me: I get bored when trying to solve difficult problems.

| I am open to trying new things. | I like to research topics that are interesting to me. | I am willing to help people whenever they ask for my help. |

Most like me: I am willing to help people whenever they ask for my help.

Least like me: I like to research topics that are interesting to me.

| I do not like to change the way something is done if the current way still works. | Before doing something, I first think carefully about it. | It is easy for me to find something else to do if someone cancels at the last minute. |

Most like me: I do not like to change the way something is done if the current way still works.

Least like me: Before doing something, I first think carefully about it.

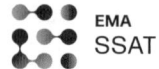

Situational Judgment

Please rate the appropriateness of each possible response from 1 (not appropriate at all) to 4 (very appropriate). You can apply the same rating to more than one response. If, for example, you believe that two of the possible responses would be 1 (not appropriate at all), you may mark them both with a 1.

After two weeks of late nights, Sarah feels overwhelmed by the demands of her Spanish class and the upcoming assessment. Sarah has been an attentive student, but Spanish does not come easy to her. She wants to meet with her Spanish teacher, but he has been ill during the week and will not return to school tomorrow. Unfortunately, this is the day before the test.

Possible Responses	1 (not appropriate at all)	2	3	4 (very appropriate)
Meet with the Spanish teacher and suggest that giving the test this week is not fair since he has been absent.		2		
Meet with the Spanish teacher and ask him if there is a way he can give her a few more days to prepare for the test.			3	
Speak to her parents and ask them to call the Spanish teacher to voice their concern about giving students a test immediately after the teacher was unavailable to students for so long.	1			
Meet with the Spanish teacher when he returns to discuss her recent progress and develop a long-term plan to improve.				4

As a member of the student council, Caroline is on a committee that plans themes for school dances. While Caroline proposes a 1960's theme for the winter formal, the other members of the committee propose a "night at the movies" theme.

Possible Responses	1 (not appropriate at all)	2	3	4 (very appropriate)
Accept the proposal of the majority of committee members.			3	
Accept the proposal of the majority of committee members, but demand that she can choose the theme for the next dance.		2		
Resign from student council because she did not get her way.	1			
Accept the proposal of the majority of committee members, but quietly convince as many students as she can not to attend the dance.		2		

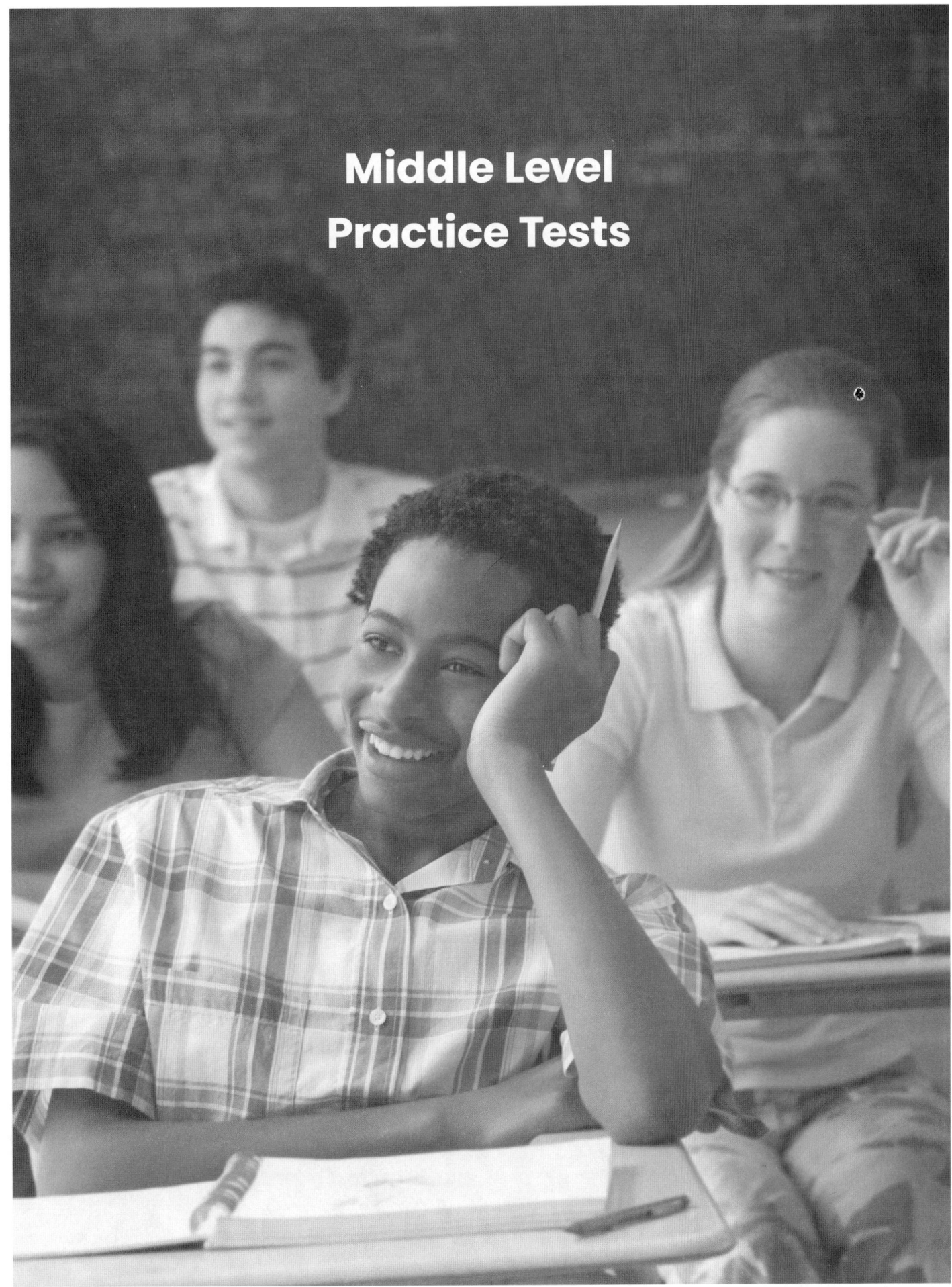

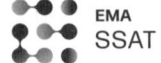

Trying Out the Middle Level SSAT

Now it's time to find out what it's actually like to take the Middle Level SSAT. Ask someone to help you set up a simulation — a re-creation of the experience that is as close as possible to actually taking the SSAT. Think of it as a dress rehearsal for the real thing. Simulating the SSAT experience can help you gain confidence and clarity about what to expect.

Remove (or photocopy) the answer sheet and use it to complete each practice test.

You can choose to do your simulation section by section or by taking an entire test from start to finish.

Here are the rules you'll need to follow to make your SSAT simulation as realistic as possible:

+ Ask your "test proctor" to keep time and tell you when to begin and end each section.
+ No talking or music is allowed during the SSAT; so, make sure the room in which you are taking the test is quiet and turn off anything that makes noise, such as your phone, iPod, or TV.
+ You will not be allowed to use any research material while taking the SSAT; so, put away your smartphone, laptop, books, dictionary, calculator, ruler, and notes.
+ Work only on one section during the time allotted. Do not go back to another section to finish unanswered questions.
+ Use sharpened #2 pencils and an eraser.
+ Fill in the answer sheet (located before each test in the book) just as you would during a regular test.

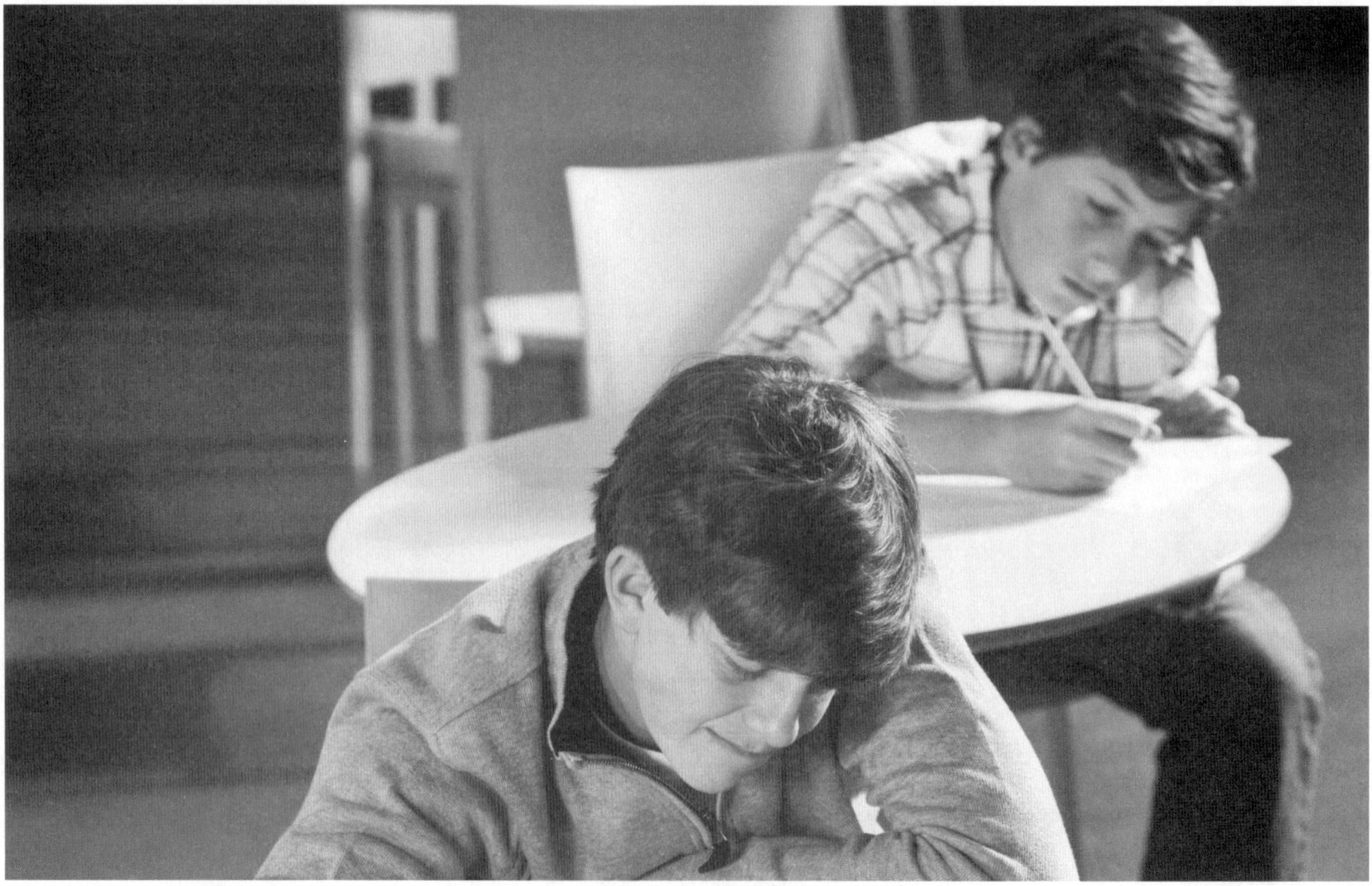

Simulating the Test: Section by Section

If your goal is to sharpen your test-taking techniques in a specific area, use the individual sections for the simulation. Review the exercises in Chapter 2 before beginning, and be sure to follow the instructions for each section carefully. Schedule the allotted time for each section, and ask the person supervising your simulation to time you, or set a timer for yourself.

As you will when you actually take the SSAT, mark your answer choices on the answer sheet.

Simulating the Test: Start to Finish

If your goal is to practice taking the entire SSAT (minus the experimental section), here's how to schedule your time blocks, including breaks:

Test Overview

Section	Number of Questions	Time Allotted to Administer Each Section
Writing Sample	1	25 minutes
Break		10 minutes
Section 1 (Quantitative)	25	30 minutes
Section 2 (Reading)	40	40 minutes
Break		10 minutes
Section 3 (Verbal)	60	30 minutes
Section 4 (Quantitative)	25	30 minutes
Totals	**151**	**2 hours, 55 minutes**

You'll see that the total testing time is 2 hours and 35 minutes. When you add in the two breaks, the total time is 2 hours and 55 minutes (these practice tests do not include an experimental section). Be sure to use your breaks for stretching, getting a drink of water, and focusing your eyes on something other than a test paper. This will help clear your mind and get you ready for the next section.

A note about special timing: Some students are granted "time and a half" accommodations, and are given 1.5 times the minutes available for each test section, including the writing sample. Students who are granted 1.5x time do not take the experimental section.

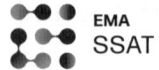

Practice Test I: Middle Level Answer Sheet

Be sure each mark completely fills the answer space.
Start with number 1 for each new section of the test.

Section 1

1 Ⓐ Ⓑ Ⓒ Ⓓ Ⓔ   6 Ⓐ Ⓑ Ⓒ Ⓓ Ⓔ   11 Ⓐ Ⓑ Ⓒ Ⓓ Ⓔ   16 Ⓐ Ⓑ Ⓒ Ⓓ Ⓔ   21 Ⓐ Ⓑ Ⓒ Ⓓ Ⓔ
2 Ⓐ Ⓑ Ⓒ Ⓓ Ⓔ   7 Ⓐ Ⓑ Ⓒ Ⓓ Ⓔ   12 Ⓐ Ⓑ Ⓒ Ⓓ Ⓔ   17 Ⓐ Ⓑ Ⓒ Ⓓ Ⓔ   22 Ⓐ Ⓑ Ⓒ Ⓓ Ⓔ
3 Ⓐ Ⓑ Ⓒ Ⓓ Ⓔ   8 Ⓐ Ⓑ Ⓒ Ⓓ Ⓔ   13 Ⓐ Ⓑ Ⓒ Ⓓ Ⓔ   18 Ⓐ Ⓑ Ⓒ Ⓓ Ⓔ   23 Ⓐ Ⓑ Ⓒ Ⓓ Ⓔ
4 Ⓐ Ⓑ Ⓒ Ⓓ Ⓔ   9 Ⓐ Ⓑ Ⓒ Ⓓ Ⓔ   14 Ⓐ Ⓑ Ⓒ Ⓓ Ⓔ   19 Ⓐ Ⓑ Ⓒ Ⓓ Ⓔ   24 Ⓐ Ⓑ Ⓒ Ⓓ Ⓔ
5 Ⓐ Ⓑ Ⓒ Ⓓ Ⓔ   10 Ⓐ Ⓑ Ⓒ Ⓓ Ⓔ   15 Ⓐ Ⓑ Ⓒ Ⓓ Ⓔ   20 Ⓐ Ⓑ Ⓒ Ⓓ Ⓔ   25 Ⓐ Ⓑ Ⓒ Ⓓ Ⓔ

Section 2

1 Ⓐ Ⓑ Ⓒ Ⓓ Ⓔ   9 Ⓐ Ⓑ Ⓒ Ⓓ Ⓔ   17 Ⓐ Ⓑ Ⓒ Ⓓ Ⓔ   25 Ⓐ Ⓑ Ⓒ Ⓓ Ⓔ   33 Ⓐ Ⓑ Ⓒ Ⓓ Ⓔ
2 Ⓐ Ⓑ Ⓒ Ⓓ Ⓔ   10 Ⓐ Ⓑ Ⓒ Ⓓ Ⓔ   18 Ⓐ Ⓑ Ⓒ Ⓓ Ⓔ   26 Ⓐ Ⓑ Ⓒ Ⓓ Ⓔ   34 Ⓐ Ⓑ Ⓒ Ⓓ Ⓔ
3 Ⓐ Ⓑ Ⓒ Ⓓ Ⓔ   11 Ⓐ Ⓑ Ⓒ Ⓓ Ⓔ   19 Ⓐ Ⓑ Ⓒ Ⓓ Ⓔ   27 Ⓐ Ⓑ Ⓒ Ⓓ Ⓔ   35 Ⓐ Ⓑ Ⓒ Ⓓ Ⓔ
4 Ⓐ Ⓑ Ⓒ Ⓓ Ⓔ   12 Ⓐ Ⓑ Ⓒ Ⓓ Ⓔ   20 Ⓐ Ⓑ Ⓒ Ⓓ Ⓔ   28 Ⓐ Ⓑ Ⓒ Ⓓ Ⓔ   36 Ⓐ Ⓑ Ⓒ Ⓓ Ⓔ
5 Ⓐ Ⓑ Ⓒ Ⓓ Ⓔ   13 Ⓐ Ⓑ Ⓒ Ⓓ Ⓔ   21 Ⓐ Ⓑ Ⓒ Ⓓ Ⓔ   29 Ⓐ Ⓑ Ⓒ Ⓓ Ⓔ   37 Ⓐ Ⓑ Ⓒ Ⓓ Ⓔ
6 Ⓐ Ⓑ Ⓒ Ⓓ Ⓔ   14 Ⓐ Ⓑ Ⓒ Ⓓ Ⓔ   22 Ⓐ Ⓑ Ⓒ Ⓓ Ⓔ   30 Ⓐ Ⓑ Ⓒ Ⓓ Ⓔ   38 Ⓐ Ⓑ Ⓒ Ⓓ Ⓔ
7 Ⓐ Ⓑ Ⓒ Ⓓ Ⓔ   15 Ⓐ Ⓑ Ⓒ Ⓓ Ⓔ   23 Ⓐ Ⓑ Ⓒ Ⓓ Ⓔ   31 Ⓐ Ⓑ Ⓒ Ⓓ Ⓔ   39 Ⓐ Ⓑ Ⓒ Ⓓ Ⓔ
8 Ⓐ Ⓑ Ⓒ Ⓓ Ⓔ   16 Ⓐ Ⓑ Ⓒ Ⓓ Ⓔ   24 Ⓐ Ⓑ Ⓒ Ⓓ Ⓔ   32 Ⓐ Ⓑ Ⓒ Ⓓ Ⓔ   40 Ⓐ Ⓑ Ⓒ Ⓓ Ⓔ

Section 3

1 Ⓐ Ⓑ Ⓒ Ⓓ Ⓔ   13 Ⓐ Ⓑ Ⓒ Ⓓ Ⓔ   25 Ⓐ Ⓑ Ⓒ Ⓓ Ⓔ   37 Ⓐ Ⓑ Ⓒ Ⓓ Ⓔ   49 Ⓐ Ⓑ Ⓒ Ⓓ Ⓔ
2 Ⓐ Ⓑ Ⓒ Ⓓ Ⓔ   14 Ⓐ Ⓑ Ⓒ Ⓓ Ⓔ   26 Ⓐ Ⓑ Ⓒ Ⓓ Ⓔ   38 Ⓐ Ⓑ Ⓒ Ⓓ Ⓔ   50 Ⓐ Ⓑ Ⓒ Ⓓ Ⓔ
3 Ⓐ Ⓑ Ⓒ Ⓓ Ⓔ   15 Ⓐ Ⓑ Ⓒ Ⓓ Ⓔ   27 Ⓐ Ⓑ Ⓒ Ⓓ Ⓔ   39 Ⓐ Ⓑ Ⓒ Ⓓ Ⓔ   51 Ⓐ Ⓑ Ⓒ Ⓓ Ⓔ
4 Ⓐ Ⓑ Ⓒ Ⓓ Ⓔ   16 Ⓐ Ⓑ Ⓒ Ⓓ Ⓔ   28 Ⓐ Ⓑ Ⓒ Ⓓ Ⓔ   40 Ⓐ Ⓑ Ⓒ Ⓓ Ⓔ   52 Ⓐ Ⓑ Ⓒ Ⓓ Ⓔ
5 Ⓐ Ⓑ Ⓒ Ⓓ Ⓔ   17 Ⓐ Ⓑ Ⓒ Ⓓ Ⓔ   29 Ⓐ Ⓑ Ⓒ Ⓓ Ⓔ   41 Ⓐ Ⓑ Ⓒ Ⓓ Ⓔ   53 Ⓐ Ⓑ Ⓒ Ⓓ Ⓔ
6 Ⓐ Ⓑ Ⓒ Ⓓ Ⓔ   18 Ⓐ Ⓑ Ⓒ Ⓓ Ⓔ   30 Ⓐ Ⓑ Ⓒ Ⓓ Ⓔ   42 Ⓐ Ⓑ Ⓒ Ⓓ Ⓔ   54 Ⓐ Ⓑ Ⓒ Ⓓ Ⓔ
7 Ⓐ Ⓑ Ⓒ Ⓓ Ⓔ   19 Ⓐ Ⓑ Ⓒ Ⓓ Ⓔ   31 Ⓐ Ⓑ Ⓒ Ⓓ Ⓔ   43 Ⓐ Ⓑ Ⓒ Ⓓ Ⓔ   55 Ⓐ Ⓑ Ⓒ Ⓓ Ⓔ
8 Ⓐ Ⓑ Ⓒ Ⓓ Ⓔ   20 Ⓐ Ⓑ Ⓒ Ⓓ Ⓔ   32 Ⓐ Ⓑ Ⓒ Ⓓ Ⓔ   44 Ⓐ Ⓑ Ⓒ Ⓓ Ⓔ   56 Ⓐ Ⓑ Ⓒ Ⓓ Ⓔ
9 Ⓐ Ⓑ Ⓒ Ⓓ Ⓔ   21 Ⓐ Ⓑ Ⓒ Ⓓ Ⓔ   33 Ⓐ Ⓑ Ⓒ Ⓓ Ⓔ   45 Ⓐ Ⓑ Ⓒ Ⓓ Ⓔ   57 Ⓐ Ⓑ Ⓒ Ⓓ Ⓔ
10 Ⓐ Ⓑ Ⓒ Ⓓ Ⓔ   22 Ⓐ Ⓑ Ⓒ Ⓓ Ⓔ   34 Ⓐ Ⓑ Ⓒ Ⓓ Ⓔ   46 Ⓐ Ⓑ Ⓒ Ⓓ Ⓔ   58 Ⓐ Ⓑ Ⓒ Ⓓ Ⓔ
11 Ⓐ Ⓑ Ⓒ Ⓓ Ⓔ   23 Ⓐ Ⓑ Ⓒ Ⓓ Ⓔ   35 Ⓐ Ⓑ Ⓒ Ⓓ Ⓔ   47 Ⓐ Ⓑ Ⓒ Ⓓ Ⓔ   59 Ⓐ Ⓑ Ⓒ Ⓓ Ⓔ
12 Ⓐ Ⓑ Ⓒ Ⓓ Ⓔ   24 Ⓐ Ⓑ Ⓒ Ⓓ Ⓔ   36 Ⓐ Ⓑ Ⓒ Ⓓ Ⓔ   48 Ⓐ Ⓑ Ⓒ Ⓓ Ⓔ   60 Ⓐ Ⓑ Ⓒ Ⓓ Ⓔ

Section 4

1 Ⓐ Ⓑ Ⓒ Ⓓ Ⓔ   6 Ⓐ Ⓑ Ⓒ Ⓓ Ⓔ   11 Ⓐ Ⓑ Ⓒ Ⓓ Ⓔ   16 Ⓐ Ⓑ Ⓒ Ⓓ Ⓔ   21 Ⓐ Ⓑ Ⓒ Ⓓ Ⓔ
2 Ⓐ Ⓑ Ⓒ Ⓓ Ⓔ   7 Ⓐ Ⓑ Ⓒ Ⓓ Ⓔ   12 Ⓐ Ⓑ Ⓒ Ⓓ Ⓔ   17 Ⓐ Ⓑ Ⓒ Ⓓ Ⓔ   22 Ⓐ Ⓑ Ⓒ Ⓓ Ⓔ
3 Ⓐ Ⓑ Ⓒ Ⓓ Ⓔ   8 Ⓐ Ⓑ Ⓒ Ⓓ Ⓔ   13 Ⓐ Ⓑ Ⓒ Ⓓ Ⓔ   18 Ⓐ Ⓑ Ⓒ Ⓓ Ⓔ   23 Ⓐ Ⓑ Ⓒ Ⓓ Ⓔ
4 Ⓐ Ⓑ Ⓒ Ⓓ Ⓔ   9 Ⓐ Ⓑ Ⓒ Ⓓ Ⓔ   14 Ⓐ Ⓑ Ⓒ Ⓓ Ⓔ   19 Ⓐ Ⓑ Ⓒ Ⓓ Ⓔ   24 Ⓐ Ⓑ Ⓒ Ⓓ Ⓔ
5 Ⓐ Ⓑ Ⓒ Ⓓ Ⓔ   10 Ⓐ Ⓑ Ⓒ Ⓓ Ⓔ   15 Ⓐ Ⓑ Ⓒ Ⓓ Ⓔ   20 Ⓐ Ⓑ Ⓒ Ⓓ Ⓔ   25 Ⓐ Ⓑ Ⓒ Ⓓ Ⓔ

Section 5

Experimental Section – See page 9 for details.

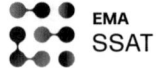

THIS PAGE INTENTIONALLY LEFT BLANK.

Writing Sample

Schools would like to get to know you better through a story you tell or an essay you write. If you choose to write a story, use the sentence presented in A to begin. Make sure that your story has a beginning, middle, and end. If you choose to write a personal essay, base your essay on the topic presented in B. Please fill in the circle next to your choice.

Ⓐ I had fifteen minutes to solve the puzzle.

Ⓑ What has been your favorite class in the past year or so? Describe the class and explain why it has been your favorite.

Use this page and the next page to complete your writing sample.

Continue on next page

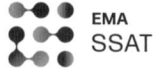

THIS PAGE INTENTIONALLY LEFT BLANK.

SECTION 1
25 Questions

Following each problem in this section, there are five suggested answers. Work each problem in your head or in the blank space provided at the right of the page. Then look at the five suggested answers and decide which one is best.

Note: Figures that accompany problems in this section are drawn as accurately as possible EXCEPT when it is stated in a specific problem that its figure is not drawn to scale.

Sample Problem:

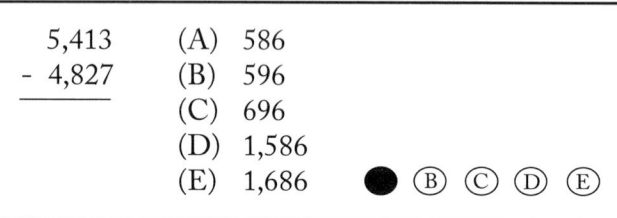

USE THIS SPACE FOR FIGURING.

1. If $n + 5 = 5$, what is the value of n?

    (A) 0
    (B) $\frac{1}{5}$
    (C) 1
    (D) 5
    (E) 10

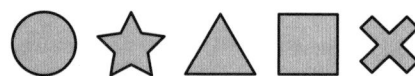

2. The sequence of shapes above repeats indefinitely as shown. Which shape is the 12th shape in the sequence?

    (A)

    (B)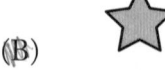

    (C)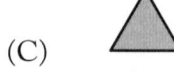

    (D)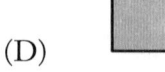

    (E)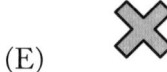

GO ON TO THE NEXT PAGE.

3. There were 20 illustrations in Julio's sketch pad. While at a museum, he drew x more illustrations in the sketch pad. Which expression represents the total number of illustrations in Julio's sketch pad after his museum visit?

   (A) $\frac{x}{20}$

   (B) $\frac{20}{x}$

   (C) $20x$

   (D) $20 - x$

   (E) $20 + x$

$$4,\blacksquare 86$$

4. The ■ in the number above represents a digit from 0 through 9. If the number is less than 4,486, what is the greatest possible value for ■?

   (A) 0
   (B) 3
   (C) 4
   (D) 7
   (E) 9

5. Which of the following is the sum of $\frac{3}{8}$ and $\frac{4}{7}$?

   (A) $\frac{1}{8}$

   (B) $\frac{3}{14}$

   (C) $\frac{7}{15}$

   (D) $\frac{33}{56}$

   (E) $\frac{53}{56}$

USE THIS SPACE FOR FIGURING.

6. Ilona goes on a 4-hour hike from her campsite to a scenic lookout. The graph shows her altitude during the hike and the time it took her to reach each corresponding altitude. Based on the graph, the altitude of the scenic outlook is how many meters above the altitude of the campsite?

   (A) 100
   (B) 200
   (C) 300
   (D) 400
   (E) 500

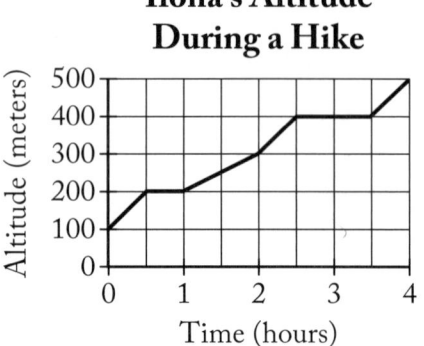

7. What is the value of $0.5 \times 23.5 \times 0.2$?

   (A) 0.0235
   (B) 0.235
   (C) 2.35
   (D) 23.5
   (E) 235

8. On a table, there are ten of each of the following types of coins: 1-cent, 5-cent, 10-cent, and 25-cent coins. If Edith needs exactly 36 cents, what is the least number of coins she must take from the table?

   (A) Two
   (B) Three
   (C) Four
   (D) Five
   (E) Six

9. What is the value of $\frac{1}{2}\left(\frac{3}{4} \times \frac{1}{3}\right)$?

   (A) $\frac{1}{8}$
   (B) $\frac{5}{24}$
   (C) $\frac{2}{9}$
   (D) $\frac{13}{24}$
   (E) $\frac{19}{12}$

GO ON TO THE NEXT PAGE.

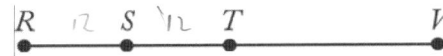

10. In the figure above, segment $\overline{ST}$ has length 12, T is the midpoint of the segment $\overline{RV}$, and S is the midpoint of segment $\overline{RT}$. What is the length of the segment $\overline{SV}$?

    (A) 12
    (B) 18
    (C) 24
    (D) 36
    (E) 48

11. Let ⓐ be defined by ⓐ = $a^2 + 1$, where a is a whole number.

    What is the value of ③ ?

    (A) 16
    (B) 10
    (C) 8
    (D) 7
    (E) 6

12. Each student at Central Middle School wears a uniform consisting of 1 shirt and 1 pair of pants. The table shows the colors available for each item of clothing. How many different uniforms are possible?

    (A) Three
    (B) Four
    (C) Seven
    (D) Ten
    (E) Twelve

Uniform Choices	
Shirt Color	Pants Color
Tan	Black
Red	Khaki
White	Navy
Yellow	

13. If n is a positive odd integer, which of the following must be an even integer?

    (A) $3n - 1$
    (B) $2n + 3$
    (C) $2n - 1$
    (D) $n + 2$
    (E) $\frac{3n}{2}$

14. Joseph's car began the week with a full tank of gasoline. During the week, he drove his car 232 miles and paid $32 for gasoline that week. At this rate, how many miles will he drive if he pays $40 for gasoline next week?

    (A) 240
    (B) 288
    (C) 290
    (D) 320
    (E) 332

15. Of the following fractions, which is closest to 37% ?

    (A) $\frac{1}{3}$
    (B) $\frac{1}{4}$
    (C) $\frac{2}{5}$
    (D) $\frac{3}{7}$
    (E) $\frac{3}{8}$

16. At Banham School, there are 20 students in each class, and 5 classes wish to form 3 clubs. Each of the students must belong to only one club, and the membership of each club may not outnumber the membership of the other clubs by more than one student. What is the least possible number of students in one club?

    (A) 15
    (B) 20
    (C) 21
    (D) 33
    (E) 34

17. The rectangle shown is divided into 6 congruent squares. What fraction of the rectangle is shaded?

    (A) $\frac{3}{8}$

    (B) $\frac{5}{8}$

    (C) $\frac{5}{9}$

    (D) $\frac{7}{12}$

    (E) $\frac{2}{3}$

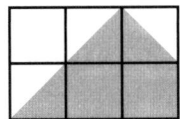

18. In a game, 2 gold pieces may be exchanged for 6 silver pieces, and 7 silver pieces may be exchanged for 42 copper pieces. At this rate, how many copper pieces may be exchanged for 5 gold pieces?

    (A) 10
    (B) 18
    (C) 36
    (D) 72
    (E) 90

19. The figure shown consists of three segments and two squares. Each square has side lengths of 2 centimeters, and AB = 6 centimeters, CD = 8 centimeters, and EF = 10 centimeters. Based on the figure, what is the length of n, in centimeters?

    (A) 18
    (B) 20
    (C) 22
    (D) 24
    (E) 26

20. Calculate: $3 + 6 \times 2^3 \div 3 + 3^2$

    (A) 21
    (B) 24
    (C) 27
    (D) 28
    (E) 33

GO ON TO THE NEXT PAGE.

21. A square card that is blank on both sides is punched with 2 small holes. The top face of the card is shown in the figure. If the card is turned facedown, which of the following orientations of the card is NOT possible?

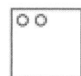

(A)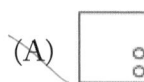

(B)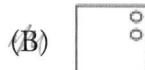

(C)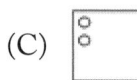

(D)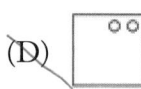

(E)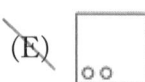

22. If a number n is even, which of the following expressions must be an integer?

(A) $\dfrac{3n}{2}$

(B) $\dfrac{3n}{4}$

(C) $\dfrac{n+4}{4}$

(D) $\dfrac{n+2}{3}$

(E) $\dfrac{3(n+1)}{2}$

23. On Monday, Aidan reads $\frac{1}{3}$ of a book, and on Tuesday, Aidan reads $\frac{1}{4}$ of the remaining pages. To complete reading the book, he must read an additional 60 pages. How many pages are in the book?

(A) 720
(B) 360
(C) 144
(D) 120
(E) 72

GO ON TO THE NEXT PAGE.

24. A square piece of paper has an area of 144 square inches. What is the circumference, in inches, of the largest circle that can be cut from the paper?

(A) 12π
(B) 24π
(C) 36π
(D) 72π
(E) 144π

25. The number 120 is increased by 50%, and the result is then decreased by 30% to give the number x. What is the value of x?

(A) 174
(B) 162
(C) 144
(D) 136
(E) 126

SECTION 2
40 Questions

Read each passage carefully and then answer the questions about it. For each question, decide on the basis of the passage which one of the choices best answers the question.

  Matthew Cuthbert ought to have been sowing his turnip seed on the big red brook field away over by Green Gables. Mrs. Rachel knew that he ought because she had heard him tell Peter Morrison the evening before in William J. Blair's store over at Carmody that he meant to sow his turnip seed the next afternoon. Peter had asked him, of course, for Matthew Cuthbert had never
Line 5 been known to volunteer information about anything in his whole life. And yet here was Matthew Cuthbert, at half-past three on the afternoon of a busy day, placidly driving over the hollow and up the hill; moreover, he wore a white collar and his best suit of clothes, which was plain proof that he was going out of Avonlea; and he had the buggy and the sorrel mare, which betokened that he was going a considerable distance. Now, where was Matthew Cuthbert going and why was he going
   10 there? Had it been any other man in Avonlea, Mrs. Rachel, deftly putting this and that together, might have given a pretty good guess as to both questions. But Matthew so rarely went from home that it must be something pressing and unusual which was taking him; he was the shyest man alive and hated to have to go among strangers or to any place where he might have to talk. Matthew, dressed up with a white collar and driving in a buggy, was something that didn't happen often. Mrs.
   15 Rachel, ponder as she might, could make nothing of it, and her afternoon's enjoyment was spoiled.

---

1. Mrs. Rachel is portrayed in the passage as a
   (A) recluse
   (B) busybody
   (C) worrywart
   (D) matchmaker
   (E) rabble-rouser

2. As it is used in line 3, the word "meant" most nearly means
   (A) signified
   (B) destined
   (C) intended
   (D) implied
   (E) foretold

3. The author uses the expression "putting this and that together" (line 10) to describe a process of
   (A) combining resources
   (B) fabricating an excuse
   (C) building a consensus
   (D) formulating a conjecture
   (E) gathering suggestions

4. As he is depicted in the passage, Matthew Cuthbert has a reputation for being
   (A) gullible
   (B) conceited
   (C) ill-tempered
   (D) irresponsible
   (E) uncommunicative

5. The passage suggests that Mrs. Rachel's enjoyment of the afternoon "was spoiled" (line 15) because
   (A) she was unable to satisfy her curiosity
   (B) she had no one to work in her fields
   (C) she had no means of leaving Avonlea
   (D) she feared for her neighbor's safety
   (E) she was overcome with jealousy

GO ON TO THE NEXT PAGE.

In 1930 an astronomer at the Lowell Observatory made an exciting discovery. Telescopic photographs revealed a sizeable body, much larger than any known comet or asteroid, orbiting the Sun in the furthest reaches of the solar system. The newly discovered object was soon hailed as the ninth planet and given the name of Pluto.

Line 5

However, toward the end of the twentieth century some astronomers began to raise doubts about Pluto's planetary status. Though substantial enough to have several moons of its own, Pluto was still much smaller than any other planet, and its eccentric orbit was tilted at a very different angle than those of its celestial siblings.

After carefully weighing the question of Pluto's planethood, the International Astronomical

10 Union in 2006 ruled that in order to be classified as a planet, an object must meet three criteria. It must orbit the Sun; it must be nearly round in shape; and it must have cleared the neighborhood around its orbit. Pluto meets the first two criteria but not the third. Unlike the eight true planets, Pluto lacks the gravitational force to drive away the multitude of icy celestial objects that share its orbital zone. For that reason, the International Astronomical Union downgraded Pluto's status to

15 that of a "dwarf planet."

6. The passage suggests that the general reaction to the discovery of Pluto was

   (A) fearful
   (B) hostile
   (C) enthusiastic
   (D) skeptical
   (E) puzzled

7. In line 6, the author uses the word "Though" to acknowledge that

   (A) Pluto had some claim to being considered a planet
   (B) there was strong popular support for Pluto's planetary status
   (C) the original classification of Pluto was made in haste
   (D) Astronomers were bitterly divided in their opinions about Pluto
   (E) Pluto did not fit the precise scientific definition of a planet

8. The author's use of metaphor in the last sentence of the second paragraph suggests that the solar system is like

   (A) an army
   (B) a family
   (C) a fleet
   (D) an atom
   (E) a machine

9. As it is used in line 10, the word "meet" most nearly means

   (A) gather
   (B) coincide
   (C) encounter
   (D) satisfy
   (E) confront

10. The words "For that reason" (line 14) refer to the fact that Pluto

    (A) is much smaller than any of the eight planets
    (B) has an eccentric and unusually tilted orbit
    (C) is located at the very edge of the solar system
    (D) allows other objects to occupy its neighborhood
    (E) is not sufficiently round in its shape

GO ON TO THE NEXT PAGE.

> At 5 a.m. on an intensely hot summer day, President John Quincy Adams left the White House by stagecoach for Quincy, Massachusetts. It was July 9, 1826, just two days short of his fifty-ninth birthday. He had been up the night before "in anxiety and apprehension, until near midnight."
> The heat made him miserable. Candlelight attracted insects. There were no screens. The day before,
>
> *Line 5* he had gotten three letters from Quincy with the news that his ninety-one-year-old father, the second president of the United States, was on his deathbed. John Quincy had "flattered" himself that his father "would survive this summer, and even other years." A rider was on his way from Baltimore to tell him he was wrong.

11. As it is used in line 3, the word "up" most nearly means
    (A) aloft
    (B) prepared
    (C) successful
    (D) cheerful
    (E) awake

12. The author suggests that Adams' "anxiety" (line 3) was due to concern about
    (A) growing old
    (B) matters of state
    (C) the summer heat
    (D) a long stagecoach ride
    (E) his father's health

13. The author mentions that there were "no screens" (line 4) in order to emphasize that Adams was
    (A) living in poverty
    (B) exposed to the public
    (C) socially uninhibited
    (D) physically vulnerable
    (E) fully informed

14. The use of the word "flattered" (line 6) suggests that Adams was
    (A) exceedingly vain
    (B) engaged in wishful thinking
    (C) manipulative and insincere
    (D) generous in his praise of others
    (E) immensely popular

15. The final sentence of the passage implies that Adams would be told that
    (A) his father had passed away
    (B) it was unsafe to travel by stagecoach
    (C) the weather in Quincy was not as bad as he feared
    (D) he had misinterpreted the letters from Quincy
    (E) it was irresponsible of him to leave the White House

> He rose at dawn, and, flushed with hope,
> Shot o'er the seething harbour-bar,
> And reached the ship, and caught the rope,
> And whistled to the morning star.
>
> Line 5 And while on deck he whistled loud,
> He heard a fierce mermaiden cry,
> "Boy, though thou art young and proud,
> I see the place where thou wilt lie.
>
> The sands and yeasty surges mix
> 10 In caves about the dreary bay,
> And on thy ribs the limpet sticks,
> And on thy heart the scrawl shall play!"
>
> "Fool!" he answered, "death is sure
> To those that stay and those that roam;
> 15 But I will never more endure
> To sit with empty hands at home.
>
> My mother clings about my neck;
> My sister clamours, 'Stay, for shame!'
> My father raves of death and wreck, —
> 20 They are all to blame, they are all to blame.
>
> God help me! save I take my part
> Of danger on the roaring sea,
> A devil rises in my heart,
> Far worse than any death to me!"

16. The first stanza (lines 1-4) depicts a boy
    (A) recklessly destroying property
    (B) reluctantly performing a chore
    (C) eagerly beginning a new adventure
    (D) merrily cavorting with his friends
    (E) sadly leaving his family

17. The third stanza (lines 9-12) presents
    (A) a grim prophecy
    (B) a bitter accusation
    (C) a heartfelt prayer
    (D) an urgent request
    (E) a stern reprimand

18. In the fourth stanza (lines 13-16), the boy indicates that he
    (A) fears death
    (B) despises idleness
    (C) regrets his choice
    (D) desires fame and fortune
    (E) recognizes his foolishness

19. In the fifth stanza (lines 17-20), the boy's family are depicted as trying to
    (A) convince him that they are innocent
    (B) understand his point of view
    (C) discourage him from carrying out his plan
    (D) make amends for their misdeeds
    (E) reward him for his courage

20. In the final stanza (lines 21-24), the boy expresses the belief that
    (A) good always triumphs over evil
    (B) he will die if he does not go to sea
    (C) the dangers of the sea are greatly exaggerated
    (D) a life without hazard is not worth living
    (E) he will return safely from his journey

GO ON TO THE NEXT PAGE.

Passing through the woods in summer, we often find beautiful bits of a low form of plant growth called fungi, branching from the trees, covering old stumps, or poking their dainty heads up through the ground at our feet. How strikingly different are fungi from other plants! They have no leaves and none of that wonderful green coloring-matter, chlorophyll, which takes carbon from the air and hydrogen and oxygen from water and forms them into food for the plant, so making it an independent being. As the fungi lack this, they must get the food already made by some other plant or animal. That is the reason we find them attached to trees, logs, anything that will furnish them with the desired food.

Line 5

21. As it is used in line 1, the word "Passing" most nearly means
    (A) transferring
    (B) extending
    (C) elapsing
    (D) undergoing
    (E) traveling

22. To describe how fungi appear "at our feet" (line 3), the author makes use of which literary device?
    (A) Onomatopoeia
    (B) Simile
    (C) Hyperbole
    (D) Personification
    (E) Alliteration

23. According to the passage, the lack of chlorophyll explains why fungi
    (A) have no leaves
    (B) grow where they do
    (C) are the color they are
    (D) are not classified as plants
    (E) are not eaten by forest animals

24. The author uses the word "independent" (line 6) to indicate that certain plants
    (A) are nutritionally self-sufficient
    (B) are unrelated to other species
    (C) are not considered part of the forest
    (D) grow freely without cultivation
    (E) thrive in isolation from other plants

25. The main purpose of the passage is to
    (A) illustrate the balance of nature
    (B) explain how plants synthesize food
    (C) distinguish fungi from other plants
    (D) identify which forest plants are edible
    (E) debunk a popular myth about fungus

GO ON TO THE NEXT PAGE.

> The plan which I adopted, and the one by which I was most successful, was that of making friends of all the little white boys whom I met in the street. As many of these as I could, I converted into teachers. With their kindly aid, obtained at different times and in different places, I finally succeeded in learning to read. When I was sent on errands, I always took my book with me, and by going one part of my errand quickly, I found time to get a lesson before my return. I used also to carry bread with me, enough of which was always in the house, and to which I was always welcome; for I was much better off in this regard than many of the poor white children in our neighborhood. This bread I used to bestow upon the hungry little urchins, who, in return, would give me that more valuable bread of knowledge. I am strongly tempted to give the names of two or three of those little boys, as a testimonial of the gratitude and affection I bear them; but prudence forbids;—not that it would injure me, but it might embarrass them; for it is almost an unpardonable offence to teach slaves to read in this Christian country.

Line 5
10

26. As revealed in the passage, the goal of the narrator's "plan" (line 1) was to

    (A) exact revenge
    (B) earn money
    (C) attain freedom
    (D) escape punishment
    (E) acquire a skill

27. According to the passage, "the hungry little urchins" (line 8) were given bread in exchange for

    (A) protection
    (B) friendship
    (C) instruction
    (D) keeping quiet
    (E) running errands

28. The narrator indicates that in regard to the "little boys" (lines 9-10) he felt

    (A) envious
    (B) superior
    (C) guilty
    (D) thankful
    (E) ambivalent

29. In line 10, the narrator uses the word "not" in order to

    (A) disprove a false allegation
    (B) clarify a potentially misleading statement
    (C) challenge a widely accepted assumption
    (D) suggest an alternative hypothesis
    (E) distinguish between two options

30. It can be inferred that at the time of the events described in the passage, the narrator was a

    (A) slave
    (B) fugitive
    (C) schoolboy
    (D) street urchin
    (E) bread peddler

GO ON TO THE NEXT PAGE.

Never did a couple set forward on the flowery path of early and well-suited marriage with a fairer prospect of felicity. It was the misfortune of my friend, however, to have embarked his property in large speculations; and he had not been married many months, when, by a succession of sudden disasters, it was swept from him, and he found himself reduced almost to penury. For a time
Line 5 he kept his situation to himself, and went about with a haggard countenance, and a breaking heart. His life was but a protracted agony; and what rendered it more insupportable was the necessity of keeping up a smile in the presence of his wife; for he could not bring himself to overwhelm her with the news. She saw, however, with the quick eyes of affection, that all was not well with him. She marked his altered looks and stifled sighs, and was not to be deceived by his sickly and vapid
10 attempts at cheerfulness. She tasked all her sprightly powers and tender blandishments to win him back to happiness; but she only drove the arrow deeper into his soul.

31. In line 2, "felicity" most likely refers to

    (A) worldly success
    (B) marital bliss
    (C) graceful speech
    (D) natural aptitude
    (E) good health

32. The author uses the word "speculations" (line 3) to describe

    (A) scientific theories
    (B) risky business ventures
    (C) jealous suspicions
    (D) unconfirmed rumors
    (E) philosophical reflections

33. Which of the following best describes the husband's "situation" (line 5)?

    (A) He is being blackmailed.
    (B) His marriage is in jeopardy.
    (C) He is in trouble with the law.
    (D) He has a serious medical condition.
    (E) He is on the brink of financial ruin.

34. According to the passage, what made the husband's life "insupportable" (line 6) was the need to

    (A) curtail his lavish lifestyle
    (B) acknowledge his mistakes
    (C) maintain a false appearance
    (D) accept his wife's pity
    (E) ask friends for help

35. As it is used in line 9, the word "marked" most nearly means

    (A) noticed
    (B) graded
    (C) labeled
    (D) defaced
    (E) accentuated

GO ON TO THE NEXT PAGE.

> But if you would see the purest, the sincerest, the most affecting piety of a parent's love, startle a young family of quails, and watch the conduct of the mother. She will not leave you. No, not she. But she will fall at your feet, uttering a noise which none but a distressed mother can make, and she will run, and flutter, and seem to try to be caught, and cheat your outstretched hand, and
>
> *Line 5* affect to be wing-broken and wounded, and yet have just strength to tumble along, until she has drawn you, fatigued, a safe distance from her threatened children and the young hopes of her heart; and then will she mount, whirring with glad strength, and away through the maze of trees you have not seen before, like a close-shot bullet, fly to her skulking infants.

36. The author uses the phrase "No, not she" (lines 2-3) to indicate that the mother quail
    (A) is too proud to move aside
    (B) shows no sign of distress
    (C) does not behave as expected
    (D) is unaware of any danger
    (E) neglects her maternal duties

37. The author uses the word "cheat" (line 4) to describe how the mother quail
    (A) feigns injury
    (B) eludes capture
    (C) flies through a maze
    (D) wearies her pursuer
    (E) disguises her voice

38. As it is used in line 6, the word "drawn" most nearly means
    (A) led
    (B) pulled
    (C) selected
    (D) stretched
    (E) portrayed

39. The simile in line 8 serves primarily to emphasize the mother quail's
    (A) ingenuity
    (B) speed
    (C) anguish
    (D) fear
    (E) elegance

40. The author describes the mother quail in a tone of
    (A) frustration
    (B) resentment
    (C) disbelief
    (D) admiration
    (E) triumph

STOP
**IF YOU FINISH BEFORE TIME IS CALLED, YOU MAY CHECK YOUR WORK ON THIS SECTION ONLY.
DO NOT TURN TO ANY OTHER SECTION IN THE TEST.**

SECTION 3
60 Questions

This section consists of two different types of questions: synonyms and analogies. There are directions and a sample question for each type.

Synonyms

Each of the following questions consists of one word followed by five words or phrases. You are to select the one word or phrase whose meaning is closest to the word in capital letters.

Sample Question:

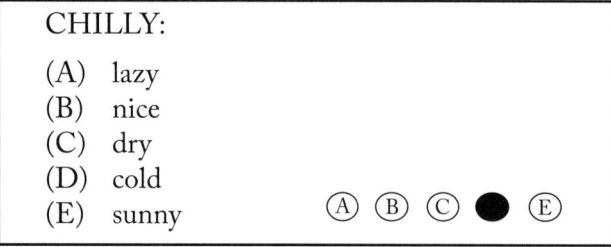

1. TRADE:
   (A) tax
   (B) rush
   (C) advise
   (D) flatten
   (E) exchange

2. CALM:
   (A) hide
   (B) soothe
   (C) drain
   (D) thicken
   (E) borrow

3. DONATE:
   (A) give
   (B) divide
   (C) confine
   (D) govern
   (E) copy

4. PRICELESS:
   (A) accurate
   (B) reckless
   (C) doubtful
   (D) invaluable
   (E) legal

5. SCARCE:
   (A) rare
   (B) evil
   (C) sudden
   (D) alarming
   (E) abandoned

6. THOROUGH:
   (A) actual
   (B) useful
   (C) careful
   (D) possible
   (E) novel

7. SYMPATHETIC:
   (A) compassionate
   (B) incompetent
   (C) straightforward
   (D) gullible
   (E) indifferent

8. AMBIANCE:
   (A) carousel
   (B) atmosphere
   (C) temperament
   (D) precaution
   (E) doubt

GO ON TO THE NEXT PAGE.

9. MEMENTO:
   (A) script
   (B) badge
   (C) speed
   (D) receipt
   (E) souvenir

10. HOAX:
    (A) maze
    (B) dream
    (C) riddle
    (D) prank
    (E) error

11. COLOSSAL:
    (A) sweet
    (B) smooth
    (C) huge
    (D) fierce
    (E) costly

12. AUTHENTIC:
    (A) written
    (B) ordinary
    (C) expert
    (D) real
    (E) ancient

13. CALAMITY:
    (A) rejection
    (B) slander
    (C) disaster
    (D) restriction
    (E) penalty

14. EMBELLISH:
    (A) adorn
    (B) boast
    (C) attack
    (D) obstruct
    (E) display

15. CONTRADICT:
    (A) destroy
    (B) exchange
    (C) reveal
    (D) impede
    (E) deny

16. EXPUNGE:
    (A) steal
    (B) uncover
    (C) erase
    (D) repel
    (E) release

17. ADHERE:
    (A) leave
    (B) climb
    (C) force
    (D) stick
    (E) hope

18. GLITCH:
    (A) error
    (B) denial
    (C) ejection
    (D) noise
    (E) lie

19. MEDLEY:
    (A) song
    (B) cure
    (C) average
    (D) mixture
    (E) reason

20. FAINT:
    (A) weak
    (B) harsh
    (C) false
    (D) blatant
    (E) insensitive

GO ON TO THE NEXT PAGE.

21. PROBABLE:
    (A) visible
    (B) restrictive
    (C) accidental
    (D) likely
    (E) curious

22. ORATION:
    (A) speech
    (B) gesture
    (C) applause
    (D) request
    (E) attitude

23. DWINDLE:
    (A) delay
    (B) rotate
    (C) shrink
    (D) steal
    (E) fail

24. TRAILBLAZER:
    (A) bodyguard
    (B) pioneer
    (C) scoundrel
    (D) tycoon
    (E) courier

25. ABSTAIN:
    (A) taunt
    (B) bother
    (C) tarnish
    (D) refrain
    (E) wonder

26. FISSURE:
    (A) disorder
    (B) eruption
    (C) entrance
    (D) branch
    (E) crack

27. RETORT:
    (A) sharp answer
    (B) naive question
    (C) deafening shout
    (D) arrogant demand
    (E) convincing argument

28. ELATION:
    (A) convenience
    (B) appearance
    (C) exclusion
    (D) accuracy
    (E) delight

29. CANDID:
    (A) popular
    (B) shallow
    (C) frank
    (D) literate
    (E) ambitious

30. ANIMOSITY:
    (A) monster
    (B) hostility
    (C) revenge
    (D) keepsake
    (E) excitement

GO ON TO THE NEXT PAGE.

Analogies

The following questions ask you to find relationships between words. For each question, select the answer choice that best completes the meaning of the sentence.

Sample Question:

Kitten is to cat as
(A) fawn is to colt
(B) puppy is to dog
(C) cow is to bull
(D) wolf is to bear
(E) hen is to rooster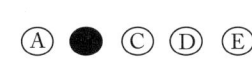

Choice (B) is the best answer because a kitten is a young cat just as a puppy is a young dog. Of all the answer choices, (B) states a relationship that is most like the relationship between kitten and cat.

---

31. Polish is to shiny as
    (A) caress is to soft
    (B) hone is to sharp
    (C) swelter is to hot
    (D) wash is to dirty
    (E) hoist is to heavy

32. Battery is to electricity as
    (A) oven is to temperature
    (B) closet is to door
    (C) bank is to money
    (D) kettle is to steam
    (E) orange is to juice

33. Composer is to score as
    (A) architect is to blueprint
    (B) customer is to receipt
    (C) traveler is to map
    (D) banker is to money
    (E) pilot is to aircraft

34. Seed is to sprout as
    (A) ball is to throw
    (B) garden is to tend
    (C) egg is to hatch
    (D) infant is to talk
    (E) rain is to trickle

35. Swarm is to bee as
    (A) ape is to monkey
    (B) herd is to buffalo
    (C) river is to fish
    (D) kennel is to dog
    (E) cocoon is to moth

36. Greedy is to wealth as
    (A) tranquil is to peace
    (B) concise is to brevity
    (C) irate is to malice
    (D) steadfast is to loyalty
    (E) vindictive is to revenge

37. Landscape is to painting as
    (A) wall is to mural
    (B) style is to clothing
    (C) tongue is to speech
    (D) car is to vehicle
    (E) blade is to grass

38. Toss is to throw as
    (A) stroll is to walk
    (B) gasp is to breathe
    (C) seek is to find
    (D) drop is to lift
    (E) dine is to eat

GO ON TO THE NEXT PAGE.

39. Glare is to light as
   (A) mud is to dirt
   (B) racket is to sound
   (C) dike is to flood
   (D) dream is to sleep
   (E) sprint is to speed

40. Duck is to bird as
   (A) iron is to metal
   (B) daisy is to rose
   (C) lake is to ocean
   (D) peak is to mountain
   (E) tree is to grove

41. Trivial is to importance as
   (A) brazen is to courage
   (B) stealthy is to thief
   (C) genial is to enemy
   (D) bland is to flavor
   (E) jealous is to love

42. Praise is to condemn as
   (A) endeavor is to fail
   (B) observe is to notice
   (C) increase is to diminish
   (D) coax is to persuade
   (E) immerse is to float

43. Comb is to hair as
   (A) fork is to meat
   (B) file is to nail
   (C) glove is to hand
   (D) glass is to water
   (E) rake is to grass

44. Blanket is to warmth as
   (A) bandage is to wound
   (B) pillow is to head
   (C) sail is to wind
   (D) curtain is to privacy
   (E) garment is to fashion

45. Incentive is to motivate as
   (A) threat is to intimidate
   (B) prohibition is to punish
   (C) reminder is to remember
   (D) feedback is to provide
   (E) challenge is to accept

46. Employee is to hire as
   (A) politician is to elect
   (B) scholar is to study
   (C) pedestrian is to walk
   (D) athlete is to win
   (E) benefactor is to donate

47. Eat is to devour as
   (A) speak is to whisper
   (B) lend is to borrow
   (C) search is to find
   (D) launch is to fly
   (E) take is to seize

48. Hangar is to airplane as
   (A) signal is to train
   (B) runway is to landing
   (C) ocean is to steamship
   (D) turnpike is to hitchhiker
   (E) garage is to automobile

49. Cold is to frigid as
   (A) doubtful is to decisive
   (B) tardy is to chronic
   (C) rigid is to flexible
   (D) happy is to ecstatic
   (E) long is to distant

50. Cast is to actor as
   (A) team is to player
   (B) battle is to soldier
   (C) party is to host
   (D) movie is to director
   (E) flock is to shepherd

GO ON TO THE NEXT PAGE.

51. Hermit is to solitude as
    (A) hostage is to ransom
    (B) braggart is to modesty
    (C) prisoner is to punishment
    (D) refugee is to protection
    (E) scapegoat is to blame

52. Enticement is to lure as
    (A) debt is to borrow
    (B) approval is to condemn
    (C) obstacle is to block
    (D) bargain is to buy
    (E) clue is to investigate

53. Shovel is to dirt as
    (A) pen is to ink
    (B) spoon is to food
    (C) drill is to hole
    (D) wrench is to bolt
    (E) needle is to stitch

54. Generous is to stingy as
    (A) modest is to shy
    (B) large is to huge
    (C) ornate is to plain
    (D) plenty is to enough
    (E) patient is to late

55. Hurdle is to overcome as
    (A) victory is to celebrate
    (B) detour is to travel
    (C) penance is to atone
    (D) danger is to rescue
    (E) problem is to solve

56. Accidental is to chance as
    (A) incompetent is to skill
    (B) prosperous is to wealth
    (C) disastrous is to recovery
    (D) inevitable is to necessity
    (E) random is to prediction

57. Palace is to residence as
    (A) crown is to headpiece
    (B) trophy is to victory
    (C) ship is to fleet
    (D) temple is to religion
    (E) queen is to realm

58. Blood is to artery as
    (A) spout is to gutter
    (B) air is to balloon
    (C) water is to river
    (D) song is to voice
    (E) current is to wire

59. Compete is to rivalry as
    (A) dabble is to amateur
    (B) converse is to dialogue
    (C) condemn is to penalty
    (D) recover is to disaster
    (E) appease is to anger

60. Splinter is to wood as
    (A) grain is to rice
    (B) slate is to stone
    (C) pearl is to oyster
    (D) shard is to glass
    (E) lump is to sugar

STOP
**IF YOU FINISH BEFORE TIME IS CALLED, YOU MAY CHECK YOUR WORK ON THIS SECTION ONLY.
DO NOT TURN TO ANY OTHER SECTION IN THE TEST.**

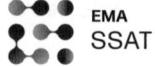

THIS PAGE INTENTIONALLY LEFT BLANK.

SECTION 4
25 Questions

Following each problem in this section, there are five suggested answers. Work each problem in your head or in the blank space provided at the right of the page. Then look at the five suggested answers and decide which one is best.

Note: Figures that accompany problems in this section are drawn as accurately as possible EXCEPT when it is stated in a specific problem that its figure is not drawn to scale.

Sample Problem:

```
  5,413      (A)  586
- 4,827      (B)  596
             (C)  696
             (D)  1,586
             (E)  1,686    ● Ⓑ Ⓒ Ⓓ Ⓔ
```

USE THIS SPACE FOR FIGURING.

1. If $x = 5$ and $y = 10$, what is the value of $2xy$?
   (A) 17
   (B) 30
   (C) 50
   (D) 60
   (E) 100

2. If 2 dozen toys are divided equally among 8 children, how many toys will each child receive? (1 dozen = 12)
   (A) 2
   (B) 3
   (C) 4
   (D) 5
   (E) 6

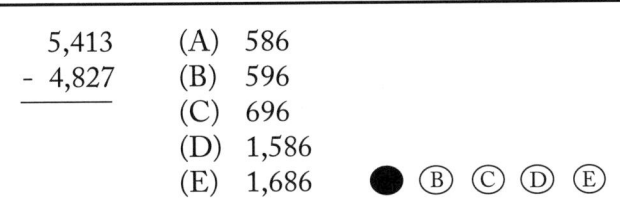

3. What is $\frac{3}{6} - \frac{1}{4}$?
   (A) $\frac{1}{12}$
   (B) $\frac{1}{6}$
   (C) $\frac{1}{4}$
   (D) $\frac{1}{2}$
   (E) 1

GO ON TO THE NEXT PAGE.

4. Javier lives 10.33 miles from school. His classmate, Gabriella, lives 6.8 miles from school. How much farther from school, in miles, does Javier live than Gabriella?

    (A) 3.53
    (B) 4.53
    (C) 5.77
    (D) 9.65
    (E) 17.13

$$\frac{1}{3}, \frac{2}{4}, \frac{3}{5}, \frac{4}{6}, \frac{5}{7}, \ldots, \frac{10}{\square}$$

5. In the sequence above, $\frac{1}{3}$ is the first term. For each term after the first, the numerator and the denominator are each 1 more than the numerator and denominator in the preceding term. What is the value of $\square$?

    (A) 12
    (B) 13
    (C) 14
    (D) 18
    (E) 30

6. In the map shown, Paul is located at the intersection of Broad Street and Main Street, and the side of each square represents one city block. Paul travels 2 city blocks east and 3 city blocks north. Which of the following points is his new location?

    (A) A
    (B) B
    (C) C
    (D) D
    (E) E

USE THIS SPACE FOR FIGURING.

STREET MAP OF MAPLE CITY

GO ON TO THE NEXT PAGE.

Practice Test I: Middle Level

USE THIS SPACE FOR FIGURING.

7. If m is 4 more than k, then k must be
   (A) $\frac{1}{4}$ of m
   (B) 4 minus m
   (C) 4 times m
   (D) 4 less than m
   (E) 4 more than m

8. Janeene has a cellphone. She pays $50 per month for her plan, plus $2 for each call she makes that is outside of her area. Her total monthly bill in September was $70. How many calls did Janeene make outside of her area in September?
   (A) 40
   (B) 22
   (C) 20
   (D) 18
   (E) 10

9. What is 16% of 75 ?
   (A) 16
   (B) 12
   (C) 9
   (D) 8
   (E) 4

10. A certain machine can process 6,000 letters in 1 hour. At this rate, how many letters can the machine process in $\frac{1}{12}$ hour?
    (A) 5,000
    (B) 4,800
    (C) 720
    (D) 500
    (E) 480

11. Of the following, which is closest to the value of $\frac{998 \times 1{,}004}{48 \times 52}$?
    (A) 40
    (B) 200
    (C) 400
    (D) 2,000
    (E) 4,000

GO ON TO THE NEXT PAGE.

USE THIS SPACE FOR FIGURING.

12. The top view of a rectangular package of 6 tightly packed balls is shown. If each ball has a radius of 2 centimeters, which of the following are closest to the dimensions, in centimeters, of the rectangular package?

    (A) 2 × 3 × 6
    (B) 4 × 6 × 6
    (C) 2 × 4 × 6
    (D) 4 × 8 × 12
    (E) 6 × 8 × 12

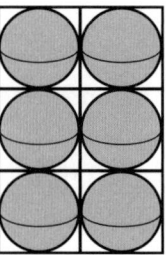

13. Which of the following lists contains only prime numbers?

    (A) 0, 1, 2, 3, 5
    (B) 1, 2, 3, 4, 5
    (C) 2, 3, 5, 7, 11
    (D) 3, 7, 11, 13, 15
    (E) 5, 9, 13 17, 23

14. Ann swims 6 laps every 5 minutes. At that rate, how many laps does she swim in one <u>hour</u>?

    (A) 72
    (B) 60
    (C) 50
    (D) 36
    (E) 30

      30, −15, 10, 35, −15, −30, 20

15. What is the median of the list above?

    (A) −15
    (B)   5
    (C) 10
    (D) 20
    (E) 35

GO ON TO THE NEXT PAGE.

16. In the figure, *ABEF* is a rectangle, and *ABCD* is a square. If *CE* = 3, and *EF* = 5, what is the area of rectangle *ABEF*?

    (A) 15
    (B) 24
    (C) 26
    (D) 31
    (E) 40

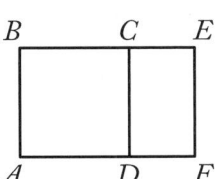

17. The cost of using a parcel service is *r* dollars for the first 3 pounds and *s* dollars for each additional pound. Which of the following expressions represents the cost, in dollars, of sending a parcel that weighs 9 pounds?

    (A) $r + 3s$
    (B) $r + 6s$
    (C) $3r + 6s$
    (D) $3r + 9s$
    (E) $9r + 9s$

18. Which of the following fractions has the least value?

    (A) $\frac{3}{4}$

    (B) $\frac{6}{11}$

    (C) $\frac{7}{15}$

    (D) $\frac{7}{16}$

    (E) $\frac{9}{16}$

GO ON TO THE NEXT PAGE.

19. The circle graph shows each part of a typical day that Marco spends on different activities. Based on the graph, how many hours does he spend per day on family time and on homework combined?

    (A) 1.92
    (B) 2.88
    (C) 4.08
    (D) 5.04
    (E) 6.00

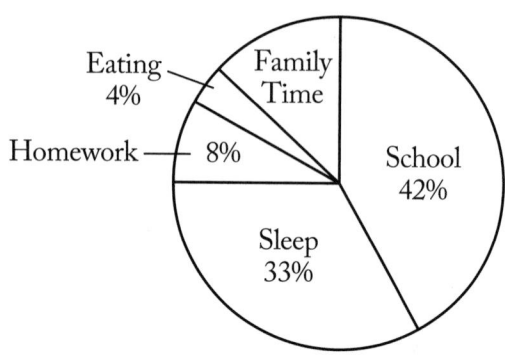

Marco's Daily Activities

---

20. If $3 + 7 \times n = 6$, what is the value of n?

    (A) -4
    (B) $\frac{3}{7}$
    (C) $\frac{3}{5}$
    (D) $\frac{9}{7}$
    (E) 2

---

21. Which of the following is equivalent to $\frac{6}{12} \div 0.2$?

    (A) 0.1
    (B) 0.4
    (C) 2.5
    (D) 10
    (E) 25

---

22. Sophie is making bows for packages and uses 1.25 meters of ribbon per bow. If she has 12 meters of ribbon and makes as many complete bows as possible, how much ribbon, in meters, will remain?

    (A) 0.60
    (B) 0.75
    (C) 0.85
    (D) 1.75
    (E) 1.85

23. In the figure shown, line *t* is parallel to line *v*, and lines *r* and *s* intersect lines *t* and *v*. What is the value of *x* ?

    (A) 150
    (B) 135
    (C) 120
    (D) 105
    (E) 95

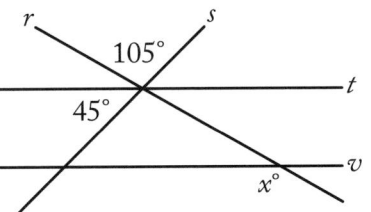

24. What is the value of $\frac{2}{3} \times \frac{1}{8} \div \frac{3}{4}$?

    (A) $\frac{1}{18}$
    (B) $\frac{1}{16}$
    (C) $\frac{1}{12}$
    (D) $\frac{1}{9}$
    (E) $\frac{1}{6}$

25. If $40 < n^2 < 50$, of the following, which is a possible value of $2n$?

    (A) 11
    (B) 14
    (C) 21
    (D) 24
    (E) 44

STOP
**IF YOU FINISH BEFORE TIME IS CALLED, YOU MAY CHECK YOUR WORK ON THIS SECTION ONLY.
DO NOT TURN TO ANY OTHER SECTION IN THE TEST.**

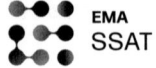

THIS PAGE INTENTIONALLY LEFT BLANK.

Practice Test II: Middle Level Answer Sheet

Be sure each mark completely fills the answer space.
Start with number 1 for each new section of the test.

Section 1

1. Ⓐ Ⓑ Ⓒ Ⓓ Ⓔ
2. Ⓐ Ⓑ Ⓒ Ⓓ Ⓔ
3. Ⓐ Ⓑ Ⓒ Ⓓ Ⓔ
4. Ⓐ Ⓑ Ⓒ Ⓓ Ⓔ
5. Ⓐ Ⓑ Ⓒ Ⓓ Ⓔ
6. Ⓐ Ⓑ Ⓒ Ⓓ Ⓔ
7. Ⓐ Ⓑ Ⓒ Ⓓ Ⓔ
8. Ⓐ Ⓑ Ⓒ Ⓓ Ⓔ
9. Ⓐ Ⓑ Ⓒ Ⓓ Ⓔ
10. Ⓐ Ⓑ Ⓒ Ⓓ Ⓔ
11. Ⓐ Ⓑ Ⓒ Ⓓ Ⓔ
12. Ⓐ Ⓑ Ⓒ Ⓓ Ⓔ
13. Ⓐ Ⓑ Ⓒ Ⓓ Ⓔ
14. Ⓐ Ⓑ Ⓒ Ⓓ Ⓔ
15. Ⓐ Ⓑ Ⓒ Ⓓ Ⓔ
16. Ⓐ Ⓑ Ⓒ Ⓓ Ⓔ
17. Ⓐ Ⓑ Ⓒ Ⓓ Ⓔ
18. Ⓐ Ⓑ Ⓒ Ⓓ Ⓔ
19. Ⓐ Ⓑ Ⓒ Ⓓ Ⓔ
20. Ⓐ Ⓑ Ⓒ Ⓓ Ⓔ
21. Ⓐ Ⓑ Ⓒ Ⓓ Ⓔ
22. Ⓐ Ⓑ Ⓒ Ⓓ Ⓔ
23. Ⓐ Ⓑ Ⓒ Ⓓ Ⓔ
24. Ⓐ Ⓑ Ⓒ Ⓓ Ⓔ
25. Ⓐ Ⓑ Ⓒ Ⓓ Ⓔ

Section 2

1. Ⓐ Ⓑ Ⓒ Ⓓ Ⓔ
2. Ⓐ Ⓑ Ⓒ Ⓓ Ⓔ
3. Ⓐ Ⓑ Ⓒ Ⓓ Ⓔ
4. Ⓐ Ⓑ Ⓒ Ⓓ Ⓔ
5. Ⓐ Ⓑ Ⓒ Ⓓ Ⓔ
6. Ⓐ Ⓑ Ⓒ Ⓓ Ⓔ
7. Ⓐ Ⓑ Ⓒ Ⓓ Ⓔ
8. Ⓐ Ⓑ Ⓒ Ⓓ Ⓔ
9. Ⓐ Ⓑ Ⓒ Ⓓ Ⓔ
10. Ⓐ Ⓑ Ⓒ Ⓓ Ⓔ
11. Ⓐ Ⓑ Ⓒ Ⓓ Ⓔ
12. Ⓐ Ⓑ Ⓒ Ⓓ Ⓔ
13. Ⓐ Ⓑ Ⓒ Ⓓ Ⓔ
14. Ⓐ Ⓑ Ⓒ Ⓓ Ⓔ
15. Ⓐ Ⓑ Ⓒ Ⓓ Ⓔ
16. Ⓐ Ⓑ Ⓒ Ⓓ Ⓔ
17. Ⓐ Ⓑ Ⓒ Ⓓ Ⓔ
18. Ⓐ Ⓑ Ⓒ Ⓓ Ⓔ
19. Ⓐ Ⓑ Ⓒ Ⓓ Ⓔ
20. Ⓐ Ⓑ Ⓒ Ⓓ Ⓔ
21. Ⓐ Ⓑ Ⓒ Ⓓ Ⓔ
22. Ⓐ Ⓑ Ⓒ Ⓓ Ⓔ
23. Ⓐ Ⓑ Ⓒ Ⓓ Ⓔ
24. Ⓐ Ⓑ Ⓒ Ⓓ Ⓔ
25. Ⓐ Ⓑ Ⓒ Ⓓ Ⓔ
26. Ⓐ Ⓑ Ⓒ Ⓓ Ⓔ
27. Ⓐ Ⓑ Ⓒ Ⓓ Ⓔ
28. Ⓐ Ⓑ Ⓒ Ⓓ Ⓔ
29. Ⓐ Ⓑ Ⓒ Ⓓ Ⓔ
30. Ⓐ Ⓑ Ⓒ Ⓓ Ⓔ
31. Ⓐ Ⓑ Ⓒ Ⓓ Ⓔ
32. Ⓐ Ⓑ Ⓒ Ⓓ Ⓔ
33. Ⓐ Ⓑ Ⓒ Ⓓ Ⓔ
34. Ⓐ Ⓑ Ⓒ Ⓓ Ⓔ
35. Ⓐ Ⓑ Ⓒ Ⓓ Ⓔ
36. Ⓐ Ⓑ Ⓒ Ⓓ Ⓔ
37. Ⓐ Ⓑ Ⓒ Ⓓ Ⓔ
38. Ⓐ Ⓑ Ⓒ Ⓓ Ⓔ
39. Ⓐ Ⓑ Ⓒ Ⓓ Ⓔ
40. Ⓐ Ⓑ Ⓒ Ⓓ Ⓔ

Section 3

1. Ⓐ Ⓑ Ⓒ Ⓓ Ⓔ
2. Ⓐ Ⓑ Ⓒ Ⓓ Ⓔ
3. Ⓐ Ⓑ Ⓒ Ⓓ Ⓔ
4. Ⓐ Ⓑ Ⓒ Ⓓ Ⓔ
5. Ⓐ Ⓑ Ⓒ Ⓓ Ⓔ
6. Ⓐ Ⓑ Ⓒ Ⓓ Ⓔ
7. Ⓐ Ⓑ Ⓒ Ⓓ Ⓔ
8. Ⓐ Ⓑ Ⓒ Ⓓ Ⓔ
9. Ⓐ Ⓑ Ⓒ Ⓓ Ⓔ
10. Ⓐ Ⓑ Ⓒ Ⓓ Ⓔ
11. Ⓐ Ⓑ Ⓒ Ⓓ Ⓔ
12. Ⓐ Ⓑ Ⓒ Ⓓ Ⓔ
13. Ⓐ Ⓑ Ⓒ Ⓓ Ⓔ
14. Ⓐ Ⓑ Ⓒ Ⓓ Ⓔ
15. Ⓐ Ⓑ Ⓒ Ⓓ Ⓔ
16. Ⓐ Ⓑ Ⓒ Ⓓ Ⓔ
17. Ⓐ Ⓑ Ⓒ Ⓓ Ⓔ
18. Ⓐ Ⓑ Ⓒ Ⓓ Ⓔ
19. Ⓐ Ⓑ Ⓒ Ⓓ Ⓔ
20. Ⓐ Ⓑ Ⓒ Ⓓ Ⓔ
21. Ⓐ Ⓑ Ⓒ Ⓓ Ⓔ
22. Ⓐ Ⓑ Ⓒ Ⓓ Ⓔ
23. Ⓐ Ⓑ Ⓒ Ⓓ Ⓔ
24. Ⓐ Ⓑ Ⓒ Ⓓ Ⓔ
25. Ⓐ Ⓑ Ⓒ Ⓓ Ⓔ
26. Ⓐ Ⓑ Ⓒ Ⓓ Ⓔ
27. Ⓐ Ⓑ Ⓒ Ⓓ Ⓔ
28. Ⓐ Ⓑ Ⓒ Ⓓ Ⓔ
29. Ⓐ Ⓑ Ⓒ Ⓓ Ⓔ
30. Ⓐ Ⓑ Ⓒ Ⓓ Ⓔ
31. Ⓐ Ⓑ Ⓒ Ⓓ Ⓔ
32. Ⓐ Ⓑ Ⓒ Ⓓ Ⓔ
33. Ⓐ Ⓑ Ⓒ Ⓓ Ⓔ
34. Ⓐ Ⓑ Ⓒ Ⓓ Ⓔ
35. Ⓐ Ⓑ Ⓒ Ⓓ Ⓔ
36. Ⓐ Ⓑ Ⓒ Ⓓ Ⓔ
37. Ⓐ Ⓑ Ⓒ Ⓓ Ⓔ
38. Ⓐ Ⓑ Ⓒ Ⓓ Ⓔ
39. Ⓐ Ⓑ Ⓒ Ⓓ Ⓔ
40. Ⓐ Ⓑ Ⓒ Ⓓ Ⓔ
41. Ⓐ Ⓑ Ⓒ Ⓓ Ⓔ
42. Ⓐ Ⓑ Ⓒ Ⓓ Ⓔ
43. Ⓐ Ⓑ Ⓒ Ⓓ Ⓔ
44. Ⓐ Ⓑ Ⓒ Ⓓ Ⓔ
45. Ⓐ Ⓑ Ⓒ Ⓓ Ⓔ
46. Ⓐ Ⓑ Ⓒ Ⓓ Ⓔ
47. Ⓐ Ⓑ Ⓒ Ⓓ Ⓔ
48. Ⓐ Ⓑ Ⓒ Ⓓ Ⓔ
49. Ⓐ Ⓑ Ⓒ Ⓓ Ⓔ
50. Ⓐ Ⓑ Ⓒ Ⓓ Ⓔ
51. Ⓐ Ⓑ Ⓒ Ⓓ Ⓔ
52. Ⓐ Ⓑ Ⓒ Ⓓ Ⓔ
53. Ⓐ Ⓑ Ⓒ Ⓓ Ⓔ
54. Ⓐ Ⓑ Ⓒ Ⓓ Ⓔ
55. Ⓐ Ⓑ Ⓒ Ⓓ Ⓔ
56. Ⓐ Ⓑ Ⓒ Ⓓ Ⓔ
57. Ⓐ Ⓑ Ⓒ Ⓓ Ⓔ
58. Ⓐ Ⓑ Ⓒ Ⓓ Ⓔ
59. Ⓐ Ⓑ Ⓒ Ⓓ Ⓔ
60. Ⓐ Ⓑ Ⓒ Ⓓ Ⓔ

Section 4

1. Ⓐ Ⓑ Ⓒ Ⓓ Ⓔ
2. Ⓐ Ⓑ Ⓒ Ⓓ Ⓔ
3. Ⓐ Ⓑ Ⓒ Ⓓ Ⓔ
4. Ⓐ Ⓑ Ⓒ Ⓓ Ⓔ
5. Ⓐ Ⓑ Ⓒ Ⓓ Ⓔ
6. Ⓐ Ⓑ Ⓒ Ⓓ Ⓔ
7. Ⓐ Ⓑ Ⓒ Ⓓ Ⓔ
8. Ⓐ Ⓑ Ⓒ Ⓓ Ⓔ
9. Ⓐ Ⓑ Ⓒ Ⓓ Ⓔ
10. Ⓐ Ⓑ Ⓒ Ⓓ Ⓔ
11. Ⓐ Ⓑ Ⓒ Ⓓ Ⓔ
12. Ⓐ Ⓑ Ⓒ Ⓓ Ⓔ
13. Ⓐ Ⓑ Ⓒ Ⓓ Ⓔ
14. Ⓐ Ⓑ Ⓒ Ⓓ Ⓔ
15. Ⓐ Ⓑ Ⓒ Ⓓ Ⓔ
16. Ⓐ Ⓑ Ⓒ Ⓓ Ⓔ
17. Ⓐ Ⓑ Ⓒ Ⓓ Ⓔ
18. Ⓐ Ⓑ Ⓒ Ⓓ Ⓔ
19. Ⓐ Ⓑ Ⓒ Ⓓ Ⓔ
20. Ⓐ Ⓑ Ⓒ Ⓓ Ⓔ
21. Ⓐ Ⓑ Ⓒ Ⓓ Ⓔ
22. Ⓐ Ⓑ Ⓒ Ⓓ Ⓔ
23. Ⓐ Ⓑ Ⓒ Ⓓ Ⓔ
24. Ⓐ Ⓑ Ⓒ Ⓓ Ⓔ
25. Ⓐ Ⓑ Ⓒ Ⓓ Ⓔ

Section 5

Experimental Section – See page 9 for details.

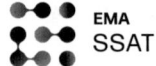

Writing Sample

Schools would like to get to know you better through a story you tell or an essay you write. If you choose to write a story, use the sentence presented in A to begin. Make sure that your story has a beginning, middle, and end. If you choose to write a personal essay, base your essay on the topic presented in B. Please fill in the circle next to your choice.

Ⓐ "Wow! That was amazing!" I said.

Ⓑ Describe one of your friends. What makes your relationship work?

Use this page and the next page to complete your writing sample.

Continue on next page

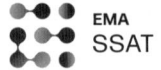

SECTION 1
25 Questions

Following each problem in this section, there are five suggested answers. Work each problem in your head or in the blank space provided at the right of the page. Then look at the five suggested answers and decide which one is best.

Note: Figures that accompany problems in this section are drawn as accurately as possible EXCEPT when it is stated in a specific problem that its figure is not drawn to scale.

Sample Problem:

5,413 - 4,827	(A) 586 (B) 596 (C) 696 (D) 1,586 (E) 1,686 ● Ⓑ Ⓒ Ⓓ Ⓔ

USE THIS SPACE FOR FIGURING.

1. Calculate: 1.001 + 2.1 + 0.05
    (A) 1.027
    (B) 1.27
    (C) 3.151
    (D) 3.16
    (E) 3.60

2. One notepad costs $0.79. Of the following, which is closest to the price of 3 of these notepads?
    (A) $2.70
    (B) $2.40
    (C) $2.10
    (D) $1.80
    (E) $1.60

GO ON TO THE NEXT PAGE.

3. In which of the following figures will a triangle be formed if points *T* and *S* are joined by a straight line?

(A)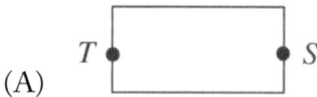

(B)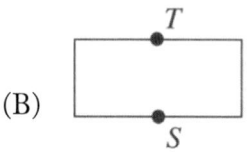

(C)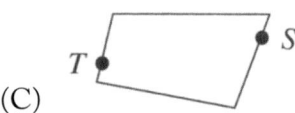

(D)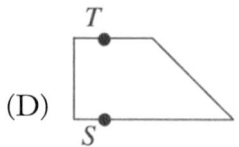

(E)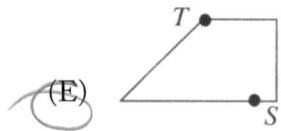

4. At a zoo, a baby rhinoceros weighs 120 pounds. A baby elephant weighs 80 pounds more than the baby rhinoceros. How much does the baby elephant weigh?

   (A) 200 pounds
   (B) 160 pounds
   (C) 120 pounds
   (D) 80 pounds
   (E) 40 pounds

5. If $17 + 17 + 17 + 17 + 17 = 5 \times n$, what is the value of n?

   (A) 5
   (B) 17
   (C) 57
   (D) 75
   (E) 85

USE THIS SPACE FOR FIGURING.

GO ON TO THE NEXT PAGE.

6. Each team in a soccer league plays 16 games during the season. A certain team has won 8 games and lost 3 games. To date, what is the greatest number of games the team can lose during the remainder of the season and still win more than $\frac{1}{2}$ of the games in the season?

   (A) 1
   (B) 2
   (C) 3
   (D) 4
   (E) 5

7. If $x - \frac{1}{10} = \frac{2}{5}$, what is the value of x?

   (A) $\frac{3}{5}$

   (B) $\frac{1}{2}$

   (C) $\frac{3}{10}$

   (D) $\frac{1}{5}$

   (E) $\frac{1}{10}$

8. Hilda polled 13 classmates on the number of hours of television watched in one week. Each response was recorded as a point in the dot plot. Which of the following is the median number of hours of television watched?

   (A) 16
   (B) 18
   (C) 20
   (D) 22
   (E) 24

Television Watched in One Week

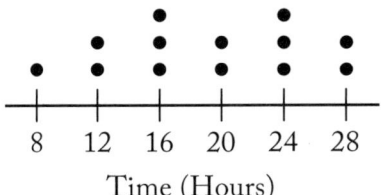

Time (Hours)

GO ON TO THE NEXT PAGE.

9. What is $3 - \frac{1}{2} + \frac{7}{3}$?

   (A) $\frac{1}{6}$

   (B) $\frac{9}{5}$

   (C) $\frac{10}{3}$

   (D) $\frac{21}{5}$

   (E) $\frac{29}{6}$

Yellow, Red, Blue, Green, White

10. Mr. Valdez has shirts in each of the colors listed above. Each day he will select a shirt color by repeating the colors above in the order shown. If he wears a yellow shirt on the first day of the month, what will be the color of the shirt he will wear on the 30th day of the month?

    (A) Blue
    (B) Green
    (C) Red
    (D) White
    (E) Yellow

11. The figure shown contains three squares. The areas of the squares are 4, 9, and 16. What is the area of the figure?

    (A) 11
    (B) 17
    (C) 21
    (D) 25
    (E) 29

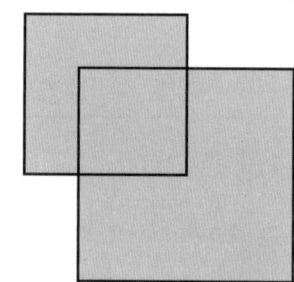

12. During a 3-mile walk, Rose walked the first mile in 10 minutes. If she continued to walk at the same rate, how long, in hours, did it take her to walk 3 miles?

    (A) $\frac{3}{4}$

    (B) $\frac{1}{2}$

    (C) $\frac{1}{3}$

    (D) $\frac{1}{4}$

    (E) $\frac{1}{6}$

GO ON TO THE NEXT PAGE.

13. If 10% of a number is 40, what is 20% of the number?
    (A) 80
    (B) 50
    (C) 20
    (D) 12
    (E) 8

14. If each of the dimensions of a rectangular prism is doubled, how will the volume of the prism be affected?
    (A) It will be 2 times the original volume.
    (B) It will be 4 times the original volume.
    (C) It will be 6 times the original volume.
    (D) It will be 8 times the original volume.
    (E) It will be 9 times the original volume.

15. The □ in the number □.3 represents a digit from 0 through 9. Which of the following fractions is equivalent to □.3 ?
    (A) $\frac{\square + 3}{10}$
    (B) $\frac{\square + 3}{100}$
    (C) $\frac{10 \times (\square + 3)}{10}$
    (D) $\frac{(10 \times \square) + 3}{10}$
    (E) $\frac{(100 \times \square) + 3}{100}$

16. Which of the following lists will contain equal numbers when each number in the list is rounded to the nearest tenth?
    (A) 4.36, 4.41, 4.46, 4.409
    (B) 5.09, 5.14, 5.149, 5.17
    (C) 6.17, 6.08, 6.09, 6.14
    (D) 7.91, 7.98, 7.88, 7.85
    (E) 8.17, 8.23, 8.18, 8.209

17. Ellen has a fish tank with a volume of 40 liters. She went to the pet store and bought 16 tiny fish for the tank. If Ellen uses a water-to-fish ratio of 4 liters to 1 fish, how many of the fish she bought will need to go into a different tank?
    (A) 4
    (B) 6
    (C) 10
    (D) 12
    (E) 24

18. Which of the following is Step 6 in the number trick shown?

    (A) Subtract 12.
    (B) Multiply by 3.
    (C) Add the number from step 1.
    (D) Subtract the number from step 1.
    (E) Subtract the number from step 1, twice.

Number Trick	
Step 1	Pick a number greater than 0.
Step 2	Multiply the number by 4.
Step 3	Then add 8.
Step 4	Take 50% of the sum.
Step 5	Then add 2.
Step 6	?
Result	The answer is 6.

$$76\%, 0.54, \tfrac{1}{2}, 35\%, \tfrac{3}{4}, 0.92$$

19. Which of the following expresses the list above in order from least to greatest?

    (A) $0.54, 0.92, \tfrac{1}{2}, \tfrac{3}{4}, 35\%, 76\%$

    (B) $\tfrac{1}{2}, \tfrac{3}{4}, 35\%, 0.54, 76\%, 0.92$

    (C) $\tfrac{1}{2}, 35\%, \tfrac{3}{4}, 0.54, 76\%, 0.92$

    (D) $35\%, 76\%, 0.54, \tfrac{1}{2}, \tfrac{3}{4}, 0.92$

    (E) $35\%, \tfrac{1}{2}, 0.54, \tfrac{3}{4}, 76\%, 0.92$

$$7x - 2(1 - x) - 3 + 4x$$

20. Which of the following is equivalent to the expression above?

    (A) $13x - 5$
    (B) $13x - 1$
    (C) $11x - 3$
    (D) $10x - 5$
    (E) $10x - 2$

21. On the first day of Luke's fitness plan, he completed 30 push-ups. On the second day, he completed 45 push-ups. What was the percent increase in the number of push-ups completed by Luke from the first to the second day?

    (A) 15%
    (B) 33%
    (C) 45%
    (D) 50%
    (E) 75%

22. The sum of three consecutive even numbers is 258. Which of the following is the least number?
   (A) 82
   (B) 84
   (C) 85
   (D) 86
   (E) 88

23. For the circle with center C, the distance from the center to any point on the circle is 6. Which of the following CANNOT be the length of a line segment with endpoints on the circle?
   (A) 13
   (B) 9
   (C) 8
   (D) 6
   (E) 4

24. Solve for x: $-23 - (-2x) = -17$
   (A) −20
   (B) −3
   (C) 3
   (D) 6
   (E) 15

25. The floor dimensions of a rectangular living room are 20 feet by 18 feet. How many square yards of carpeting are needed to cover the floor? (1 yard = 3 feet)
   (A) 40
   (B) 45
   (C) 90
   (D) 240
   (E) 360

STOP

IF YOU FINISH BEFORE TIME IS CALLED, YOU MAY CHECK YOUR WORK ON THIS SECTION ONLY.
DO NOT TURN TO ANY OTHER SECTION IN THE TEST.

SECTION 2
40 Questions

Read each passage carefully and then answer the questions about it. For each question, decide on the basis of the passage which one of the choices best answers the question.

In colonial New York and Boston, as well as in the smaller towns, women artisans and merchants made or sold everything from dry goods to china, furniture, and hardware. This was especially true after 1760, with the extension of the market for many items manufactured in the home. Women usually ran taverns and coffeehouses. Others were carpenters, cabinetmakers,
Line 5 braziers, soapmakers, cutlers, ropemakers, and even blacksmiths. The hardier of these occupations had generally been inherited from deceased husbands.

Women were also more active on the professional level, and for the same reasons: a short-handed country could not disdain womanpower, and in the Colonial era these occupations required little formal education. Women frequently taught in the common schools. Nurses and midwives
10 had more patients than they could handle, and they and other women did a flourishing business by offering their services as doctors.

---

1. What is the primary reason the author gives for the involvement of women in the colonial economy?
   (A) A desire for financial independence
   (B) Advances in technology
   (C) A labor shortage
   (D) The growth of the population
   (E) Men going off to war

2. As it is used in line 4, the word "ran" most nearly means
   (A) sprinted
   (B) extended
   (C) campaigned
   (D) managed
   (E) fled

3. In line 5, the word "hardier" probably means
   (A) weightier
   (B) more strenuous
   (C) more complex
   (D) more time-consuming
   (E) requiring more education

4. The author mentions all of the following occupations for women EXCEPT
   (A) blacksmith
   (B) doctor
   (C) carpenter
   (D) glassblower
   (E) soapmaker

5. The author would most likely agree with which of the following statements about Colonial times?
   (A) Some occupations, such as medicine and teaching, required extensive education.
   (B) There were fewer women in the marketplace after 1760.
   (C) It was essential that women made what they sold.
   (D) The women of New York and Boston had better jobs than those of smaller towns.
   (E) There was an increase in the number of professional women.

GO ON TO THE NEXT PAGE.

In the late 1970s, the Food and Drug Administration (FDA) approved the first vaccine that successfully prevented pneumococcal pneumonia. Researchers found that the rate that pneumonia occurs increases as we get older. In 2012, the FDA approved a new vaccine for adults 50 and older. This vaccine protects against thirteen strains of pneumococcal bacteria, which cause
Line 5   meningitis, pneumonia, and ear infections. The FDA said that 300,000 adults 50 years and older are hospitalized every year for pneumococcal pneumonia. Initial distribution was being aimed at persons over 65.

"Despite the wide use of antibiotics, pneumonia today is the sixth leading cause of death in the United States," an FDA representative said. "The type of pneumonia against which the vaccine
10   protects accounts for a major portion of these deaths. The vaccine is effective in at least 80 percent of the people who receive it." Still, all these years later, the vaccine is a safe and effective way to prevent pneumonia.

6. The passage is primarily about
   (A) medical researchers
   (B) pneumococcal bacteria
   (C) a vaccine for pneumonia
   (D) illness in the United States
   (E) the Food and Drug Administration

7. The passage suggests that the vaccine approved in the late 1970s probably
   (A) reduced the number of deaths from pneumonia
   (B) made the use of antibiotics obsolete
   (C) increased the authority of the FDA
   (D) provided protection against illnesses other than pneumonia
   (E) increased health expenses for people in the United States

8. As it is used in line 4, the word "strains" most nearly means
   (A) pressures
   (B) exertions
   (C) melodies
   (D) injuries
   (E) types

9. The attitude of the "FDA representative" (line 9) toward use of the pneumococcal pneumonia vaccine is best described as
   (A) cautious
   (B) critical
   (C) fanatical
   (D) supportive
   (E) ambivalent

10. The style of the passage is most like that found in
    (A) a textbook
    (B) an almanac
    (C) a news article
    (D) an encyclopedia
    (E) an advertisement

GO ON TO THE NEXT PAGE.

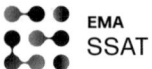

With the invention of new diving equipment, scientists have been able to study animals such as the octopus in their ocean habitats. Investigators have given tests to octopuses and found that their intelligence is high compared to that of other mollusks.

In one interesting test, a live lobster was placed in a glass jar. In the mouth of the jar there
Line 5   was a cork stopper in which a small hole had been drilled. The jar was taken to sea and put in front of the entrance to the dwelling of an octopus. Octopuses like to eat lobsters, so in spite of the fact that it was surrounded by cameras, lights, and interested divers, the octopus came out and threw itself upon the lobster. When it discovered that it could not reach its prey, it turned red with anger and surprise, for the octopus shows its emotions by changing color.

10   Normally, the octopus would have been able to paralyze its victim with the poison from its salivary glands. But it could see the lobster was still moving around inside the jar. It became very impatient and began to explore the jar. The octopus then found the hole in the cork stopper and squeezed its arm inside. When the tip of the arm touched the lobster and the lobster moved, the octopus looked electrified. It seemed to realize that the stopper could be moved and in a few minutes
15   it had pulled the stopper out of the jar with one arm and collected the lobster with two others.

11. The major purpose of the experiment described in the passage was to
    (A) test how the octopus solves problems
    (B) discover how the octopus poisons its victims
    (C) study the emotions displayed by an octopus
    (D) discover whether the octopus attacks lobsters
    (E) observe how the octopus behaves when surrounded by divers

12. According to the passage, what was the octopus' first reaction to the lobster in the jar?
    (A) Exploring the jar
    (B) Pulling out the cork
    (C) Eating the lobster
    (D) Throwing itself on the jar
    (E) Pushing its arm through the hole

13. According to the passage, the octopus shows its emotions by
    (A) changing color
    (B) waving its arms
    (C) hiding in caves
    (D) secreting poison
    (E) attacking its enemies

14. The passage implies that the octopus came out of its home because it
    (A) was attracted by the lights
    (B) wanted to eat the lobster
    (C) was frightened by the cameras
    (D) was interested in the scientists
    (E) had been coaxed by the divers

15. The main purpose of the passage is to
    (A) explain how scientists observe animals in inaccessible locations
    (B) demonstrate the workings of nature's food chain
    (C) compare the predatory habits of two different sea creatures
    (D) debunk a popular myth about the octopus
    (E) give an illustration of the octopus' superior intelligence

GO ON TO THE NEXT PAGE.

> I wandered lonely as a cloud
> That floats on high o'er vales and hills,
> When all at once I saw a crowd,
> A host, of golden daffodils,
> Line 5 Beside the lake, beneath the trees,
> Fluttering and dancing in the breeze.
>
> Continuous as the stars that shine
> And twinkle on the Milky Way,
> They stretched in never-ending line
> 10 Along the margin of a bay.
> Ten thousand saw I at a glance,
> Tossing their heads in sprightly dance.
>
> The waves beside them danced, but they
> Outdid the sparkling waves in glee.
> 15 A poet could not but be gay,
> In such a jocund company.
> I gazed—and gazed—but little thought
> What wealth the show to me had brought.
>
> For oft, when on my couch I lie
> 20 In vacant or in pensive mood,
> They flash upon that inward eye
> Which is the bliss of solitude,
> And then my heart with pleasure fills,
> And dances with the daffodils.

16. The figure of speech represented in line 12 is
    (A) simile
    (B) irony
    (C) hyperbole
    (D) alliteration
    (E) personification

17. The tone of the poem is best described as
    (A) humorous
    (B) mournful
    (C) chatty
    (D) joyful
    (E) detached

18. In line 16, "jocund" most nearly means
    (A) fancy
    (B) cheerful
    (C) sincere
    (D) imaginary
    (E) noisy

19. The poet uses the word "vacant" (line 20) to describe
    (A) a daydream
    (B) an illness
    (C) loneliness
    (D) his heart
    (E) his home

20. Which of the following best describes the main idea of the poem?
    (A) You should always be envious of the beauty of nature.
    (B) Flowers can often remind you of unpleasant past events.
    (C) Ocean waves can remind you of flowers moving with a breeze.
    (D) Gazing at the Milky Way can never replace the joy that flowers can bring.
    (E) Nature provides so much joy that even the memory of it can make you happy.

GO ON TO THE NEXT PAGE.

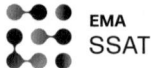

As Earth whirls along its endless journey through space, it has a companion that is always beside it—the moon. The moon is a small celestial body. It is only about one-fourth as big as Earth.

The moon is our nearest neighbor in space. The stars are billions of miles away. The sun is millions of miles away. But the moon is only about 239,000 miles away. That makes the moon truly
Line 5   a next-door neighbor.

In a way, the moon "belongs" to Earth. Just as Earth moves around the Sun, the moon moves around the Earth. It is held in place by the tug of Earth's stronger gravity. A celestial body that is held by another this way is called a satellite. The moon is Earth's satellite.

The moon is a ball of gray rock, some of which is covered with dust. It has no air or water—
10   and, of course, no plants or animals. Its whole surface is nothing but mountains and plains of rock. When we look up at a full moon, we often see dark patches. These dark patches are the lowlands. They seem to form a shadowy face, which people have named "the man in the moon." The brighter parts of the moon are the highlands.

In ancient times, many people worshipped the moon. The Romans, who thought the moon
15   was a goddess, named it Luna. Our word *lunar* means "of the moon."

21. Why does the author think that the moon "belongs" (line 6) to the Earth?

    (A) The moon could not exist without the Earth.
    (B) One can see the man in the moon from Earth.
    (C) Ancient Romans considered it a goddess.
    (D) It is a satellite of the Earth.
    (E) It is Earth's nearest neighbor.

22. According to the passage, which of the following can be found on the moon?

    (A) air
    (B) water
    (C) plants
    (D) animals
    (E) mountains

23. According to the passage, the face of the "man in the moon" (line 12) is formed by

    (A) mountains
    (B) lowlands
    (C) craters
    (D) forests
    (E) seas

24. The author's main purpose for writing the passage is most likely to

    (A) describe the origin of the word "lunar"
    (B) dispel myths about the man in the moon
    (C) inform the reader about the moon
    (D) compare the moon and the Earth
    (E) explain why the ancient Romans worshipped the moon

25. Which of the following statements is NOT asserted or implied in the passage?

    (A) The moon is Earth's satellite.
    (B) The moon is composed of the same materials as Earth.
    (C) The moon's lowlands appear dark from the Earth.
    (D) The moon is four times smaller than Earth.
    (E) The moon is closer to the Earth than anything else in space.

GO ON TO THE NEXT PAGE.

> One day the minister's wife rushed in where Spencervale people had feared to tread, went boldly to Old Lady Lloyd, and asked her if she wouldn't come to their Sewing Circle, which met fortnightly on Saturday afternoons.
>
> "We are filling a box to send to our Trinidad missionary," said the minister's wife, "and we should be so pleased to have you come, Miss Lloyd."
>
> The Old Lady was on the point of refusing rather haughtily. Not that she was opposed to missions—or sewing circles either—quite the contrary; but she knew that each member of the Circle was expected to pay ten cents a week for the purpose of procuring sewing materials; and the poor Old Lady really did not see how she could afford it. But a sudden thought checked her refusal before it reached her lips.

Line 5

10

26. The first paragraph implies that the people of Spencervale find Old Lady Lloyd to be

    (A) eccentric
    (B) intimidating
    (C) fascinating
    (D) bothersome
    (E) congenial

27. The passage implies that the main purpose of the Sewing Circle's project is

    (A) charitable
    (B) educational
    (C) commercial
    (D) political
    (E) artistic

28. In the passage, Old Lady Lloyd is depicted as

    (A) shy but cordial
    (B) modest but accomplished
    (C) impoverished but proud
    (D) anxious and fretful
    (E) curious and intrusive

29. In line 6, the narrator uses the expression "Not that . . ." to introduce

    (A) a needed clarification
    (B) a logical conclusion
    (C) contradictory evidence
    (D) an alternative viewpoint
    (E) a dissenting opinion

30. As it is used in line 9, the word "checked" most nearly means

    (A) inspected
    (B) marked
    (C) deposited
    (D) verified
    (E) stopped

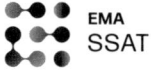

Until the nineteenth century very little was known about the ancient history of Egypt. The brief statements of Hebrew writers in the Old Testament and some stories preserved by the Greeks were all that historians had to go on. There were also the writings that the ancient Egyptians themselves had carved in stone, but these were mysterious hieroglyphics written in a long forgotten
Line 5   language that no one could read.

But about 1800 A.D. some soldiers of Napoleon in Egypt, while laying foundations for a fort at the Rosetta mouth of the Nile, found a curious slab of black rock. This "Rosetta Stone" bore three inscriptions: one of these was in Greek, one in the ancient hieroglyphs of the pyramids, and the third in a later Egyptian writing, called demotic, which had likewise been forgotten. A French
10 scholar, Champollion, shrewdly hypothesized that the three inscriptions all told the same story and therefore would each contain words similar in meaning to the words in the other two inscriptions. In 1822 he proved this to be true. Then, working from the Greek, he found the meanings of the hieroglyphics and so learned to read the long-forgotten language of old Egypt.

31. The passage is mainly about
    (A) how Hebrew and Greek writers viewed the ancient Egyptians
    (B) how the Rosetta Stone was discovered
    (C) how the Egyptians lived in ancient times
    (D) how the ancient Egyptian language was deciphered
    (E) how historians reacted to the discovery of the Rosetta Stone

32. As used in line 3, the expression "go on" most nearly means
    (A) continue
    (B) learn from
    (C) talk at length
    (D) move forward
    (E) happen

33. In the passage, Champollion is characterized as
    (A) temperamental
    (B) benevolent
    (C) ambitious
    (D) devious
    (E) clever

34. It can be inferred from the passage that Champollion
    (A) was a soldier in Napoleon's army
    (B) claimed possession of the Rosetta Stone for France
    (C) had studied the hieroglyphics of the pyramids
    (D) could read the ancient Greek language
    (E) published French translations of the inscriptions

35. The passage as a whole implies that Champollion's achievement resulted in
    (A) a revival of ancient Egyptian as a living language
    (B) enhanced prestige for French universities
    (C) a deeper understanding of the ancient history of Egypt
    (D) popular fascination with the culture of ancient Egypt
    (E) a new theory about the construction of the pyramids

GO ON TO THE NEXT PAGE.

On the 31st of August, 1846, I left Concord in Massachusetts for Bangor and the backwoods of Maine, by way of the railroad and steamboat. I was intending to accompany a relative of mine engaged in the lumber-trade in Bangor, as far as a dam on the west branch of the Penobscot, in which property he was interested. From this place, which is about one hundred miles by the river above Bangor, thirty miles from the Houlton military road, and five miles beyond the last log-hut, I proposed to make excursions to Mount Ktaadn, the second highest mountain in New England, about thirty miles distant, and to some of the lakes of the Penobscot, either alone or with such company as I might pick up there. It is unusual to find a camp so far in the woods at that season, when lumbering operations have ceased. I was glad to avail myself of the circumstance of a gang of men being employed there at that time repairing the injuries caused by the great freshet in the spring. The mountain may be approached more easily and directly on horseback and on foot from the northeast side, by the Aroostook road, and the Wassataquoik River, but in that case you see much less of the wilderness, none of the glorious river and lake scenery, and have no experience of the batteau and the boat man's life. I was fortunate also in the season of the year. In the summer myriads of black flies, mosquitoes, and midges make travelling in the woods almost impossible; but now their reign was nearly over.

36. According to the passage, which of the following occurred in the spring?

    (A) The author met his relative.
    (B) There were damaging floods.
    (C) The author travelled by train.
    (D) Insects interfered with travel.
    (E) Lumbering operations ceased.

37. As it is used in line 8, the phrase "pick up" most nearly means

    (A) lift
    (B) learn
    (C) detect
    (D) acquire
    (E) increase

38. The author indicates that when he encountered a "gang of men" (line 10) in the woods he was

    (A) justifiably annoyed
    (B) deeply puzzled
    (C) pleasantly surprised
    (D) mildly amused
    (E) somewhat fearful

39. The author indicates that he preferred to approach the "mountain" (line 11) by boat because

    (A) he disliked riding horses
    (B) he wanted to avoid insects
    (C) doing so made for an easier journey
    (D) doing so made for a shorter journey
    (E) doing so provided a more scenic route

40. To describe the period of time during which "black flies, mosquitoes, and midges" (line 15) dominate the woods, the author uses which of the following literary devices?

    (A) Metaphor
    (B) Onomatopoeia
    (C) Simile
    (D) Irony
    (E) Allusion

STOP
**IF YOU FINISH BEFORE TIME IS CALLED, YOU MAY CHECK YOUR WORK ON THIS SECTION ONLY.
DO NOT TURN TO ANY OTHER SECTION IN THE TEST.**

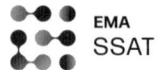

SECTION 3
60 Questions

This section consists of two different types of questions: synonyms and analogies. There are directions and a sample question for each type.

Synonyms

Each of the following questions consists of one word followed by five words or phrases. You are to select the one word or phrase whose meaning is closest to the word in capital letters.

Sample Question:

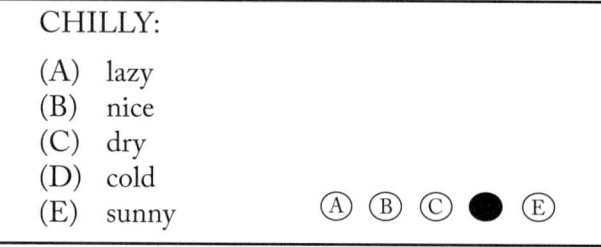

1. EMPHASIZE:
   (A) insert
   (B) stress
   (C) enlarge
   (D) force
   (E) create

2. COMMERCE:
   (A) trade
   (B) humor
   (C) advertisement
   (D) transportation
   (E) supply

3. LUMINOUS:
   (A) wealthy
   (B) beneficial
   (C) heavy
   (D) smooth
   (E) glowing

4. RESTRICT:
   (A) punish
   (B) interrupt
   (C) limit
   (D) capture
   (E) eliminate

5. EXCURSION:
   (A) reason
   (B) outing
   (C) delivery
   (D) upheaval
   (E) surplus

6. PROPHECY:
   (A) prayer
   (B) miracle
   (C) boast
   (D) prediction
   (E) command

7. HAZARD:
   (A) disaster
   (B) poison
   (C) danger
   (D) ambush
   (E) accident

8. EERIE:
   (A) silent
   (B) hesitant
   (C) spooky
   (D) exciting
   (E) suspect

GO ON TO THE NEXT PAGE.

9. DISCLOSE:
   (A) begin
   (B) erase
   (C) learn
   (D) expel
   (E) reveal

10. VALOR:
    (A) wealth
    (B) praise
    (C) pride
    (D) bravery
    (E) truth

11. CODDLE:
    (A) cheat
    (B) waver
    (C) confuse
    (D) pamper
    (E) delay

12. COARSE:
    (A) crude
    (B) stingy
    (C) bold
    (D) plain
    (E) angry

13. ROBUST:
    (A) dishonest
    (B) penniless
    (C) colossal
    (D) vigorous
    (E) significant

14. CONVERGE:
    (A) meet
    (B) spin
    (C) change
    (D) talk
    (E) fade

15. AMPLE:
    (A) timely
    (B) popular
    (C) worthy
    (D) expensive
    (E) abundant

16. PETITION:
    (A) roster
    (B) request
    (C) recurrence
    (D) protest
    (E) ballot

17. ALLURE:
    (A) refer
    (B) permit
    (C) trick
    (D) entice
    (E) invent

18. OBSOLETE:
    (A) stubborn
    (B) outdated
    (C) undeniable
    (D) nostalgic
    (E) impractical

19. WRITHE:
    (A) scribble
    (B) wash
    (C) complain
    (D) cringe
    (E) squirm

20. ADVERSE:
    (A) bizarre
    (B) sideways
    (C) infamous
    (D) unfavorable
    (E) straightforward

GO ON TO THE NEXT PAGE.

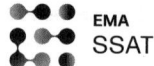

21. SPECTER:
    (A) ghost
    (B) display
    (C) telescope
    (D) guardian
    (E) range

22. SUBTERRANEAN:
    (A) frigid
    (B) southern
    (C) underground
    (D) incompetent
    (E) unobtainable

23. CONJECTURE:
    (A) summon
    (B) guess
    (C) defame
    (D) plead
    (E) discard

24. WARY:
    (A) fatigued
    (B) hopeful
    (C) cautious
    (D) slender
    (E) menacing

25. VANQUISH:
    (A) disappear
    (B) conquer
    (C) neglect
    (D) release
    (E) deceive

26. PERPETUAL:
    (A) rapid
    (B) resistant
    (C) everlasting
    (D) enormous
    (E) bothersome

27. ABATE:
    (A) entrap
    (B) inhabit
    (C) embarrass
    (D) diminish
    (E) agree

28. INCENTIVE:
    (A) decision
    (B) reputation
    (C) agreement
    (D) observance
    (E) motivation

29. PLACID:
    (A) smug
    (B) tranquil
    (C) ordinary
    (D) feeble
    (E) wise

30. HOMAGE:
    (A) honor
    (B) debt
    (C) habitat
    (D) trait
    (E) status

GO ON TO THE NEXT PAGE.

Analogies
The following questions ask you to find relationships between words. For each question, select the answer choice that best completes the meaning of the sentence.

Sample Question:

> Kitten is to cat as
> (A) fawn is to colt
> (B) puppy is to dog
> (C) cow is to bull
> (D) wolf is to bear
> (E) hen is to rooster

Choice (B) is the best answer because a kitten is a young cat just as a puppy is a young dog. Of all the answer choices, (B) states a relationship that is most like the relationship between kitten and cat.

---

31. Closet is to clothing as
    (A) fireplace is to wood
    (B) window is to drapery
    (C) foyer is to entrance
    (D) basement is to house
    (E) cupboard is to food

32. Alarming is to concern as
    (A) hilarious is to amusement
    (B) marital is to wedding
    (C) unruly is to discipline
    (D) drowsy is to sleep
    (E) inept is to skill

33. Yawn is to boredom as
    (A) enrage is to anger
    (B) expect is to surprise
    (C) smile is to laughter
    (D) shrug is to shoulder
    (E) wince is to pain

34. Show is to see as
    (A) hide is to find
    (B) ask is to give
    (C) know is to learn
    (D) tell is to hear
    (E) earn is to take

35. Roof is to house as
    (A) icing is to cake
    (B) chair is to table
    (C) heel is to boot
    (D) page is to book
    (E) street is to city

36. Clarify is to clear as
    (A) change is to stable
    (B) liberate is to free
    (C) eat is to hungry
    (D) rejoice is to happy
    (E) offend is to rude

37. Enroll is to college as
    (A) graduate is to diploma
    (B) coach is to team
    (C) elect is to office
    (D) enlist is to army
    (E) teach is to class

38. Bone is to skeleton as
    (A) blood is to vein
    (B) girder is to steel
    (C) meter is to poem
    (D) painting is to sketch
    (E) word is to sentence

GO ON TO THE NEXT PAGE.

39. Sad is to sorrow as
    (A) foolish is to laughter
    (B) thirsty is to beverage
    (C) uncertain is to doubt
    (D) envious is to hatred
    (E) lost is to location

40. Bead is to necklace as
    (A) boxcar is to train
    (B) square is to checkerboard
    (C) wrist is to bracelet
    (D) branch is to tree
    (E) sand is to beach

41. Mural is to paint as
    (A) statue is to stand
    (B) lecture is to listen
    (C) poem is to interpret
    (D) graffiti is to write
    (E) poster is to advertise

42. Ecstatic is to happy as
    (A) miserly is to rich
    (B) precious is to valuable
    (C) punctual is to tardy
    (D) notorious is to famous
    (E) frail is to hardy

43. Shoe is to foot as
    (A) nail is to finger
    (B) shield is to armor
    (C) tire is to wheel
    (D) umbrella is to rain
    (E) oar is to boat

44. Unsightly is to beauty as
    (A) wicked is to virtue
    (B) foolish is to humor
    (C) audible is to sound
    (D) sick is to remedy
    (E) sour is to flavor

45. Inform is to knowledge as
    (A) conceal is to truth
    (B) accuse is to guilt
    (C) embolden is to courage
    (D) pacify is to anger
    (E) appreciate is to value

46. Fragile is to break as
    (A) stubborn is to yield
    (B) crooked is to straighten
    (C) sharp is to hone
    (D) level is to slant
    (E) portable is to carry

47. River is to stream as
    (A) aisle is to church
    (B) canyon is to cliff
    (C) boulevard is to street
    (D) mountain is to foot
    (E) dock is to harbor

48. Err is to mistake as
    (A) try is to effort
    (B) ask is to answer
    (C) lack is to supply
    (D) weep is to pity
    (E) owe is to payment

49. Echo is to sound as
    (A) wave is to ocean
    (B) gust is to wind
    (C) reflection is to light
    (D) circle is to shape
    (E) period is to time

50. Culprit is to guilty as
    (A) rival is to jealous
    (B) dupe is to deceptive
    (C) braggart is to humble
    (D) celebrity is to famous
    (E) fiend is to afraid

GO ON TO THE NEXT PAGE.

51. Tapestry is to wall as
    (A) pane is to window
    (B) threshold is to door
    (C) chandelier is to ceiling
    (D) clothing is to dresser
    (E) carpet is to floor

52. Aspire is to ambition as
    (A) dare is to courage
    (B) regret is to mistake
    (C) infer is to truth
    (D) doubt is to conviction
    (E) appease is to anger

53. Arena is to game as
    (A) sanctuary is to refuge
    (B) cafeteria is to menu
    (C) warehouse is to merchandise
    (D) studio is to artist
    (E) cinema is to movie

54. Lenient is to forgive as
    (A) anxious is to relax
    (B) content is to complain
    (C) meddlesome is to interfere
    (D) heroic is to admire
    (E) suspect is to accuse

55. Valiant is to cowardly as
    (A) cheery is to bleak
    (B) angry is to hostile
    (C) humid is to cold
    (D) unique is to obvious
    (E) open is to ajar

56. Doodle is to draw as
    (A) lurk is to wait
    (B) rest is to work
    (C) wander is to travel
    (D) whisper is to speak
    (E) stumble is to fall

57. Fence is to enclose as
    (A) gate is to enter
    (B) pillar is to support
    (C) roof is to slant
    (D) stair is to climb
    (E) road is to pave

58. Continuous is to interrupt as
    (A) illegible is to write
    (B) accidental is to intend
    (C) familiar is to accustom
    (D) patient is to await
    (E) reverent is to pray

59. Teach is to learn as
    (A) seize is to take
    (B) sow is to reap
    (C) remind is to forget
    (D) think is to believe
    (E) lend is to borrow

60. Mask is to face as
    (A) alibi is to crime
    (B) armor is to battle
    (C) alias is to name
    (D) mythology is to legend
    (E) hoax is to chicanery

STOP
**IF YOU FINISH BEFORE TIME IS CALLED, YOU MAY CHECK YOUR WORK ON THIS SECTION ONLY.
DO NOT TURN TO ANY OTHER SECTION IN THE TEST.**

SECTION 4
25 Questions

Following each problem in this section, there are five suggested answers. Work each problem in your head or in the blank space provided at the right of the page. Then look at the five suggested answers and decide which one is best.

Note: Figures that accompany problems in this section are drawn as accurately as possible EXCEPT when it is stated in a specific problem that its figure is not drawn to scale.

Sample Problem:

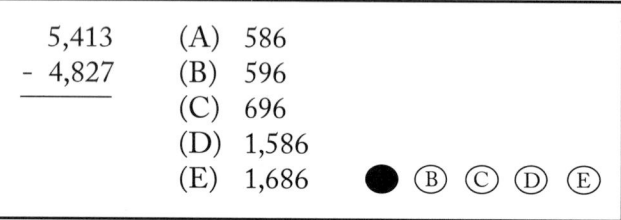

USE THIS SPACE FOR FIGURING.

1. There are 150 calories in a $\frac{1}{2}$-cup serving of a certain cereal. How many calories are in a 1-cup serving of the cereal?
   (A) 75
   (B) 225
   (C) 300
   (D) 450
   (E) 600

2. What is 5.01 − 3.22 ?
   (A) 1.79
   (B) 1.89
   (C) 2.21
   (D) 2.79
   (E) 2.89

3. Of the following sums, which has a value that is closest to 39 + 18 + 42 ?
   (A) 30 + 10 + 30
   (B) 30 + 10 + 40
   (C) 40 + 10 + 40
   (D) 40 + 20 + 40
   (E) 40 + 20 + 50

GO ON TO THE NEXT PAGE.

Practice Test II: Middle Level

USE THIS SPACE FOR FIGURING.

4. The perimeter of a square is 2 feet. What is the length, in feet, of each side of the square?

   (A) $\frac{1}{4}$

   (B) $\frac{1}{2}$

   (C) 1

   (D) 4

   (E) 8

5. If $500 + 100 + x + y = 668$, what does $x + y$ equal?
   (A) 8
   (B) 60
   (C) 68
   (D) 600
   (E) 1,268

6. A length of 2.5 meters is equivalent to a length of how many millimeters?
   (A) 0.0025
   (B) 0.25
   (C) 25
   (D) 250
   (E) 2,500

7. If $x = 6$ and $y = 10$, what is the value of $\frac{2x}{y+2}$?

   (A) 2

   (B) 1

   (C) $\frac{5}{2}$

   (D) $\frac{6}{7}$

   (E) $\frac{3}{5}$

GO ON TO THE NEXT PAGE.

8. Lisa is 16 years old, and Josh is half as old as Lisa. How old will Josh be when Lisa is 20 years old?
   - (A) 4
   - (B) 6
   - (C) 8
   - (D) 10
   - (E) 12

9. What is the value of $\frac{3}{7} \times \frac{21}{6}$?
   - (A) $\frac{1}{6}$
   - (B) $\frac{6}{49}$
   - (C) 1
   - (D) $\frac{3}{2}$
   - (E) $\frac{49}{6}$

10. The number 25 is 3 more than $\frac{1}{2}$ the number n. What is the value of n?
    - (A) 11
    - (B) 22
    - (C) 44
    - (D) 47
    - (E) 56

11. Compute: $-3 + 2 \times 15 - 7$
    - (A) 20
    - (B) 13
    - (C) -8
    - (D) -22
    - (E) -40

Practice Test II: Middle Level

USE THIS SPACE FOR FIGURING.

12. The ratio of the number of red pieces to the number of blue pieces in a game is 2:3. Which of the following could be the total number of red and blue pieces in the game?

    (A) 6
    (B) 8
    (C) 9
    (D) 10
    (E) 12

13. Compute: $\frac{1}{3} \div \frac{1}{3}$

    (A) 0

    (B) $\frac{1}{9}$

    (C) $\frac{1}{3}$

    (D) 1

    (E) 9

14. In the square shown, M is the midpoint of side $\overline{AB}$. What percent of the square is shaded?

    (A) 25%
    (B) 33%
    (C) 50%
    (D) 66%
    (E) 75%

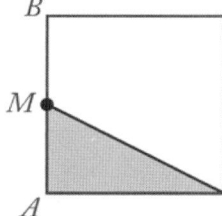

15. What is $\frac{1}{2}$ of $\frac{1}{6}$?

    (A) 3

    (B) $\frac{1}{3}$

    (C) $\frac{1}{4}$

    (D) $\frac{1}{8}$

    (E) $\frac{1}{12}$

GO ON TO THE NEXT PAGE.

USE THIS SPACE FOR FIGURING.

16. A group of 4 people hire a taxi to take them to the airport. The company charges a fixed cost of $40 for 2 people, and $5 for each additional person. If the group chooses to split the cost equally, how much will each person pay?

    (A) $10.00
    (B) $11.25
    (C) $12.50
    (D) $21.25
    (E) $22.50

17. If $\frac{n}{3}$ is a whole number, which of the following could be the value of n?

    (A) 343
    (B) 353
    (C) 403
    (D) 473
    (E) 483

18. The figure shows two parallel lines intersected by a transversal line. What is the value of x?

    (A) 40
    (B) 50
    (C) 80
    (D) 100
    (E) 160

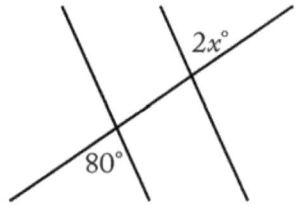

19. Last month, the mean weight of 3 dogs was 44 kilograms. By the end of this month, the weight for 2 of the dogs had increased by 3 kilograms each, and the third dog's weight had stayed the same. What was the mean weight of the 3 dogs, in kilograms, at the end of this month?

    (A) 45
    (B) 46
    (C) 47
    (D) 50
    (E) 53

GO ON TO THE NEXT PAGE.

USE THIS SPACE FOR FIGURING.

20. How many eighths are in 2.375 ?
    (A) 19
    (B) 13
    (C) 8
    (D) 5
    (E) 3

21. The temperature was $(x + 3)$ degrees Fahrenheit in the morning. By the evening, the temperature had doubled, and then decreased by 5 degrees Fahrenheit. Which of the following expressions represents the temperature, in degrees Fahrenheit, in the evening?
    (A) $2x - 4$
    (B) $2x - 2$
    (C) $2x - 1$
    (D) $2x + 1$
    (E) $2x + 2$

22. Which of the following figures can be formed by intersecting a plane and a cube?
    I. A point
    II. A triangle
    III. A rectangle

    (A) I only
    (B) II only
    (C) III only
    (D) II and III only
    (E) I, II, and III

GO ON TO THE NEXT PAGE.

23. The table shows the original and current prices for five tablets. Based on the table, the original price of which tablet was reduced by 25% to give the current price?

    (A) P
    (B) Q
    (C) R
    (D) S
    (E) T

Tablet	Original Price	Current Price
P	$550	$525
Q	$500	$400
R	$600	$150
S	$300	$275
T	$400	$300

24. If a positive whole number n is multiplied by a number less than 1, the answer MUST be

    (A) greater than n
    (B) less than n
    (C) less than 1
    (D) between 0 and 1
    (E) 0

25. Donny and Travis are building a sand castle. While Donny works on the castle, Travis digs a moat around the castle in the shape of a circle, as shown. The inner circle has a diameter of 24 inches. The moat has a width of 4 inches. Based on the figure, what is the circumference, in inches, of the outer circle?

    (A) 24π
    (B) 28π
    (C) 32π
    (D) 56π
    (E) 64π

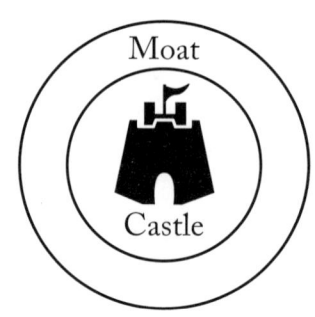

STOP
IF YOU FINISH BEFORE TIME IS CALLED, YOU MAY CHECK YOUR WORK ON THIS SECTION ONLY. DO NOT TURN TO ANY OTHER SECTION IN THE TEST.

Practice Test III: Middle Level Answer Sheet

Be sure each mark completely fills the answer space.
Start with number 1 for each new section of the test.

Section 1

1 Ⓐ Ⓑ Ⓒ Ⓓ Ⓔ   6 Ⓐ Ⓑ Ⓒ Ⓓ Ⓔ   11 Ⓐ Ⓑ Ⓒ Ⓓ Ⓔ   16 Ⓐ Ⓑ Ⓒ Ⓓ Ⓔ   21 Ⓐ Ⓑ Ⓒ Ⓓ Ⓔ
2 Ⓐ Ⓑ Ⓒ Ⓓ Ⓔ   7 Ⓐ Ⓑ Ⓒ Ⓓ Ⓔ   12 Ⓐ Ⓑ Ⓒ Ⓓ Ⓔ   17 Ⓐ Ⓑ Ⓒ Ⓓ Ⓔ   22 Ⓐ Ⓑ Ⓒ Ⓓ Ⓔ
3 Ⓐ Ⓑ Ⓒ Ⓓ Ⓔ   8 Ⓐ Ⓑ Ⓒ Ⓓ Ⓔ   13 Ⓐ Ⓑ Ⓒ Ⓓ Ⓔ   18 Ⓐ Ⓑ Ⓒ Ⓓ Ⓔ   23 Ⓐ Ⓑ Ⓒ Ⓓ Ⓔ
4 Ⓐ Ⓑ Ⓒ Ⓓ Ⓔ   9 Ⓐ Ⓑ Ⓒ Ⓓ Ⓔ   14 Ⓐ Ⓑ Ⓒ Ⓓ Ⓔ   19 Ⓐ Ⓑ Ⓒ Ⓓ Ⓔ   24 Ⓐ Ⓑ Ⓒ Ⓓ Ⓔ
5 Ⓐ Ⓑ Ⓒ Ⓓ Ⓔ   10 Ⓐ Ⓑ Ⓒ Ⓓ Ⓔ   15 Ⓐ Ⓑ Ⓒ Ⓓ Ⓔ   20 Ⓐ Ⓑ Ⓒ Ⓓ Ⓔ   25 Ⓐ Ⓑ Ⓒ Ⓓ Ⓔ

Section 2

1 Ⓐ Ⓑ Ⓒ Ⓓ Ⓔ   9 Ⓐ Ⓑ Ⓒ Ⓓ Ⓔ   17 Ⓐ Ⓑ Ⓒ Ⓓ Ⓔ   25 Ⓐ Ⓑ Ⓒ Ⓓ Ⓔ   33 Ⓐ Ⓑ Ⓒ Ⓓ Ⓔ
2 Ⓐ Ⓑ Ⓒ Ⓓ Ⓔ   10 Ⓐ Ⓑ Ⓒ Ⓓ Ⓔ   18 Ⓐ Ⓑ Ⓒ Ⓓ Ⓔ   26 Ⓐ Ⓑ Ⓒ Ⓓ Ⓔ   34 Ⓐ Ⓑ Ⓒ Ⓓ Ⓔ
3 Ⓐ Ⓑ Ⓒ Ⓓ Ⓔ   11 Ⓐ Ⓑ Ⓒ Ⓓ Ⓔ   19 Ⓐ Ⓑ Ⓒ Ⓓ Ⓔ   27 Ⓐ Ⓑ Ⓒ Ⓓ Ⓔ   35 Ⓐ Ⓑ Ⓒ Ⓓ Ⓔ
4 Ⓐ Ⓑ Ⓒ Ⓓ Ⓔ   12 Ⓐ Ⓑ Ⓒ Ⓓ Ⓔ   20 Ⓐ Ⓑ Ⓒ Ⓓ Ⓔ   28 Ⓐ Ⓑ Ⓒ Ⓓ Ⓔ   36 Ⓐ Ⓑ Ⓒ Ⓓ Ⓔ
5 Ⓐ Ⓑ Ⓒ Ⓓ Ⓔ   13 Ⓐ Ⓑ Ⓒ Ⓓ Ⓔ   21 Ⓐ Ⓑ Ⓒ Ⓓ Ⓔ   29 Ⓐ Ⓑ Ⓒ Ⓓ Ⓔ   37 Ⓐ Ⓑ Ⓒ Ⓓ Ⓔ
6 Ⓐ Ⓑ Ⓒ Ⓓ Ⓔ   14 Ⓐ Ⓑ Ⓒ Ⓓ Ⓔ   22 Ⓐ Ⓑ Ⓒ Ⓓ Ⓔ   30 Ⓐ Ⓑ Ⓒ Ⓓ Ⓔ   38 Ⓐ Ⓑ Ⓒ Ⓓ Ⓔ
7 Ⓐ Ⓑ Ⓒ Ⓓ Ⓔ   15 Ⓐ Ⓑ Ⓒ Ⓓ Ⓔ   23 Ⓐ Ⓑ Ⓒ Ⓓ Ⓔ   31 Ⓐ Ⓑ Ⓒ Ⓓ Ⓔ   39 Ⓐ Ⓑ Ⓒ Ⓓ Ⓔ
8 Ⓐ Ⓑ Ⓒ Ⓓ Ⓔ   16 Ⓐ Ⓑ Ⓒ Ⓓ Ⓔ   24 Ⓐ Ⓑ Ⓒ Ⓓ Ⓔ   32 Ⓐ Ⓑ Ⓒ Ⓓ Ⓔ   40 Ⓐ Ⓑ Ⓒ Ⓓ Ⓔ

Section 3

1 Ⓐ Ⓑ Ⓒ Ⓓ Ⓔ   13 Ⓐ Ⓑ Ⓒ Ⓓ Ⓔ   25 Ⓐ Ⓑ Ⓒ Ⓓ Ⓔ   37 Ⓐ Ⓑ Ⓒ Ⓓ Ⓔ   49 Ⓐ Ⓑ Ⓒ Ⓓ Ⓔ
2 Ⓐ Ⓑ Ⓒ Ⓓ Ⓔ   14 Ⓐ Ⓑ Ⓒ Ⓓ Ⓔ   26 Ⓐ Ⓑ Ⓒ Ⓓ Ⓔ   38 Ⓐ Ⓑ Ⓒ Ⓓ Ⓔ   50 Ⓐ Ⓑ Ⓒ Ⓓ Ⓔ
3 Ⓐ Ⓑ Ⓒ Ⓓ Ⓔ   15 Ⓐ Ⓑ Ⓒ Ⓓ Ⓔ   27 Ⓐ Ⓑ Ⓒ Ⓓ Ⓔ   39 Ⓐ Ⓑ Ⓒ Ⓓ Ⓔ   51 Ⓐ Ⓑ Ⓒ Ⓓ Ⓔ
4 Ⓐ Ⓑ Ⓒ Ⓓ Ⓔ   16 Ⓐ Ⓑ Ⓒ Ⓓ Ⓔ   28 Ⓐ Ⓑ Ⓒ Ⓓ Ⓔ   40 Ⓐ Ⓑ Ⓒ Ⓓ Ⓔ   52 Ⓐ Ⓑ Ⓒ Ⓓ Ⓔ
5 Ⓐ Ⓑ Ⓒ Ⓓ Ⓔ   17 Ⓐ Ⓑ Ⓒ Ⓓ Ⓔ   29 Ⓐ Ⓑ Ⓒ Ⓓ Ⓔ   41 Ⓐ Ⓑ Ⓒ Ⓓ Ⓔ   53 Ⓐ Ⓑ Ⓒ Ⓓ Ⓔ
6 Ⓐ Ⓑ Ⓒ Ⓓ Ⓔ   18 Ⓐ Ⓑ Ⓒ Ⓓ Ⓔ   30 Ⓐ Ⓑ Ⓒ Ⓓ Ⓔ   42 Ⓐ Ⓑ Ⓒ Ⓓ Ⓔ   54 Ⓐ Ⓑ Ⓒ Ⓓ Ⓔ
7 Ⓐ Ⓑ Ⓒ Ⓓ Ⓔ   19 Ⓐ Ⓑ Ⓒ Ⓓ Ⓔ   31 Ⓐ Ⓑ Ⓒ Ⓓ Ⓔ   43 Ⓐ Ⓑ Ⓒ Ⓓ Ⓔ   55 Ⓐ Ⓑ Ⓒ Ⓓ Ⓔ
8 Ⓐ Ⓑ Ⓒ Ⓓ Ⓔ   20 Ⓐ Ⓑ Ⓒ Ⓓ Ⓔ   32 Ⓐ Ⓑ Ⓒ Ⓓ Ⓔ   44 Ⓐ Ⓑ Ⓒ Ⓓ Ⓔ   56 Ⓐ Ⓑ Ⓒ Ⓓ Ⓔ
9 Ⓐ Ⓑ Ⓒ Ⓓ Ⓔ   21 Ⓐ Ⓑ Ⓒ Ⓓ Ⓔ   33 Ⓐ Ⓑ Ⓒ Ⓓ Ⓔ   45 Ⓐ Ⓑ Ⓒ Ⓓ Ⓔ   57 Ⓐ Ⓑ Ⓒ Ⓓ Ⓔ
10 Ⓐ Ⓑ Ⓒ Ⓓ Ⓔ   22 Ⓐ Ⓑ Ⓒ Ⓓ Ⓔ   34 Ⓐ Ⓑ Ⓒ Ⓓ Ⓔ   46 Ⓐ Ⓑ Ⓒ Ⓓ Ⓔ   58 Ⓐ Ⓑ Ⓒ Ⓓ Ⓔ
11 Ⓐ Ⓑ Ⓒ Ⓓ Ⓔ   23 Ⓐ Ⓑ Ⓒ Ⓓ Ⓔ   35 Ⓐ Ⓑ Ⓒ Ⓓ Ⓔ   47 Ⓐ Ⓑ Ⓒ Ⓓ Ⓔ   59 Ⓐ Ⓑ Ⓒ Ⓓ Ⓔ
12 Ⓐ Ⓑ Ⓒ Ⓓ Ⓔ   24 Ⓐ Ⓑ Ⓒ Ⓓ Ⓔ   36 Ⓐ Ⓑ Ⓒ Ⓓ Ⓔ   48 Ⓐ Ⓑ Ⓒ Ⓓ Ⓔ   60 Ⓐ Ⓑ Ⓒ Ⓓ Ⓔ

Section 4

1 Ⓐ Ⓑ Ⓒ Ⓓ Ⓔ   6 Ⓐ Ⓑ Ⓒ Ⓓ Ⓔ   11 Ⓐ Ⓑ Ⓒ Ⓓ Ⓔ   16 Ⓐ Ⓑ Ⓒ Ⓓ Ⓔ   21 Ⓐ Ⓑ Ⓒ Ⓓ Ⓔ
2 Ⓐ Ⓑ Ⓒ Ⓓ Ⓔ   7 Ⓐ Ⓑ Ⓒ Ⓓ Ⓔ   12 Ⓐ Ⓑ Ⓒ Ⓓ Ⓔ   17 Ⓐ Ⓑ Ⓒ Ⓓ Ⓔ   22 Ⓐ Ⓑ Ⓒ Ⓓ Ⓔ
3 Ⓐ Ⓑ Ⓒ Ⓓ Ⓔ   8 Ⓐ Ⓑ Ⓒ Ⓓ Ⓔ   13 Ⓐ Ⓑ Ⓒ Ⓓ Ⓔ   18 Ⓐ Ⓑ Ⓒ Ⓓ Ⓔ   23 Ⓐ Ⓑ Ⓒ Ⓓ Ⓔ
4 Ⓐ Ⓑ Ⓒ Ⓓ Ⓔ   9 Ⓐ Ⓑ Ⓒ Ⓓ Ⓔ   14 Ⓐ Ⓑ Ⓒ Ⓓ Ⓔ   19 Ⓐ Ⓑ Ⓒ Ⓓ Ⓔ   24 Ⓐ Ⓑ Ⓒ Ⓓ Ⓔ
5 Ⓐ Ⓑ Ⓒ Ⓓ Ⓔ   10 Ⓐ Ⓑ Ⓒ Ⓓ Ⓔ   15 Ⓐ Ⓑ Ⓒ Ⓓ Ⓔ   20 Ⓐ Ⓑ Ⓒ Ⓓ Ⓔ   25 Ⓐ Ⓑ Ⓒ Ⓓ Ⓔ

Section 5

Experimental Section – See page 9 for details.

THIS PAGE INTENTIONALLY LEFT BLANK.

Writing Sample

Schools would like to get to know you better through a story you tell or an essay you write. If you choose to write a story, use the sentence presented in A to begin. Make sure that your story has a beginning, middle, and end. If you choose to write a personal essay, base your essay on the topic presented in B. Please fill in the circle next to your choice.

Ⓐ "How did you find it?" my friend asked.

Ⓑ Describe a time you failed at something and tell what you learned from it.

Use this page and the next page to complete your writing sample.

Continue on next page

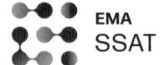

Practice Test III: Middle Level

SECTION 1
25 Questions

Following each problem in this section, there are five suggested answers. Work each problem in your head or in the blank space provided at the right of the page. Then look at the five suggested answers and decide which one is best.

Note: Figures that accompany problems in this section are drawn as accurately as possible EXCEPT when it is stated in a specific problem that its figure is not drawn to scale.

Sample Problem:

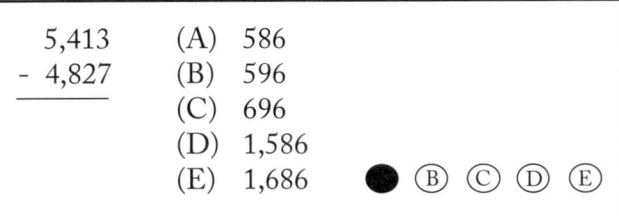

USE THIS SPACE FOR FIGURING.

1. What number is halfway between 19 and 25 ?

    (A) 19.5
    (B) 20
    (C) 21
    (D) 22
    (E) 23

2. Tony has 80 cents. If balloons cost 18 cents, what is the greatest number of balloons he can buy with this money?

    (A) 4
    (B) 5
    (C) 6
    (D) 8
    (E) 10

3. If $\frac{2}{4} = \frac{4}{x}$, what is the value of x ?

    (A) 6
    (B) 8
    (C) 10
    (D) 12
    (E) 16

GO ON TO THE NEXT PAGE.

4. Segments $\overline{AE}$, $\overline{BF}$, $\overline{CF}$, and $\overline{DG}$ are shown on a grid with unit squares. Which of the following lists the segments in order from shortest to longest?

   (A) $\overline{CF}, \overline{BF}, \overline{DG}, \overline{AE}$
   (B) $\overline{CF}, \overline{DG}, \overline{BF}, \overline{AE}$
   (C) $\overline{DG}, \overline{BF}, \overline{CF}, \overline{AE}$
   (D) $\overline{DG}, \overline{CF}, \overline{BF}, \overline{AE}$
   (E) $\overline{DG}, \overline{CF}, \overline{AE}, \overline{BF}$

5. When shipped from a certain publisher, magazines are packaged in bundles of 15. If a delivery van has bundles from the publisher only, which of the following could be the total number of magazines in the van?

   (A) 402
   (B) 403
   (C) 410
   (D) 415
   (E) 420

6. What is the value of 6.4 − 1.8 + 2.4 ?

   (A) 2.2
   (B) 5.8
   (C) 7.0
   (D) 7.8
   (E) 10.6

7. A pitcher that is $\frac{2}{3}$ full contains 6 cups of juice. How many cups of juice does the pitcher hold when it is full?

   (A) 4
   (B) 8
   (C) 9
   (D) 12
   (E) 18

Practice Test III: Middle Level

USE THIS SPACE FOR FIGURING.

8. The first number in a sequence is 1, the second number is 2, and each number after the second is the sum of the two preceding numbers. What is the 6th number of the sequence?

   (A) 6
   (B) 8
   (C) 9
   (D) 13
   (E) 21

9. In which of the following figures could the area of the shaded region be less than $\frac{1}{2}$ of the total area of the figure?

(A)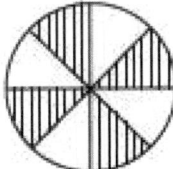

(B)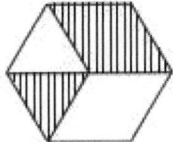

(C)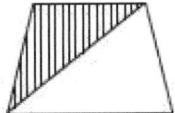

(D)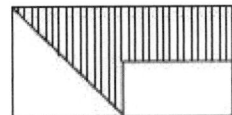

(E)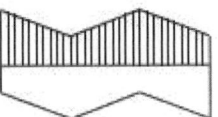

GO ON TO THE NEXT PAGE.

10. At a social gathering, 3 large pizzas are ordered and each pizza is cut into 12 slices. If each person takes exactly 2 slices and there are 10 slices remaining, how many people are at the gathering?

    (A) 10
    (B) 13
    (C) 18
    (D) 26
    (E) 52

11. The ratio of 3 to 7 is the same as which of the following ratios?

    (A) 9 to 28
    (B) 9 to 14
    (C) 12 to 28
    (D) 12 to 21
    (E) 14 to 6

12. The sum of the ages of 3 children is 28. What will be the sum of their ages 4 years from now?

    (A) 40
    (B) 37
    (C) 35
    (D) 32
    (E) 31

13. All of the measures of the angles of a certain triangle are less than 90°. Which of the following could NOT be used to classify the triangle?

    (A) Acute
    (B) Obtuse
    (C) Scalene
    (D) Isosceles
    (E) Equilateral

USE THIS SPACE FOR FIGURING.

GO ON TO THE NEXT PAGE.

Practice Test III: Middle Level

USE THIS SPACE FOR FIGURING.

14. At a carnival, rides cost $5 each and games cost $2 each. Alicia brings $35 with her to the carnival and goes on 4 rides. How many games can she play with the remaining money?

   (A) 3
   (B) 5
   (C) 6
   (D) 7
   (E) 8

15. The number 12 is 20% of the number k. What is the value of k?

   (A) 6
   (B) 24
   (C) 48
   (D) 50
   (E) 60

16. If $3(x - 2) = 3$, what is the value of x?

   (A) −1
   (B) 0
   (C) 1
   (D) 2
   (E) 3

17. What is the value of $\frac{5}{8}$ divided by $\frac{2}{5}$?

   (A) $\frac{1}{4}$
   (B) $\frac{16}{25}$
   (C) $\frac{25}{16}$
   (D) 1
   (E) 4

GO ON TO THE NEXT PAGE.

USE THIS SPACE FOR FIGURING.

18. In the triangle shown, what is the value of x?
    (A) 23
    (B) 26
    (C) 28
    (D) 30
    (E) 32

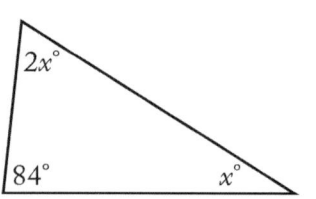

19. The bar graph shows the monthly sales, in dollars, for a small online business. Of the following, which is closest to the percent by which sales increased from February to March?
    (A) 50%
    (B) 75%
    (C) 100%
    (D) 125%
    (E) 150%

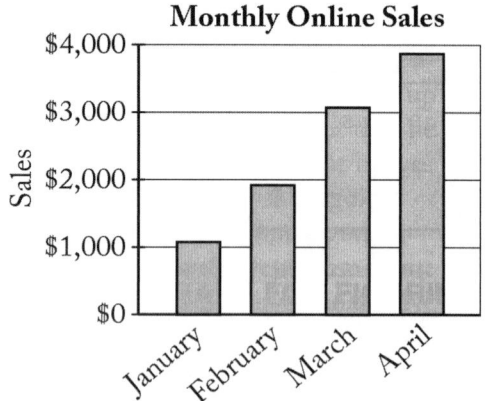

20. What is the value of $\frac{1}{3}\left(2 + \frac{2}{5}\right)$?
    (A) $\frac{4}{15}$
    (B) $\frac{5}{8}$
    (C) $\frac{4}{5}$
    (D) $\frac{16}{15}$
    (E) $\frac{42}{15}$

21. How many yards are in 20 miles?
    (1 mile = 5,280 feet and 1 yard = 3 feet)
    (A) 316,800
    (B) 35,200
    (C) 3,520
    (D) 792
    (E) 88

GO ON TO THE NEXT PAGE.

22. The figure shown consists of a rectangle and a right triangle. What is the area of the figure?

    (A) 62
    (B) 72
    (C) 74
    (D) 76
    (E) 84

USE THIS SPACE FOR FIGURING.

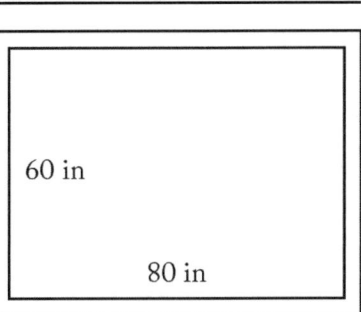

23. If 3 times a number x is less than 21, which of the following CANNOT be the value of x?

    (A) 8
    (B) 6
    (C) 4
    (D) 2
    (E) 0

24. The figure shows a large painting with a wooden frame. The width of the frame is 4 inches. What is the outer perimeter of the frame, in inches?

    (A) 148
    (B) 156
    (C) 280
    (D) 296
    (E) 312

25. If $4x = x - 15$, what is the value of x?

    (A) −18
    (B) −12
    (C) −10
    (D) −5
    (E) −3

STOP

IF YOU FINISH BEFORE TIME IS CALLED, YOU MAY CHECK YOUR WORK ON THIS SECTION ONLY. DO NOT TURN TO ANY OTHER SECTION IN THE TEST.

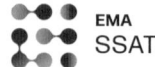

SECTION 2
40 Questions

Read each passage carefully and then answer the questions about it. For each question, decide on the basis of the passage which one of the choices best answers the question.

The backbone of the single-humped camel is not curved upward in the middle, as many people suppose. It is as straight as the backbone of a horse. Humps on camels are composed mostly of fat, and they vary in size according to the physical condition of the animal. When camels are worked too hard and not fed enough, their humps shrivel up and become flabby. Much of their
Line 5   ability to travel long distances over the desert without food and water is due to reabsorption of the extra fat carried in the humps. Thus the hump serves as a sort of food supply department from which the camel receives nourishment in time of famine. Similarly, in certain breeds of sheep, extra fat is stored in the tail.

1. The author's primary purpose in the passage is to
   (A) compare camels to horses
   (B) give information about camels' humps
   (C) describe different kinds of camels
   (D) relate a myth about camels' humps
   (E) explain why traveling in the desert is hazardous

2. According to the author, many people suppose that
   (A) the backbones of most mammals are curved upward in the middle
   (B) a horse has a hump like that of a camel
   (C) the backbone of a single-humped camel is curved upward in the middle
   (D) a camel is a kind of horse
   (E) the backbone of a camel is surrounded by fat

3. The author states that the size of a camel's hump depends primarily on which of the following?
   (A) Where the camel lives
   (B) The physical condition of the camel
   (C) How much water the camel drinks
   (D) The age of the camel
   (E) How far the camel travels

4. The author states that the camel's hump serves the same function as what part of certain breeds of sheep?
   (A) The tail
   (B) The fat
   (C) The backbone
   (D) The wool
   (E) The stomach

5. According to the passage, the hump on a camel's back helps the camel
   (A) travel far in the desert without food and water
   (B) carry heavier burdens than other animals
   (C) keep warm on cold nights in the desert
   (D) move faster than a horse
   (E) protect itself when it is attacked by other animals

6. The author calls the camel's hump a "food supply department" (line 6) in order to show that the hump
   (A) is a good place for carrying extra feedbags
   (B) is the only edible part of a camel
   (C) helps a camel locate hidden food supplies
   (D) warns a camel when famine is approaching
   (E) stores fat which can be reabsorbed by the camel as food

GO ON TO THE NEXT PAGE.

(From a parent's letter to a child away at school)

You must study in order to be frank with the world; frankness is the child of honesty and courage. Say just what you mean to do on every occasion and take it for granted that what you mean to do is right. If a friend asks you a favor, you should grant it if it is reasonable; if not, tell your friend plainly why you cannot. You will wrong both your friend and yourself by equivocation of any kind. Never do a wrong thing to make a friend or keep one; friendship that requires you to do wrong is dearly purchased at a sacrifice. Deal kindly but firmly with all your classmates; you will find it the policy which wears best... If you have any fault to find with anyone, tell that person, not others, of what you complain; there is no more dangerous experiment than that of undertaking to be one thing before a person's face and another behind his or her back. We should live, act, and say nothing to the injury of anyone. It is not only best as a matter of principle, but it is the path of peace and honor.

Line 5

10

7. What is the author probably trying to do?
   (A) Threaten
   (B) Condemn
   (C) Advise
   (D) Predict
   (E) Praise

8. The main topic of the passage is how to
   (A) interact with people
   (B) study efficiently
   (C) avoid danger
   (D) refuse requests
   (E) find fault with others

9. According to the passage, if a friend were to ask a favor, one should
   (A) agree to do it even if it is inconvenient
   (B) do it but ask for a favor in return
   (C) do it since a friend is asking
   (D) ask others whether one should do it
   (E) do it if what is being asked is not wrong

10. The author considers which of the following to be a dangerous experiment?
    (A) Studying at the expense of friendship
    (B) Hypocrisy toward others
    (C) Excessive kindness
    (D) Asking too many favors
    (E) Being overly honest with classmates

11. The author would most likely say that before one can be frank, it is important to
    (A) express sympathy whenever possible
    (B) discuss friends with others
    (C) overlook the faults of others
    (D) be firm in what one believes
    (E) do what friends want one to do

12. In line 1 the word "frank" most nearly means
    (A) outgoing
    (B) innocent
    (C) tactless
    (D) straightforward
    (E) abrupt

GO ON TO THE NEXT PAGE.

Boxwood was for many years the favorite wood for making flutes, recorders, oboes, and clarinets; it was the hardest, finest-grained wood readily available in Europe. Its disadvantage was a pronounced tendency to warp, and bent boxwood instruments can be seen in any large collection of old instruments. Boxwood is practically unobtainable in large enough dimensions for making
Line 5   instruments nowadays.

If the wooden instrument business had developed in North America, it seems likely that the commonly used wood might have been hard maple. That wood is also adversely affected by moisture and is not so dense as boxwood, but it has a fine grain and machines well. The suitability of maple, along with its availability in quite large dimensions, makes it almost the only wood that can be used for some instruments.

13. The passage is primarily about
    (A) the many uses of boxwood and maple
    (B) two woods suitable for making instruments
    (C) necessity of making instruments from hardwoods
    (D) collecting old wooden instruments
    (E) the development of the wooden instrument industry

14. The passage implies that boxwood
    (A) is not adversely affected by moisture
    (B) does not last as well as maple
    (C) is now readily obtainable in Europe
    (D) is the only wood used for some kinds of instruments
    (E) does not commonly grow in North America

15. The passage mentions all of the following properties of boxwood EXCEPT its
    (A) color
    (B) grain
    (C) scarcity
    (D) hardness
    (E) popularity

16. The author apparently considers the warping of boxwood instruments
    (A) a disgrace to their manufacturers
    (B) an indication of hard use
    (C) an unfortunate characteristic
    (D) a harmless phenomenon
    (E) an index of their quality

17. The passage was probably intended as
    (A) a tribute to the woodworkers of the past
    (B) an advertisement about wooden instruments
    (C) advice for collectors of old wooden instruments
    (D) a plea for conservation of endangered kinds of trees and woods
    (E) information about the manufacture of wooden instruments

Like many human endeavors, the Pony Express was born out of long-frustrated need. By 1860 almost half a million Americans lived west of the Rocky Mountains. Aside from the lures of land and gold, the primary concern was for news from home, those settled states east of the Missouri River.

Line 5 Here he comes! . . . nearer and nearer . . . and man and horse rush past us and are gone in a flash!

Thus a famous writer, from a westbound stage, beheld a Pony Express rider, and thus the rider galloped into history.

In spite of the legendary full-tilt gallop, the fact is that the rider had to average only ten
10 miles an hour, that in darkness or going uphill he slowed for safety or to spare the horse, as that he usually arrived on time.

The development of the Pony Express, like other episodes that have become epic, looms taller than truth, a buckaroo stew of fact and legend. And even facts have a legendary flavor.

18. According to the passage, people who were waiting for news from home lived

   (A) east of the Missouri River
   (B) in the Rocky Mountains
   (C) in the settled states
   (D) west of the Rocky Mountains
   (E) in the unsettled states of the East

19. The passage implies that the Pony Express rider rode

   (A) with great care
   (B) with great fear
   (C) to compete with other riders
   (D) only in the dark for safety
   (E) only through towns

20. From the information in the passage, we can be certain that the "famous writer" (line 7)

   (A) was once a Pony Express rider
   (B) wrote about the Pony Express rider
   (C) saw many Pony Express riders
   (D) wrote many stories about the West
   (E) thought historians misunderstood the role of the Pony Express

21. According to the passage, the original purpose of the Pony Express was to

   (A) provide a sporting event for competition and entertainment
   (B) help new settlers find home sites in the West
   (C) enable gold prospectors to communicate with one another
   (D) help people communicate with their families and friends
   (E) convey news of employment prospects to new settlers

22. In line 10 the word "spare" most nearly means

   (A) swap
   (B) reform
   (C) conserve
   (D) shortchange
   (E) cure

GO ON TO THE NEXT PAGE.

> For their physical survival human beings require food and other organic materials that are provided by green plants using the energy of sunlight. Humans also require pure water and air as well as space for wholesome living. Like other animals, in order to maintain reasonable vigor, humans need exercise, recreation, and time to unwind. These needs, as well as all biological experi-
> *Line 5* ence, suggest that humans will have to adjust their numbers to the capacity of their environment. There is no instance known to science in which any organism can increase in number indefinitely without coming to terms with physical limitations. If humans are exceptions, they are truly unique ones.

23. The passage is primarily about the
    (A) uniqueness of humans as a species
    (B) environmental limits to expansion of the human population
    (C) significant differences between humans and other species
    (D) biological requirements for human survival
    (E) pleasures of interacting with the environment

24. This passage is most likely to appear in:
    (A) an encyclopedia entry
    (B) a novel
    (C) an almanac
    (D) a memoir
    (E) a popular science article

25. In line 7, "coming to terms with" most nearly means
    (A) completing
    (B) encompassing
    (C) moving away from
    (D) adjusting to
    (E) conquering

In Europe in the eleventh century, peace and personal security were advanced by growth of the institution we know as "feudalism." In essence, feudalism was a means of carrying on some kind of government on a local basis where no organized state existed. Authority fell into the hands of persons usually called "counts." The count was the most important person of a region covering
Line 5 a few hundred square miles. To build up his own position and strengthen himself for war against other counts, he would try to maintain control over the lesser nobles in his county and keep them from fighting each other. They became his vassals, and he became their "lord." The lord protected the vassals and assured them justice and firm tenure of their land. The vassal agreed to serve the lord as a soldier for a certain number of days in the year. The vassal also owed it to the lord to
10 attend and advise him, to sit in his court in the judging of disputes. Lord and vassal were joined in a kind of contract. Each owed something to the other. It was out of this mutual or contractual character of feudalism that ideas of constitutional government later developed.

26. The passage is primarily about
    (A) the decline of Europe in the eleventh century
    (B) European feudal wars between counts and vassals
    (C) the use and abuse of contracts and constitutions
    (D) the rise of law courts in Europe
    (E) the nature and development of European feudalism

27. According to the passage, a lord was expected to
    (A) ensure the vassals' right to maintain their own land
    (B) provide workers for the vassals' land
    (C) sit in another lord's court
    (D) set up a constitutional government
    (E) abide by the decisions made by his vassals

28. The passage refers to all of the following aspects of eleventh-century Europe EXCEPT the
    (A) judging of disputes in court
    (B) lord-vassal relationship
    (C) place of religion in a feudal society
    (D) foreshadowing of constitutional government
    (E) division of land into counties

29. The passage implies that a vassal would no longer owe allegiance to a count who
    (A) disagreed with the vassal in a court dispute
    (B) forced the vassal to make war on another count
    (C) failed to protect the vassal's holdings
    (D) organized a state
    (E) made a contract with another vassal

30. The passage is most likely taken from
    (A) a psychology journal
    (B) a history textbook
    (C) a political campaign speech
    (D) the diary of a feudal lord
    (E) an advertisement for a European tour

GO ON TO THE NEXT PAGE.

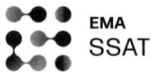

> Of all the land snails, none wears as bright a shell as "the gem of the Everglades"—the *Liguus fasciatus.*
>
> They have no taste for leaves and do not harm the tree. Parading up and down a tree trunk, the tree snail scrapes off minute algae, fungi, and lichens with a rasplike tongue called a radula. The snail moves by rippling contractions of the muscles on the surface of its large "foot." Its head, located on the front of the foot, has two pairs of retractable tentacles.
>
> Liguus is most active during late spring through early summer. At its snail's pace (up to 4 1/2 inches a minute) Liguus roams about 25 feet a day.
>
> Little by little the snail secretes a calcareous substance that hardens into shell. During its first growing season, the snail adds two or three whorls to its shell; that amount is halved each following year until the shell is between 2 and 3 inches long. The average life span of a snail is 3 to 4 years.

Line 5 / 10

31. The passage describes the snail's "foot" (line 5) as
    (A) calcareous
    (B) muscular
    (C) rasplike
    (D) bright
    (E) retractable

32. According to the passage, "radula" (line 4) is another name for the snail's
    (A) tongue
    (B) foot
    (C) head
    (D) shell
    (E) tentacles

33. The passage suggests that the age of a snail can be determined by the
    (A) hardness of its shell
    (B) color of its shell
    (C) slowness of its movements
    (D) length of its tentacles
    (E) number of whorls on its shell

34. All of the following are accurate descriptions of *Liguus fasciatus* EXCEPT that it
    (A) is a tree-climbing land snail
    (B) is called "the gem of the Everglades"
    (C) does not eat foliage
    (D) is harmful to trees
    (E) has a bright shell

35. The passage says that compared to other snails, *Liguus fasciatus*
    (A) grows the largest shell
    (B) lives the longest
    (C) has the most colorful shell
    (D) moves the fastest
    (E) has the most comfortable dwelling place

GO ON TO THE NEXT PAGE.

After graduating from the Chicago Medical College of Northwestern University, Dr. Daniel Hale Williams began practicing medicine in Chicago in 1883. A dedicated physician and skillful surgeon, Dr. Williams' reputation grew rapidly and both Black and White patients soon flocked to him.

Line 5   Dr. Williams felt keenly the need for a hospital where Black interns, nurses, and physicians could train; in 1890 he launched a drive to found a hospital. Provident Hospital, incorporated early in 1891, was the first hospital in the United States founded or fully controlled by Blacks. Under Dr. Williams' exacting leadership, Provident set high standards, had an integrated staff and patients, built a good reputation, and soon became a mecca for Black interns, nurses, and patients from all over the United States.

It was at Provident that Dr. Williams performed the world's first successful heart surgery. On July 9, 1893, he boldly opened the chest and sewed the pericardial sac of a man who had been stabbed. Medical thinking of the day demanded that heart punctures be left, either to heal themselves or to prove fatal. Dr. Williams dared to do the unthinkable operation, risking his reputation and the hospital's to save the patient. The operation succeeded and the patient lived another twenty years. Operating without any of today's modern devices, techniques, and experience, Dr. Daniel Hale Williams took the first step that led to the spectacular heart transplants of many years later.

36. The author's primary purpose is to
    (A) describe the accomplishments of a brilliant doctor
    (B) persuade people to donate money for medical research
    (C) demonstrate how to establish a hospital
    (D) describe how to acquire medical expertise
    (E) indicate that heart transplants are safe

37. The passage implies that the kind of heart operation performed by Dr. Williams was
    (A) in keeping with medical practice of the 1890s
    (B) only successful on puncture wounds to the heart
    (C) not performed again for twenty years
    (D) a courageous undertaking
    (E) the first ever attempted with anesthesia

38. The author's tone can best be described as
    (A) informal
    (B) neutral
    (C) respectful
    (D) despondent
    (E) cautious

39. The passage is most likely taken from a
    (A) textbook on surgery
    (B) college catalog
    (C) doctor's diary
    (D) listing of medical colleges
    (E) book of biographical sketches

40. In line 8, "exacting" most nearly means
    (A) accurate
    (B) rough
    (C) critical
    (D) demanding
    (E) insightful

STOP
**IF YOU FINISH BEFORE TIME IS CALLED, YOU MAY CHECK YOUR WORK ON THIS SECTION ONLY.
DO NOT TURN TO ANY OTHER SECTION IN THE TEST.**

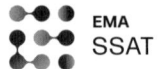

SECTION 3
60 Questions

This section consists of two different types of questions: synonyms and analogies. There are directions and a sample question for each type.

Synonyms
Each of the following questions consists of one word followed by five words or phrases. You are to select the one word or phrase whose meaning is closest to the word in capital letters.

Sample Question:

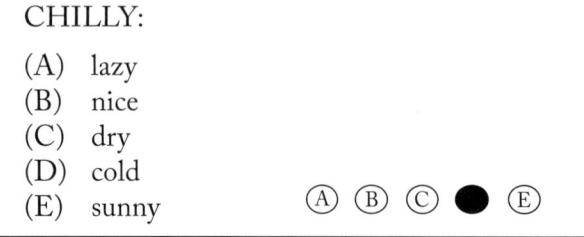

1. CONVERSATION:
    (A) change
    (B) mixture
    (C) appointment
    (D) discussion
    (E) rotation

2. QUARANTINE:
    (A) isolation
    (B) disease
    (C) observation
    (D) therapy
    (E) banishment

3. PROPOSE:
    (A) bestow
    (B) overcome
    (C) question
    (D) suggest
    (E) reveal

4. ABUNDANT:
    (A) plentiful
    (B) repetitive
    (C) frantic
    (D) obvious
    (E) precious

5. INVESTIGATE:
    (A) conceal
    (B) accuse
    (C) examine
    (D) prove
    (E) capture

6. APPROPRIATE:
    (A) suitable
    (B) successful
    (C) professional
    (D) customary
    (E) competent

7. JEER:
    (A) refuse
    (B) block
    (C) scoff
    (D) desert
    (E) ignore

8. TRADITION:
    (A) technique
    (B) training
    (C) celebration
    (D) ancestry
    (E) custom

GO ON TO THE NEXT PAGE.

9. PERPETUAL:
   (A) swift
   (B) unending
   (C) tedious
   (D) complete
   (E) reckless

10. PRESTIGE:
    (A) bliss
    (B) wealth
    (C) haste
    (D) status
    (E) reward

11. MODIFY:
    (A) update
    (B) alter
    (C) transport
    (D) soften
    (E) exchange

12. WILY:
    (A) eager
    (B) frantic
    (C) random
    (D) flexible
    (E) cunning

13. ENVELOP:
    (A) send
    (B) wrap
    (C) design
    (D) hinder
    (E) change

14. CASCADE:
    (A) waterfall
    (B) iceberg
    (C) pageant
    (D) pinnacle
    (E) barrel

15. EXTRACT:
    (A) remove
    (B) breathe
    (C) overload
    (D) abandon
    (E) dissolve

16. PERFORATE:
    (A) detach
    (B) obstruct
    (C) replace
    (D) puncture
    (E) scrape

17. GIMMICK:
    (A) halting speech
    (B) devious trick
    (C) careless error
    (D) clever prank
    (E) sticky surface

18. DRUDGERY:
    (A) filth
    (B) nonsense
    (C) cheating
    (D) sadness
    (E) toil

19. ADVERSARY:
    (A) lawyer
    (B) celebration
    (C) opponent
    (D) criminal
    (E) contest

20. OBSCURE:
    (A) clumsy
    (B) stubborn
    (C) dainty
    (D) vague
    (E) harmful

GO ON TO THE NEXT PAGE.

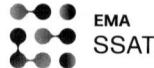

21. TOLERATE:
    (A) allow
    (B) understand
    (C) donate
    (D) confront
    (E) encourage

22. STAUNCH:
    (A) putrid
    (B) violent
    (C) steadfast
    (D) obedient
    (E) plump

23. ARID:
    (A) sharp
    (B) breezy
    (C) dry
    (D) fresh
    (E) plain

24. HOODWINK:
    (A) gamble
    (B) sleep
    (C) deceive
    (D) steal
    (E) escape

25. MALFUNCTION:
    (A) disapproval
    (B) failure
    (C) exposure
    (D) scandal
    (E) falsehood

26. QUALM:
    (A) decree
    (B) obligation
    (C) captivity
    (D) violation
    (E) misgiving

27. VIGILANT:
    (A) alert
    (B) angry
    (C) patient
    (D) fearful
    (E) smart

28. SIMULATE:
    (A) pause
    (B) include
    (C) hinder
    (D) reform
    (E) feign

29. PREMONITION:
    (A) introduction
    (B) forewarning
    (C) discovery
    (D) conspiracy
    (E) opening

30. COLLABORATE:
    (A) pass sentence
    (B) settle down
    (C) forge ahead
    (D) work together
    (E) build up

GO ON TO THE NEXT PAGE.

Analogies
The following questions ask you to find relationships between words. For each question, select the answer choice that best completes the meaning of the sentence.

Sample Question:

Kitten is to cat as
(A) fawn is to colt
(B) puppy is to dog
(C) cow is to bull
(D) wolf is to bear
(E) hen is to rooster

(A) ● (C) (D) (E)

Choice (B) is the best answer because a kitten is a young cat just as a puppy is a young dog. Of all the answer choices, (B) states a relationship that is most like the relationship between kitten and cat.

---

31. Shoe is to moccasin as
    (A) glove is to leather
    (B) collar is to coat
    (C) fragrance is to nose
    (D) gem is to ruby
    (E) hair is to head

32. Chick is to egg as
    (A) dog is to litter
    (B) cat is to kitten
    (C) fish is to school
    (D) bat is to cave
    (E) moth is to cocoon

33. Strum is to banjo as
    (A) sit is to piano
    (B) hum is to tune
    (C) strike is to chord
    (D) blow is to trumpet
    (E) practice is to scale

34. Menu is to food as
    (A) glossary is to vocabulary
    (B) catalog is to merchandise
    (C) directory is to telephone
    (D) agenda is to meeting
    (E) roster is to team

35. Thank is to gratitude as
    (A) learn is to knowledge
    (B) threaten is to fear
    (C) promise is to honesty
    (D) allay is to anger
    (E) pardon is to mercy

36. Prospector is to gold as
    (A) soldier is to army
    (B) proofreader is to error
    (C) accountant is to bank
    (D) singer is to melody
    (E) chemist is to laboratory

37. Grid is to line as
    (A) comb is to tooth
    (B) square is to angle
    (C) net is to string
    (D) shoe is to lace
    (E) road is to curve

38. Clothe is to garment as
    (A) arm is to weapon
    (B) sell is to money
    (C) invite is to party
    (D) build is to house
    (E) hire is to skill

GO ON TO THE NEXT PAGE.

39. Modesty is to humble as
    (A) wealth is to generous
    (B) sorrow is to pathetic
    (C) doubt is to confident
    (D) courage is to valiant
    (E) optimism is to naive

40. Stomp is to step as
    (A) stand is to sit
    (B) lift is to move
    (C) shove is to push
    (D) dive is to fall
    (E) slap is to flinch

41. Chisel is to marble as
    (A) camera is to film
    (B) pencil is to paper
    (C) brush is to paint
    (D) footprint is to snow
    (E) trimmer is to hedge

42. Numeric is to number as
    (A) verbal is to word
    (B) chronic is to disease
    (C) female is to gender
    (D) acute is to angle
    (E) valid is to reason

43. Sundial is to clock as
    (A) scale is to weight
    (B) ruler is to yardstick
    (C) milestone is to speedometer
    (D) thermometer is to degree
    (E) abacus is to calculator

44. Immigrant is to country as
    (A) explorer is to frontier
    (B) employee is to occupation
    (C) convert is to religion
    (D) voter is to party
    (E) member is to club

45. Herald is to proclaim as
    (A) pupil is to teach
    (B) sentry is to guard
    (C) citizen is to vote
    (D) orphan is to adopt
    (E) outcast is to shun

46. Sand is to glass as
    (A) wood is to paper
    (B) cow is to milk
    (C) crust is to bread
    (D) stitch is to clothing
    (E) lead is to pencil

47. Rub is to friction as
    (A) pour is to liquid
    (B) squeeze is to pressure
    (C) throw is to distance
    (D) boil is to temperature
    (E) drop is to gravity

48. Reek is to odor as
    (A) shine is to light
    (B) wince is to pain
    (C) cook is to flavor
    (D) blare is to sound
    (E) gaze is to view

49. Shack is to mansion as
    (A) tent is to camp
    (B) locomotive is to train
    (C) kitchen is to restaurant
    (D) grocery is to market
    (E) jalopy is to limousine

50. Clamp is to hold as
    (A) ladder is to lean
    (B) nail is to pound
    (C) lever is to lift
    (D) board is to cut
    (E) cement is to mix

GO ON TO THE NEXT PAGE.

51. Chat is to converse as
    (A) browse is to look
    (B) win is to compete
    (C) listen is to obey
    (D) lend is to borrow
    (E) lull is to sleep

52. Atrocious is to bad as
    (A) infinite is to complete
    (B) gaunt is to thin
    (C) short is to small
    (D) visible is to legible
    (E) fancy is to plain

53. Fickle is to change as
    (A) broken is to repair
    (B) mute is to speak
    (C) hesitant is to fail
    (D) fretful is to worry
    (E) random is to predict

54. Evict is to residence as
    (A) besiege is to fortress
    (B) abandon is to ship
    (C) resign is to position
    (D) banish is to country
    (E) transfer is to school

55. Bashful is to socialize as
    (A) punctual is to begin
    (B) impatient is to wait
    (C) fearless is to harm
    (D) jealous is to envy
    (E) suspicious is to blame

56. Braggart is to boastful as
    (A) fanatic is to ardent
    (B) coward is to courageous
    (C) pessimist is to angry
    (D) nomad is to lonesome
    (E) miser is to wealthy

57. Remind is to remember as
    (A) learn is to understand
    (B) reject is to accept
    (C) convince is to believe
    (D) travel is to arrive
    (E) perform is to rehearse

58. Feeble is to vigor as
    (A) optional is to choice
    (B) notorious is to fame
    (C) profound is to depth
    (D) liberal is to freedom
    (E) awkward is to grace

59. Applaud is to approval as
    (A) achieve is to success
    (B) express is to emotion
    (C) salute is to command
    (D) renege is to promise
    (E) beckon is to invitation

60. Taboo is to permissible as
    (A) gruesome is to squeamish
    (B) stalwart is to robust
    (C) dispensable is to essential
    (D) pitiful is to sympathetic
    (E) prosperous is to wealthy

STOP

**IF YOU FINISH BEFORE TIME IS CALLED, YOU MAY CHECK YOUR WORK ON THIS SECTION ONLY.
DO NOT TURN TO ANY OTHER SECTION IN THE TEST.**

SECTION 4
25 Questions

Following each problem in this section, there are five suggested answers. Work each problem in your head or in the blank space provided at the right of the page. Then look at the five suggested answers and decide which one is best.

Note: Figures that accompany problems in this section are drawn as accurately as possible EXCEPT when it is stated in a specific problem that its figure is not drawn to scale.

Sample Problem:

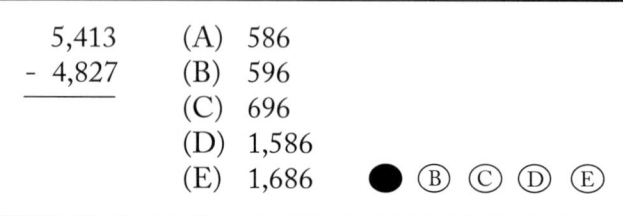

USE THIS SPACE FOR FIGURING.

1. If $2n = 12$, what is the value of n?
   (A) 6
   (B) 10
   (C) 12
   (D) 14
   (E) 24

2. In the number 137.26, which of the following digits is in the tenths place?
   (A) 1
   (B) 2
   (C) 3
   (D) 6
   (E) 7

GO ON TO THE NEXT PAGE.

3. Each week, Carmen saves 25% of her weekly allowance. Which of the following circle graphs best represents her savings?

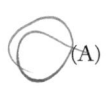 (A)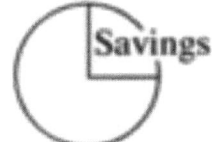

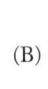 (B)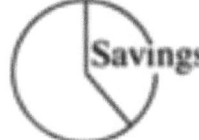

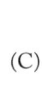 (C)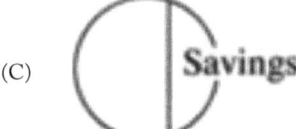

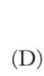 (D)

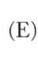 (E)

3, 6, 12, ...

4. In the sequence above, 3 is the first number and each number after the first is 2 times the preceding number. Which of the following is a number in the sequence?

(A) 30
(B) 60
(C) 144
(D) 192
(E) 248

GO ON TO THE NEXT PAGE.

USE THIS SPACE FOR FIGURING.

5. What is the value of $\frac{1}{3} + \frac{2}{6} + \frac{3}{9}$?

   (A) $\frac{1}{27}$

   (B) $\frac{2}{3}$

   (C) $\frac{8}{9}$

   (D) $\frac{17}{18}$

   (E) 1

3, 4, 5, 1, 3, 6, 4, 6

6. Each of the numbers in the list above shows the number of hours of TV that Ling watched per week over the course of 8 weeks. What is the mean number of hours of TV Ling watched per week?

   (A) 1
   (B) 2
   (C) 3
   (D) 4
   (E) 5

---

7. If $\frac{2}{5}$ of a number n is 50, then $\frac{4}{5}$ of n is

   (A) 20
   (B) 40
   (C) 60
   (D) 80
   (E) 100

---

8. In triangle ABC shown, if $AB = BC$, what is the perimeter of the triangle?

   (A) 11
   (B) 15
   (C) 16
   (D) 17
   (E) 30

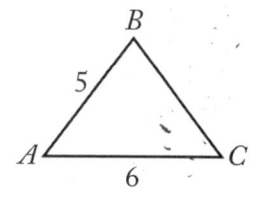

GO ON TO THE NEXT PAGE.

9. Of the following, which is closest to 79.6 − 2.12 ?
   (A) 50
   (B) 60
   (C) 68
   (D) 70
   (E) 78

10. It takes Marcia 80 minutes to hike uphill on a trail from her car to the campsite and $\frac{1}{4}$ of that time to hike downhill to her car from the campsite. What is the time it takes, in minutes, to hike to her car from the campsite?
    (A) 20
    (B) 40
    (C) 100
    (D) 120
    (E) 320

11. Which of the following can be used to create the figure shown without overlap?

(A)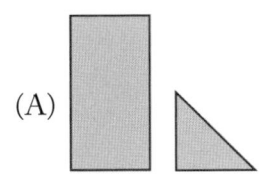

(B)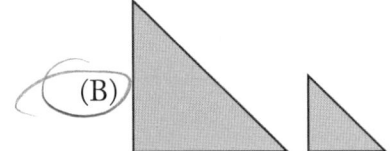

(C)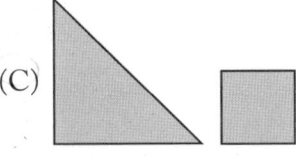

(D)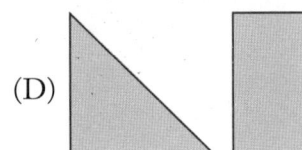

(E)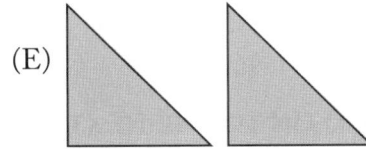

GO ON TO THE NEXT PAGE.

12. Sarah has 8 stamps and Elsa has 20. How many stamps must Elsa give Sarah so that both Sarah and Elsa have the same number of stamps?

    (A) 3
    (B) 6
    (C) 7
    (D) 8
    (E) 10

13. Which of the following is less than $\frac{1}{2}$?

    (A) $\frac{2}{6}$
    (B) $\frac{5}{10}$
    (C) $\frac{7}{14}$
    (D) $\frac{10}{18}$
    (E) $\frac{12}{24}$

14. What is the greatest common factor of 36 and 72 ?

    (A) 6
    (B) 9
    (C) 12
    (D) 36
    (E) 72

15. There are x fish for sale in a pet store, and 12 of them are goldfish. In terms of x, how many of the fish in the pet store are not goldfish?

    (A) $\frac{x}{12}$
    (B) $\frac{12}{x}$
    (C) $12 - x$
    (D) $x - 12$
    (E) $x + 12$

Practice Test III: Middle Level

USE THIS SPACE FOR FIGURING.

16. What is the value of 93 − 3 + 12 ÷ 3 ?
    (A) 34
    (B) 81
    (C) 86
    (D) 88
    (E) 94

17. Nodí has read $\frac{1}{6}$ of a book. If he has read 24 pages of the book, how many more pages must he read to finish the book?
    (A) 4
    (B) 20
    (C) 28
    (D) 120
    (E) 144

18. What is 10.9 times 0.4 ?
    (A) 0.436
    (B) 4.36
    (C) 43.6
    (D) 436
    (E) 4,360

19. In a group of 100 high school students, $\frac{1}{5}$ of the students are ninth graders, and $\frac{1}{4}$ of the other students are tenth graders. How many of the students in the group are neither ninth graders nor tenth graders?
    (A) 20
    (B) 40
    (C) 60
    (D) 75
    (E) 80

GO ON TO THE NEXT PAGE.

20. What is the value of $\frac{20}{3}$ divided by 4 ?

   (A) $\frac{3}{80}$

   (B) $\frac{3}{5}$

   (C) $\frac{5}{3}$

   (D) $\frac{15}{4}$

   (E) $\frac{80}{3}$

21. Chaim has $4,500 in a savings account. If last year he had $5,000 in the savings account, by what percent did the money in the account decrease from last year to now?

   (A) 11%
   (B) 10%
   (C) 9%
   (D) 5%
   (E) 1%

22. In the figure shown, line k intersects parallel lines l and m. What is the value of x ?

   (A) 15
   (B) 20
   (C) 25
   (D) 30
   (E) 35

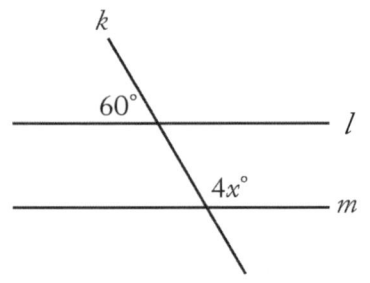

23. Which of the following is equivalent to $4(2x + 3 - x)$?

   (A) $10x$
   (B) $16x$
   (C) $4x + 12$
   (D) $7x + 3$
   (E) $12x + 12$

GO ON TO THE NEXT PAGE.

24. If $a = -2$ and $b = 3$, what is the value of $b - 4a$?
    - (A) −5
    - (B) −3
    - (C) 2
    - (D) 9
    - (E) 11

25. The length of rectangle A is 6 times the length of rectangle B. The width of rectangle A is $\frac{4}{3}$ the width of rectangle B. If the area of rectangle A is x times the area of rectangle B, what is the value of x ?
    - (A) $\frac{9}{2}$
    - (B) 6
    - (C) 8
    - (D) $\frac{20}{3}$
    - (E) 12

STOP

IF YOU FINISH BEFORE TIME IS CALLED, YOU MAY CHECK YOUR WORK ON THIS SECTION ONLY.
DO NOT TURN TO ANY OTHER SECTION IN THE TEST.

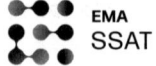

Practice Test IV: Middle Level Answer Sheet

Be sure each mark completely fills the answer space.
Start with number 1 for each new section of the test.

Section 1

1 ⒶⒷⒸⒹⒺ	6 ⒶⒷⒸⒹⒺ	11 ⒶⒷⒸⒹⒺ	16 ⒶⒷⒸⒹⒺ	21 ⒶⒷⒸⒹⒺ
2 ⒶⒷⒸⒹⒺ	7 ⒶⒷⒸⒹⒺ	12 ⒶⒷⒸⒹⒺ	17 ⒶⒷⒸⒹⒺ	22 ⒶⒷⒸⒹⒺ
3 ⒶⒷⒸⒹⒺ	8 ⒶⒷⒸⒹⒺ	13 ⒶⒷⒸⒹⒺ	18 ⒶⒷⒸⒹⒺ	23 ⒶⒷⒸⒹⒺ
4 ⒶⒷⒸⒹⒺ	9 ⒶⒷⒸⒹⒺ	14 ⒶⒷⒸⒹⒺ	19 ⒶⒷⒸⒹⒺ	24 ⒶⒷⒸⒹⒺ
5 ⒶⒷⒸⒹⒺ	10 ⒶⒷⒸⒹⒺ	15 ⒶⒷⒸⒹⒺ	20 ⒶⒷⒸⒹⒺ	25 ⒶⒷⒸⒹⒺ

Section 2

1 ⒶⒷⒸⒹⒺ	9 ⒶⒷⒸⒹⒺ	17 ⒶⒷⒸⒹⒺ	25 ⒶⒷⒸⒹⒺ	33 ⒶⒷⒸⒹⒺ
2 ⒶⒷⒸⒹⒺ	10 ⒶⒷⒸⒹⒺ	18 ⒶⒷⒸⒹⒺ	26 ⒶⒷⒸⒹⒺ	34 ⒶⒷⒸⒹⒺ
3 ⒶⒷⒸⒹⒺ	11 ⒶⒷⒸⒹⒺ	19 ⒶⒷⒸⒹⒺ	27 ⒶⒷⒸⒹⒺ	35 ⒶⒷⒸⒹⒺ
4 ⒶⒷⒸⒹⒺ	12 ⒶⒷⒸⒹⒺ	20 ⒶⒷⒸⒹⒺ	28 ⒶⒷⒸⒹⒺ	36 ⒶⒷⒸⒹⒺ
5 ⒶⒷⒸⒹⒺ	13 ⒶⒷⒸⒹⒺ	21 ⒶⒷⒸⒹⒺ	29 ⒶⒷⒸⒹⒺ	37 ⒶⒷⒸⒹⒺ
6 ⒶⒷⒸⒹⒺ	14 ⒶⒷⒸⒹⒺ	22 ⒶⒷⒸⒹⒺ	30 ⒶⒷⒸⒹⒺ	38 ⒶⒷⒸⒹⒺ
7 ⒶⒷⒸⒹⒺ	15 ⒶⒷⒸⒹⒺ	23 ⒶⒷⒸⒹⒺ	31 ⒶⒷⒸⒹⒺ	39 ⒶⒷⒸⒹⒺ
8 ⒶⒷⒸⒹⒺ	16 ⒶⒷⒸⒹⒺ	24 ⒶⒷⒸⒹⒺ	32 ⒶⒷⒸⒹⒺ	40 ⒶⒷⒸⒹⒺ

Section 3

1 ⒶⒷⒸⒹⒺ	13 ⒶⒷⒸⒹⒺ	25 ⒶⒷⒸⒹⒺ	37 ⒶⒷⒸⒹⒺ	49 ⒶⒷⒸⒹⒺ
2 ⒶⒷⒸⒹⒺ	14 ⒶⒷⒸⒹⒺ	26 ⒶⒷⒸⒹⒺ	38 ⒶⒷⒸⒹⒺ	50 ⒶⒷⒸⒹⒺ
3 ⒶⒷⒸⒹⒺ	15 ⒶⒷⒸⒹⒺ	27 ⒶⒷⒸⒹⒺ	39 ⒶⒷⒸⒹⒺ	51 ⒶⒷⒸⒹⒺ
4 ⒶⒷⒸⒹⒺ	16 ⒶⒷⒸⒹⒺ	28 ⒶⒷⒸⒹⒺ	40 ⒶⒷⒸⒹⒺ	52 ⒶⒷⒸⒹⒺ
5 ⒶⒷⒸⒹⒺ	17 ⒶⒷⒸⒹⒺ	29 ⒶⒷⒸⒹⒺ	41 ⒶⒷⒸⒹⒺ	53 ⒶⒷⒸⒹⒺ
6 ⒶⒷⒸⒹⒺ	18 ⒶⒷⒸⒹⒺ	30 ⒶⒷⒸⒹⒺ	42 ⒶⒷⒸⒹⒺ	54 ⒶⒷⒸⒹⒺ
7 ⒶⒷⒸⒹⒺ	19 ⒶⒷⒸⒹⒺ	31 ⒶⒷⒸⒹⒺ	43 ⒶⒷⒸⒹⒺ	55 ⒶⒷⒸⒹⒺ
8 ⒶⒷⒸⒹⒺ	20 ⒶⒷⒸⒹⒺ	32 ⒶⒷⒸⒹⒺ	44 ⒶⒷⒸⒹⒺ	56 ⒶⒷⒸⒹⒺ
9 ⒶⒷⒸⒹⒺ	21 ⒶⒷⒸⒹⒺ	33 ⒶⒷⒸⒹⒺ	45 ⒶⒷⒸⒹⒺ	57 ⒶⒷⒸⒹⒺ
10 ⒶⒷⒸⒹⒺ	22 ⒶⒷⒸⒹⒺ	34 ⒶⒷⒸⒹⒺ	46 ⒶⒷⒸⒹⒺ	58 ⒶⒷⒸⒹⒺ
11 ⒶⒷⒸⒹⒺ	23 ⒶⒷⒸⒹⒺ	35 ⒶⒷⒸⒹⒺ	47 ⒶⒷⒸⒹⒺ	59 ⒶⒷⒸⒹⒺ
12 ⒶⒷⒸⒹⒺ	24 ⒶⒷⒸⒹⒺ	36 ⒶⒷⒸⒹⒺ	48 ⒶⒷⒸⒹⒺ	60 ⒶⒷⒸⒹⒺ

Section 4

1 ⒶⒷⒸⒹⒺ	6 ⒶⒷⒸⒹⒺ	11 ⒶⒷⒸⒹⒺ	16 ⒶⒷⒸⒹⒺ	21 ⒶⒷⒸⒹⒺ
2 ⒶⒷⒸⒹⒺ	7 ⒶⒷⒸⒹⒺ	12 ⒶⒷⒸⒹⒺ	17 ⒶⒷⒸⒹⒺ	22 ⒶⒷⒸⒹⒺ
3 ⒶⒷⒸⒹⒺ	8 ⒶⒷⒸⒹⒺ	13 ⒶⒷⒸⒹⒺ	18 ⒶⒷⒸⒹⒺ	23 ⒶⒷⒸⒹⒺ
4 ⒶⒷⒸⒹⒺ	9 ⒶⒷⒸⒹⒺ	14 ⒶⒷⒸⒹⒺ	19 ⒶⒷⒸⒹⒺ	24 ⒶⒷⒸⒹⒺ
5 ⒶⒷⒸⒹⒺ	10 ⒶⒷⒸⒹⒺ	15 ⒶⒷⒸⒹⒺ	20 ⒶⒷⒸⒹⒺ	25 ⒶⒷⒸⒹⒺ

Section 5

1 ⒶⒷⒸⒹⒺ	5 ⒶⒷⒸⒹⒺ	9 ⒶⒷⒸⒹⒺ	13 ⒶⒷⒸⒹⒺ
2 ⒶⒷⒸⒹⒺ	6 ⒶⒷⒸⒹⒺ	10 ⒶⒷⒸⒹⒺ	14 ⒶⒷⒸⒹⒺ
3 ⒶⒷⒸⒹⒺ	7 ⒶⒷⒸⒹⒺ	11 ⒶⒷⒸⒹⒺ	15 ⒶⒷⒸⒹⒺ
4 ⒶⒷⒸⒹⒺ	8 ⒶⒷⒸⒹⒺ	12 ⒶⒷⒸⒹⒺ	16 ⒶⒷⒸⒹⒺ

Experimental Section – See page 9 for details.

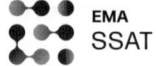

THIS PAGE INTENTIONALLY LEFT BLANK.

Writing Sample

Schools would like to get to know you better through a story you tell or an essay you write. If you choose to write a story, use the sentence presented in A to begin. Make sure that your story has a beginning, middle, and end. If you choose to write a personal essay, base your essay on the topic presented in B. Please fill in the circle next to your choice.

Ⓐ I looked around and thought, "What am I doing here?"

Ⓑ What was one of the most difficult choices you've ever had to make? Describe the situation and explain the outcome.

Use this page and the next page to complete your writing sample.

Continue on next page

THIS PAGE INTENTIONALLY LEFT BLANK.

SECTION 1
25 Questions

Following each problem in this section, there are five suggested answers. Work each problem in your head or in the blank space provided at the right of the page. Then look at the five suggested answers and decide which one is best.

Note: Figures that accompany problems in this section are drawn as accurately as possible EXCEPT when it is stated in a specific problem that its figure is not drawn to scale.

Sample Problem:

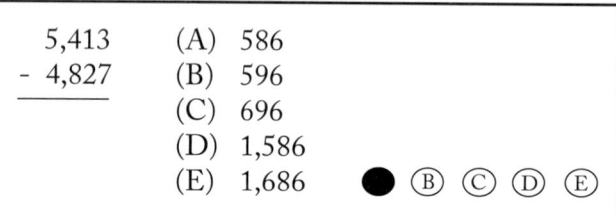

---

1. What is the value of $\frac{4}{1} + \frac{5}{10} + \frac{2}{100} + \frac{7}{1,000}$?

    (A) 45.27
    (B) 4.527
    (C) 4.5027
    (D) 4.0527
    (E) 0.4527

    4.527

USE THIS SPACE FOR FIGURING.

---

2. What is the perimeter of the triangle shown?

    (A) 4
    (B) 6
    (C) 9
    (D) 12
    (E) 13

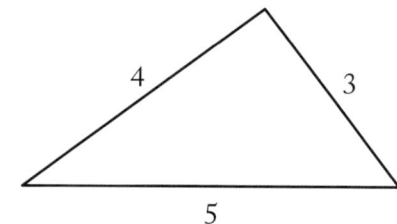

---

3. If $\frac{1}{3}$ of a number equals 24, which of the following equals $\frac{2}{3}$ of the number?

    (A) 48
    (B) 36
    (C) 32
    (D) 16
    (E) 12

GO ON TO THE NEXT PAGE.

4. According to the table, how many days was the temperature in Rapid City greater than or equal to 40°F?
   (A) 9
   (B) 10
   (C) 11
   (D) 19
   (E) 20

Temperatures in April 2019 in Rapid City, South Dakota

Average Daily Temperature	Number of Days
20°F through 29°F	3
30°F through 39°F	7
40°F through 49°F	9
50°F through 59°F	10
60°F through 69°F	1

5. Simplify: $\frac{3}{7} \times \frac{50}{9} \times \frac{21}{5}$
   (A) $\frac{1}{10}$
   (B) $\frac{9}{10}$
   (C) $\frac{10}{9}$
   (D) 10
   (E) 90

6. For rectangle $ABCD$, what is the value of x?
   (A) 15
   (B) 30
   (C) 60
   (D) 90
   (E) 150

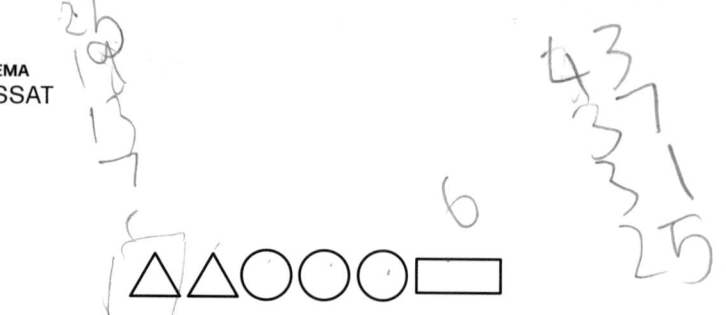

USE THIS SPACE FOR FIGURING.

7. A sequence is generated by repeating the six shapes above, in that order. What are the 42nd and 43rd shapes in the sequence?

(A)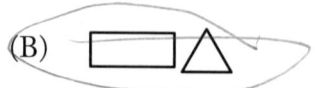

(B) ▭ △

(C) △ △

(D) △ ○

(E) ○ ○

8. Which of the following routes from Padua to Radnor to Skillman is shortest?

(A)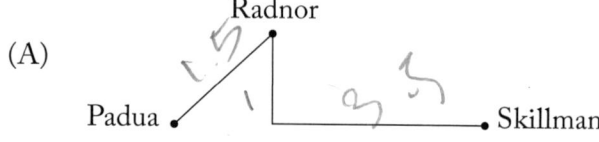

(B)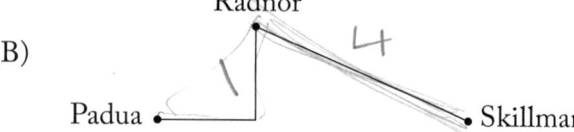

(C)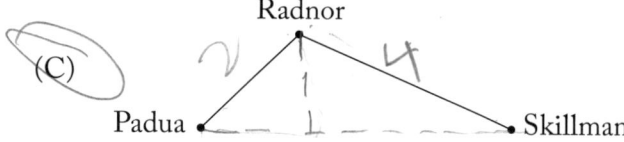

(D)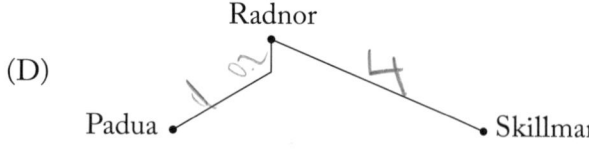

(E)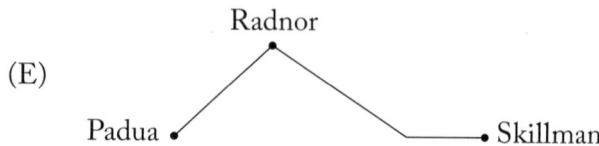

GO ON TO THE NEXT PAGE.

9. Which of the following is NOT equal to $9 \times 8 \times 7 \times 6$?
   (A) 72×42
   (B) 56×54
   (C) 42×56
   (D) 36×84
   (E) 28×108

10. At a bakery on Tuesday, $\frac{1}{5}$ of the customers each bought a pie with cookie crust. Of the customers who bought a pie with cookie crust, $\frac{2}{3}$ bought a pie with pudding filling. What fraction of the customers bought a pie with cookie crust and pudding filling?
    (A) $\frac{2}{15}$
    (B) $\frac{3}{8}$
    (C) $\frac{3}{10}$
    (D) $\frac{7}{15}$
    (E) $\frac{13}{15}$

$$4 - 2y > -12$$

11. Of the following, which is the greatest possible integer value of y that satisfies the inequality above?
    (A) 9
    (B) 7
    (C) 3
    (D) 1
    (E) −5

12. Anya is exactly 4 years older than her two 6-year old twin brothers. Every year on their birthday, Anya and the twins each receive a birthday cake, and the number of candles on each cake is equal to the age of the child who receives it. How many candles will be needed for their birthday cakes next year?

    (A) 16
    (B) 19
    (C) 22
    (D) 25
    (E) 29

13. What is $7 \div \frac{14}{21}$?

    (A) $\frac{1}{3}$
    (B) $\frac{2}{21}$
    (C) 3
    (D) $\frac{14}{3}$
    (E) $\frac{21}{2}$

14. When the beads in a bag were distributed equally to some children, there were 3 beads left over. If there were 84 beads in the bag, which of the following could be the number of children?

    (A) 9
    (B) 8
    (C) 7
    (D) 6
    (E) 5

15. A rectangular solid has length 5 inches, width 5 inches, and height 6 inches. What is the total surface area, in square inches, of the solid?

    (A) 170
    (B) 160
    (C) 150
    (D) 145
    (E) 140

GO ON TO THE NEXT PAGE.

Practice Test IV: Middle Level

USE THIS SPACE FOR FIGURING.

16. Of the following, which is the best estimate of 7.809 × 101.02 ?

   (A) 78,100
   (B) 8,000
   (C) 7,800
   (D) 800
   (E) 700

17. At eight years old, Renee's height was 50 inches. At twelve years old, her height was 60 inches. What was the percent increase in Renee's height from when she was eight years old to when she was twelve years old?

   (A) 10%
   (B) 17%
   (C) 20%
   (D) 67%
   (E) 83%

18. Of 4 numbers, the least is 20 and the greatest is 42. Which of the following could be the mean of the 4 numbers?

   (A) 38
   (B) 36
   (C) 25
   (D) 24
   (E) 22

19. A cookie company packs 30 cookies in each box and 20 boxes in each case. In the morning, the company receives an order to pack and ship 8 cases of cookies. By noon, all but one of the cases are completely packed. The number of cookies packed by noon falls within which of the following ranges?

   (A) Between 160 and 240
   (B) Between 240 and 500
   (C) Between 600 and 850
   (D) Between 4,200 and 4,800
   (E) Between 4,800 and 5,400

GO ON TO THE NEXT PAGE.

20. If n is a positive whole number, of the following, which represents the greatest number?

   (A) $\frac{n}{2} - \frac{n}{3}$
   (B) $\frac{n}{3} - \frac{n}{2}$
   (C) $\frac{n}{3} - \frac{n}{4}$
   (D) $\frac{n}{4} - \frac{n}{3}$
   (E) $\frac{n}{4} - \frac{n}{5}$

21. For a party, Mel bought 3 cups of chocolate ice cream for every 2 cups of vanilla ice cream. What fraction of the cups bought contained chocolate ice cream?

   (A) $\frac{1}{2}$
   (B) $\frac{1}{3}$
   (C) $\frac{2}{3}$
   (D) $\frac{2}{5}$
   (E) $\frac{3}{5}$

22. If $3a + b = 12$, which of the following is equal to a?

   (A) $\frac{b}{3} - 4$
   (B) $4 - b$
   (C) $4 - \frac{b}{3}$
   (D) $4 + \frac{b}{3}$
   (E) $12 - \frac{b}{3}$

23. A train travels at an average rate of 90 meters per second. At this rate, how many kilometers will the train travel in 3 hours?

   (A) 16.2
   (B) 32.4
   (C) 97.2
   (D) 324
   (E) 972

24. Simplify: $(3ab + 2a + 1) - (-2ab + 2a - 1)$
    (A) $5ab$
    (B) $ab + 2$
    (C) $ab + 4a$
    (D) $5ab + 2$
    (E) $5ab + 4a$

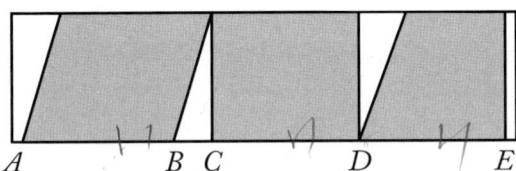

25. Inside the rectangle above is a shaded parallelogram, rectangle, and trapezoid. If $AB = CD = DE$, which of the following figures have the same area?
    (A) None of the figures
    (B) The parallelogram and the rectangle
    (C) The parallelogram and the trapezoid
    (D) The rectangle and the trapezoid
    (E) All of the figures

STOP
IF YOU FINISH BEFORE TIME IS CALLED, YOU MAY CHECK YOUR WORK ON THIS SECTION ONLY.
DO NOT TURN TO ANY OTHER SECTION IN THE TEST.

SECTION 2
40 Questions

Read each passage carefully and then answer the questions about it. For each question, decide on the basis of the passage which one of the choices best answers the question.

> The indescribable glory of the Gothic cathedral is its sculpture. The old churches are drenched with sculpture. It is estimated that the cathedral at Chartres, north of Paris, displays 10,000 carvings; they do not look as if they were added to the building like the frosted figures on a wedding cake, but as if they were a part of the building and as necessary as the arches and windows.

1. According to the passage, the outstanding feature of the cathedral at Chartres is the

    (A) age of its stonework
    (B) whiteness of the interior
    (C) location of the building
    (D) grandeur of its windows and arches
    (E) nature and number of its sculptures

2. The author indicates that the "carvings" (line 2) appear to be

    (A) purely decorative
    (B) stylistically varied
    (C) integral to the cathedral
    (D) too numerous to count
    (E) more beautiful than arches

3. The author uses the expression "frosted figures" (line 3) to create which literary device?

    (A) Onomatopoeia
    (B) Simile
    (C) Personification
    (D) Hyperbole
    (E) Oxymoron

"And now tell me about it." Mannering took notepaper from a drawer.
Sheila's glance strayed through the window and caught a little motorboat moored below. She braced herself and began to talk. He scribbled on the notepaper.
"And nobody knows about all this? Am I the first person you've managed to tell?"

Line 5   She heard herself saying calmly, "I did say something to someone. One of your guests."
"One of my guests?" Mannering stood up.
He was gone—with frank haste. Sheila sprang to her feet. She had about two minutes. She picked up the telephone. Nothing happened. The instrument had been cut off. But somewhere in the castle there might be guests still. She ran to the door.

10   Locked. Sheila ran to the window, opened it and was on the terrace. There was a guard at either end, and these converged on her instantly. Sheila ran straight forward and leapt the balustrade.
She landed on a lower terrace, and the drop was sufficient to give her a nasty jar. But she scrambled up. There were shouts behind. She ran down the steps and jumped into the motorboat.
She realized that it had controls exactly like those of a car. She cast off.

4. The passage is primarily concerned with
   (A) a discovery
   (B) an escape
   (C) a rescue
   (D) a negotiation
   (E) a confession

5. Mannering leaves the room "with frank haste" (line 7) most likely because he wants to
   (A) give Sheila a chance to be alone
   (B) find the guest to whom Sheila had talked
   (C) say goodbye to his departing guests
   (D) find out why the telephone was cut off
   (E) move his motorboat out of sight

6. In the passage Sheila is portrayed as
   (A) resourceful
   (B) befuddled
   (C) negligent
   (D) dishonest
   (E) obedient

7. As it is used in line 13, "sufficient" most nearly means
   (A) loud enough
   (B) slow enough
   (C) mild enough
   (D) long enough
   (E) straight enough

8. The mood of the passage is best described as
   (A) somber
   (B) comical
   (C) tense
   (D) sedate
   (E) eerie

GO ON TO THE NEXT PAGE.

Sounds too high for humans to hear are audible to dogs. The upper limit of human hearing is about 20,000 hertz (cycles per second), of canine hearing about 40,000 hertz, and of mice hearing about 80,000 hertz. The lower limit of human hearing is about 125 hertz at normal levels of intensity. Are any animals able to hear even lower sounds than humans can?

Line 5   It seems likely that all animals whose heads are larger than a human being's have this ability. Three investigators recently tested the hearing range of an Indian elephant. They found that Lois could not hear sounds higher than 12,000 hertz but could hear sounds as low as 16 hertz at levels of intensity that were inaudible to human beings. The investigators concluded that the range of hearing in animals is in inverse proportion, not to the size of the ear, but to the size of the skull, which is related to the distance between the ears.

9. The author uses the word "high" (line 1) in reference to
    (A) status
    (B) altitude
    (C) volume
    (D) pitch
    (E) emotion

10. According to the passage, the range of human hearing at normal levels of intensity is about
    (A) 16 to 125 hertz
    (B) 100 to 12,000 hertz
    (C) 125 to 20,000 hertz
    (D) 20,000 to 40,000 hertz
    (E) 40,000 to 80,000 hertz

11. In line 5, "this ability" refers to
    (A) making audible sounds
    (B) communicating with sounds
    (C) distinguishing high from low sounds
    (D) understanding human speech
    (E) hearing sounds below the human limit

12. It can be inferred from the passage that "Lois" (line 7) is the name of
    (A) an elephant
    (B) a canine subject
    (C) a human subject
    (D) an investigator
    (E) a recording device

13. According to the passage, an animal's range of hearing is proportionate to
    (A) the overall weight of the animal
    (B) the distance between the animal's ears
    (C) the size of the animal's ears
    (D) the range of sounds the animal produces
    (E) the volume of the animal's brain

GO ON TO THE NEXT PAGE.

There are several kinds of stories, but only one that is difficult to tell—the humorous. The humorous story is very different from the comic story. The humorous story depends for its effect upon the manner of the telling; the comic story upon the matter.

The humorous story may be spun out to great length, and wander around all it pleases, and arrive nowhere in particular, but the comic story must be brief and end with a point. The humorous story bubbles gently along; the other bursts.

The humorous story is strictly a work of art, and only an artist can tell it. No art is necessary in telling the comic story; anybody can do it. The humorous story is told gravely; the teller conceals that he or she even dimly suspects that there is anything funny about it.

The teller of a comic story tells you beforehand that it is funny, tells it with eager delight, and is the first person to laugh when the tale is told. And sometimes, if the story has had good success, the teller will gladly repeat the "nub" of it and glance around from face to face collecting applause, and then repeat it again. It is a pathetic thing to see.

Very often, of course, the rambling and disjointed humorous story finishes with a nub, point, snapper, or whatever you like to call it. Then the listener must be alert, for in many cases the teller will divert attention from that nub by dropping it in a carefully casual and indifferent way, with the pretense that he or she does not know it is a nub.

Artemus Ward used that trick a good deal; then when the audience belatedly caught the joke, he would look up with innocent surprise, as if wondering what they found to laugh at.

14. The primary purpose of the first four paragraphs (lines 1–13) is to

    (A) distinguish humorous from comic stories
    (B) outline the history of storytelling
    (C) explain how to write a humorous story
    (D) catalogue various kinds of stories
    (E) analyze a story into its component parts

15. According to the passage, in comparison with a comic story, a humorous story is more

    (A) condensed
    (B) rambling
    (C) instructive
    (D) realistic
    (E) absurd

16. According to the author, a humorous story should be told

    (A) hurriedly
    (B) sarcastically
    (C) haltingly
    (D) enthusiastically
    (E) soberly

17. Another term for the "nub" (line 12) of a comic story is

    (A) set-up
    (B) tone
    (C) punch line
    (D) plot
    (E) diversion

18. The author indicates that successful tellers of humorous stories often

    (A) burst out unexpectedly with the snapper
    (B) chuckle throughout the story
    (C) clearly restate the point of the story
    (D) focus attention on the nub of the story
    (E) appear bewildered by the audience's laughter

GO ON TO THE NEXT PAGE.

Most caffeine research has focused on adults; less is known about the stimulant's possible effects on the young. Children seldom drink much coffee, but they can be exposed to significant amounts of caffeine in soft drinks and iced tea, especially relative to their body weight.

In a 1978 report, the Federation of American Societies for Experimental Biology (FASEB) reviewed estimates of caffeine intake among American youngsters. Adjusted for body weight, the average caffeine intake of the various age groups ranged from 36 to 58 percent of the average dose for adults. However, the top 10 percent in each age group had estimated intakes 3 to 10 times higher than the group average. Surprisingly, the highest intake occurred in the 1-to-5 age group.

The scientific committee of the FASEB expressed concern about possible behavioral effects of caffeine on children. "The estimated levels of caffeine intake at these ages are near those levels that are known to affect the central nervous system in adults," said the committee. But available evidence, they noted, was insufficient to judge whether such stimulation was a hazard.

Two subsequent studies at the National Institute of Mental Health offer some tentative evidence that caffeinism, or "coffee nerves," occurs in children as well as in adults. The studies each involved only about 20 boys and must be considered preliminary. But they appear to support the FASEB's suspicion that children who consume several caffeinated soft drinks daily experience jumpiness, insomnia, and other effects seen in adult coffee drinkers.

19. In line 7, "the top 10 percent" refers to
    (A) the oldest children studied
    (B) the healthiest children studied
    (C) the children who drank the most coffee
    (D) the children who exhibited the worst symptoms of caffeinism
    (E) the children who consumed the largest amounts of caffeine

20. The tone of the statement quoted in lines 10–11 is best described as
    (A) optimistic
    (B) humorous
    (C) combative
    (D) cautionary
    (E) sorrowful

21. The fourth paragraph (lines 13–17) answers which of the following questions?
    (A) How does the average intake of caffeine among children compare with that of adults?
    (B) What effects can caffeine have on children?
    (C) Why do adults and children exhibit similar symptoms of caffeinism?
    (D) What foods contain caffeine?
    (E) How much caffeine should children consume?

22. In the last paragraph (lines 13–17), the author implies that
    (A) the FASEB has overstated its claims about caffeine intake and behavioral consequences
    (B) the study conducted by the National Institute of Mental Health should have examined adults as well as children
    (C) more study is needed before research on the effects of caffeine on children can be considered conclusive
    (D) caffeine research conducted thus far is meaningless because of the small group of subjects
    (E) the effects of caffeine should be studied by medical doctors rather than by biologists

The dogs of London, Flush soon discovered, are strictly divided into different classes. Some are chained dogs, some run wild. Some take their airings in carriages and drink from purple jars; others are unkempt and uncollared and pick up a living in the gutter. Dogs, therefore, Flush began to suspect, differ; some are high, others low; and his suspicions were confirmed by snatches of talk
Line 5 held in passing with the dogs of Wimpole Street. "See that scallywag? A mere mongrel! . . . By gad, that's a fine Spaniel. One of the best in Britain! . . . Pity his ears aren't a shade more curly . . . There's a topknot for you! . . ."

Flush knew before the summer had passed that there is no equality among dogs; there are high dogs and low dogs. Which then was he? No sooner had Flush got home than he examined
10 himself carefully in the looking-glass. Heaven be praised, he was a fine specimen! His head was smooth; his eyes were prominent but not goggled; his feet were feathered with long hair; he was the equal of the best-bred cocker in Wimpole Street. He noted with approval the purple jar from which he drank—such are the privileges of rank; he bent his head quietly to have the chain fixed to his collar—such are its penalties. When about this time Miss Barrett observed him staring in
15 the glass, she was mistaken. He was a philosopher, she thought, meditating the difference between appearance and reality. On the contrary, he was an aristocrat considering his points.

23. In the first paragraph, "the dogs of Wimpole Street" (lines 5–6) are portrayed as

    (A) unkempt
    (B) snobbish
    (C) courteous
    (D) reckless
    (E) clever

24. According to the passage, which trait does Flush have that makes him high class?

    (A) Curly ears
    (B) A shiny coat
    (C) A topknot
    (D) Goggled eyes
    (E) Feathered feet

25. It can be inferred from the passage that after examining himself in the looking glass Flush felt a sense of

    (A) superiority
    (B) accomplishment
    (C) anxiety
    (D) outrage
    (E) shame

26. According to the passage, one of the "penalties" (line 14) Flush faces is being deprived of

    (A) food
    (B) shelter
    (C) affection
    (D) freedom
    (E) grooming

27. According to the passage, when Miss Barrett saw Flush looking in a mirror, she thought he was

    (A) vain
    (B) spying
    (C) contemplative
    (D) confused
    (E) distraught

28. The tone of the passage is best described as

    (A) foreboding
    (B) impassioned
    (C) melancholy
    (D) apologetic
    (E) fanciful

GO ON TO THE NEXT PAGE.

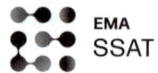

The Chickasaws were fierce warriors who once inhabited northeast Mississippi. Though fewer in number, they commanded respect from their neighbors, the Choctaws. The folklore of both tribes agreed that they had long ago been one people who had crossed the Mississippi River together, always traveling in obedience to a magic pole which pointed the way they should go. Perhaps, ironically, they originally came from that Oklahoma territory to which they were later exiled.

  One Choctaw legend has it that the united people crossed the river at the Fourth Bluff, where a quarrel arose. One faction walked out of the council and thus acquired the name "Chickasaws" or "Rebels." Another Choctaw story keeps the people united until they reached the Yazoo River, where they built a sacrificial mound known as Nunih Wai-ya. The Chickasaw version is that they separated before crossing the Mississippi and that the Chickasaws then proceeded eastward till the magic pole stood upright near Tuscumbia, Alabama. Three years later the whimsical pole again leaned eastward and the tribe journeyed to the Atlantic Ocean, where evidence of their presence still exists near Savannah, Georgia. But a plague struck, the tribe was decimated, and the people retreated to Tuscumbia, where the rash pole stood meekly upright till it rotted.

Line 5, 10

29. The passage represents the Chickasaws as
    (A) formidable in war
    (B) oppressed by their enemies
    (C) living under a curse
    (D) disdainful of tradition
    (E) hospitable to strangers

30. According to the passage, the Chickasaws first crossed the Mississippi River because they
    (A) were fleeing a plague
    (B) had outgrown their homeland
    (C) had quarreled with their neighbors
    (D) were in search of a lost tribe
    (E) were following supernatural guidance

31. According to the passage, Nunih Wai-ya was
    (A) a fortress
    (B) a battle monument
    (C) an abandoned city
    (D) a place of worship
    (E) a burial site

32. Throughout the passage, the author uses which literary device to describe the "magic pole"?
    (A) Simile
    (B) Personification
    (C) Alliteration
    (D) Understatement
    (E) Onomatopoeia

33. The passage indicates that the Chickasaws
    (A) rebelled against the Choctaws before crossing the Mississippi River
    (B) grew in number after crossing the Mississippi River
    (C) stole the magic pole from the Choctaws
    (D) reached the Atlantic Ocean during the course of their travels
    (E) were exiled finally to a location near Savannah, Georgia

GO ON TO THE NEXT PAGE.

In my dreams, however strange it may sound, I dream at the same time of children and of an independent life, which should be both comfortable and beautiful. The question of woman's fate interests me tremendously. This interest lives in me somehow fundamentally; it is called forth neither by writing nor conversation, but has taken root in me of its own accord.

Line 5   Is it necessary to add that I believe with all my heart and mind that women have absolutely equal rights with men, because I consider them in no wise men's intellectual inferior?

This year I have added to the books on social subjects, some that are concerned with the feminist question, and I shall read them with great enjoyment.

Of course, comparatively speaking, women have not asserted themselves up to now as
10   capable individuals. There are many empty coquettes as well as spiritual nonentities among them, but, all the same, it is of note that now in all professions women appear who work on a level with men.

Are there also no empty-headed men? Oh many! Do not men themselves encourage the defects of women by considering them only as amusing playthings? I speak, of course, in general.
15   There are exceptions but, taken on an average, they are in the minority.

Does the education of woman prepare her for the serious tasks of life? The evil of this education is rooted far back in the centuries. Give women scope and opportunity, and they will be no worse than men.

Yes, woman must have all the rights, and in time she can earn them fully. At present we have still
20   many women who are satisfied with their empty lives, but if we raise the standard, and improve the social conditions of her life, woman will also rise. Even now there are many among them who would be capable of leading a conscious existence successfully. Give them that possibility. When people criticize a woman in my presence, I never feel at ease, and I realize that they are wrong, but I have not the courage to dispute with them; I lack arguments and only mentally say to myself, "Wait!"

34. The author uses the word "strange" (line 1) to describe
    (A) an unfamiliar landscape
    (B) an eccentric personality
    (C) a supernatural occurrence
    (D) a seeming contradiction
    (E) a foreign language

35. According to the passage, the author's interest in the fate of women is the result of
    (A) an education rooted far back in the centuries
    (B) her extensive reading of feminist literature
    (C) her dissatisfaction with her own life
    (D) the kinship she feels with professional women
    (E) a spontaneous inner urge

GO ON TO THE NEXT PAGE.

36. The author implies that a person's "rights" (line 6) are based on
    (A) property
    (B) intelligence
    (C) ancestry
    (D) occupation
    (E) gender

37. The author uses the expression "Of course" (line 9) to
    (A) acknowledge a shortcoming
    (B) convey an expectation
    (C) accept a proposal
    (D) draw an inference
    (E) confirm a principle

38. The author indicates that if given "scope and opportunity" (line 17), women will
    (A) be as successful as men
    (B) make better leaders than men
    (C) be more adept in business than men
    (D) take jobs away from men
    (E) oppress men as they have been oppressed

39. The author indicates that she does not challenge people who criticize women primarily because she
    (A) secretly agrees with the criticisms
    (B) is waiting for someone else to speak out
    (C) knows that she is too young to voice her opinions
    (D) has been told not to interfere
    (E) feels she cannot do so successfully

40. Throughout the passage, the author conveys her beliefs by means of
    (A) similes
    (B) poetic imagery
    (C) rhetorical questions
    (D) hyperbole
    (E) anecdotes

STOP

**IF YOU FINISH BEFORE TIME IS CALLED, YOU MAY CHECK YOUR WORK ON THIS SECTION ONLY.
DO NOT TURN TO ANY OTHER SECTION IN THE TEST.**

SECTION 3
60 Questions

This section consists of two different types of questions: synonyms and analogies. There are directions and a sample question for each type.

Synonyms

Each of the following questions consists of one word followed by five words or phrases. You are to select the one word or phrase whose meaning is closest to the word in capital letters.

Sample Question:

CHILLY:
(A) lazy
(B) nice
(C) dry
(D) cold
(E) sunny

Ⓐ Ⓑ Ⓒ ● Ⓔ

---

1. ASTONISHED:
   (A) aged
   (B) talented
   (C) plump
   (D) surprised
   (E) tired

2. NOMINATE:
   (A) understand
   (B) pamper
   (C) bargain
   (D) excuse
   (E) propose

3. CERTIFY:
   (A) appoint temporarily
   (B) substitute willingly
   (C) confirm officially
   (D) replace unconditionally
   (E) allow hesitantly

4. PRECAUTION:
   (A) optimism
   (B) safeguard
   (C) removal
   (D) confidence
   (E) delicacy

5. SEQUENCE:
   (A) motion to adjourn
   (B) plan of attack
   (C) order of succession
   (D) room for growth
   (E) point of reference

6. FUMBLE:
   (A) depart hastily
   (B) destroy completely
   (C) move unnecessarily
   (D) handle clumsily
   (E) react instinctively

7. CAPSIZE:
   (A) occupy
   (B) protect
   (C) free
   (D) inspire
   (E) overturn

8. HOAX:
   (A) problem
   (B) omission
   (C) force
   (D) excess
   (E) fraud

GO ON TO THE NEXT PAGE.

9. BRAWL:
   (A) sneak attack
   (B) noisy fight
   (C) defiant attitude
   (D) impolite refusal
   (E) sudden drop

10. MEDDLE:
    (A) encounter
    (B) surround
    (C) outline
    (D) deflect
    (E) interfere

11. SWELTERING:
    (A) uncomfortably hot
    (B) intensely boring
    (C) unusually dirty
    (D) extremely sad
    (E) very painful

12. CIRCUMFERENCE:
    (A) separation from
    (B) area under
    (C) distance around
    (D) path through
    (E) placement opposite

13. DETAIN:
    (A) prepare
    (B) disturb
    (C) separate
    (D) delay
    (E) grow

14. LUBRICATE:
    (A) dissolve
    (B) illuminate
    (C) grease
    (D) dampen
    (E) twist

15. CANDOR:
    (A) frankness
    (B) sacrifice
    (C) quantity
    (D) illusion
    (E) sympathy

16. DIMINISHED:
    (A) basic
    (B) reduced
    (C) joined
    (D) vertical
    (E) repeated

17. TRIVIAL:
    (A) delightful
    (B) unseen
    (C) illegal
    (D) unimportant
    (E) tangled

18. EVOLVE:
    (A) endure
    (B) evict
    (C) develop
    (D) launch
    (E) permit

19. IRRITATE:
    (A) confirm
    (B) debate
    (C) annoy
    (D) protect
    (E) applaud

20. BLOCKADE:
    (A) make preparations
    (B) assume command
    (C) take captive
    (D) prevent passage
    (E) ignore warnings

GO ON TO THE NEXT PAGE.

21. RETROSPECT:
    (A) hindsight
    (B) retreat
    (C) supervision
    (D) memorization
    (E) tribute

22. CONFER:
    (A) proceed
    (B) increase
    (C) consult
    (D) evade
    (E) agree

23. EXPENDITURE:
    (A) amount inherited
    (B) property sold
    (C) cash borrowed
    (D) goods donated
    (E) money paid out

24. IMPROMPTU:
    (A) compulsory
    (B) unplanned
    (C) punctual
    (D) vigorous
    (E) illicit

25. WITHER:
    (A) shrivel
    (B) endure
    (C) flee
    (D) tremble
    (E) decide

26. CONGENIAL:
    (A) nervous
    (B) courageous
    (C) modest
    (D) pitiable
    (E) friendly

27. MESMERIZE:
    (A) deceive
    (B) frustrate
    (C) spellbind
    (D) recall
    (E) dishevel

28. HOSPITABLE:
    (A) cordial
    (B) parallel
    (C) weak
    (D) useful
    (E) diseased

29. VIGILANT:
    (A) heavy
    (B) menacing
    (C) alert
    (D) sane
    (E) handsome

30. HAPHAZARD:
    (A) careless
    (B) harmful
    (C) powerless
    (D) unconvincing
    (E) mysterious

GO ON TO THE NEXT PAGE.

Analogies

The following questions ask you to find relationships between words. For each question, select the answer choice that best completes the meaning of the sentence.

Sample Question:

Kitten is to cat as
(A) fawn is to colt
(B) puppy is to dog
(C) cow is to bull
(D) wolf is to bear
(E) hen is to rooster

Choice (B) is the best answer because a kitten is a young cat just as a puppy is a young dog. Of all the answer choices, (B) states a relationship that is most like the relationship between kitten and cat.

---

31. Goose is to flock as
    (A) rabbit is to bunny
    (B) wolf is to pack
    (C) duck is to litter
    (D) turtle is to tortoise
    (E) child is to parent

32. Bowling is to lane as
    (A) baseball is to bat
    (B) basketball is to court
    (C) diamond is to field
    (D) soccer is to ball
    (E) tennis is to racquet

33. Skin is to potato as
    (A) stalk is to celery
    (B) pit is to olive
    (C) pole is to bean
    (D) vine is to cucumber
    (E) shell is to almond

34. Courthouse is to law as
    (A) church is to religion
    (B) jail is to crime
    (C) bank is to vault
    (D) library is to collection
    (E) restaurant is to server

35. Needle is to sew as
    (A) blanket is to crochet
    (B) thread is to snip
    (C) hair is to braid
    (D) loom is to weave
    (E) craft is to embroider

36. Dim is to dark as
    (A) chilly is to snowy
    (B) warm is to hot
    (C) quiet is to noisy
    (D) stormy is to windy
    (E) icy is to slippery

37. Nod is to approval as
    (A) ask is to favor
    (B) blink is to eye
    (C) wave is to greeting
    (D) jump is to exercise
    (E) laugh is to joke

38. Closet is to clothing as
    (A) lobby is to hall
    (B) floor is to carpet
    (C) pantry is to food
    (D) paper is to pencil
    (E) attic is to roof

GO ON TO THE NEXT PAGE.

39. Bright is to lightning as
    (A) loud is to thunder
    (B) steep is to hill
    (C) strong is to odor
    (D) temperate is to weather
    (E) stationary is to cloud

40. Drum is to stick as
    (A) nail is to hammer
    (B) log is to saw
    (C) grass is to mower
    (D) ball is to tee
    (E) bolt is to nut

41. Dessert is to meal as
    (A) sand is to shore
    (B) cream is to milk
    (C) finale is to performance
    (D) plant is to root
    (E) medicine is to symptom

42. Joking is to serious as
    (A) smug is to justified
    (B) deceptive is to honest
    (C) suspicious is to guilty
    (D) angry is to provoked
    (E) insulting is to impolite

43. Driver is to bus as
    (A) engineer is to train
    (B) passenger is to airplane
    (C) commuter is to taxi
    (D) balloonist is to parachute
    (E) pedestrian is to sidewalk

44. Music is to composer as
    (A) money is to cashier
    (B) drama is to audience
    (C) photography is to model
    (D) merchandise is to buyer
    (E) apparel is to designer

45. Glue is to paper as
    (A) pour is to oil
    (B) stitch is to thread
    (C) wind is to clock
    (D) weld is to metal
    (E) dig is to ditch

46. Veteran is to soldier as
    (A) professor is to scholar
    (B) lecturer is to scientist
    (C) alumnus is to student
    (D) dentist is to physician
    (E) litigator is to lawyer

47. Letter is to write as
    (A) brush is to paint
    (B) knife is to cut
    (C) picture is to draw
    (D) fatigue is to sleep
    (E) heat is to burn

48. Chapter is to book as
    (A) student is to faculty
    (B) experiment is to laboratory
    (C) story is to author
    (D) juice is to glass
    (E) course is to curriculum

49. Sandal is to shoe as
    (A) pullover is to sweater
    (B) pocket is to jeans
    (C) robe is to pajamas
    (D) button is to jacket
    (E) hood is to raincoat

50. Cane is to walk as
    (A) hair is to comb
    (B) lens is to see
    (C) door is to open
    (D) knee is to bend
    (E) plow is to push

GO ON TO THE NEXT PAGE.

51. Celestial is to sky as
    (A) distant is to star
    (B) terrestrial is to alien
    (C) solar is to sun
    (D) liquid is to water
    (E) atmospheric is to cloud

52. Moth is to fabric as
    (A) termite is to wood
    (B) corn is to scarecrow
    (C) snake is to venom
    (D) butterfly is to cocoon
    (E) mosquito is to picnic

53. Sonnet is to poem as
    (A) salt is to shaker
    (B) foot is to shoe
    (C) chimney is to roof
    (D) steak is to chop
    (E) cedar is to wood

54. Spontaneous is to forethought as
    (A) immature is to youth
    (B) explosive is to fire
    (C) erroneous is to mistake
    (D) accidental is to intent
    (E) elementary is to education

55. Eminent is to obscurity as
    (A) joyous is to frivolity
    (B) brilliant is to education
    (C) deficient is to enhancement
    (D) hasty is to immediacy
    (E) affluent is to poverty

56. Magnify is to large as
    (A) speak is to silent
    (B) lift is to heavy
    (C) acquire is to greedy
    (D) elevate is to high
    (E) carry is to portable

57. Thesaurus is to word as
    (A) bibliography is to title
    (B) science is to experiment
    (C) printer is to ink
    (D) symphony is to orchestra
    (E) dictionary is to book

58. Surgeon is to operate as
    (A) chef is to serve
    (B) orator is to speak
    (C) singer is to compose
    (D) therapist is to injure
    (E) attorney is to investigate

59. Moor is to boat as
    (A) pave is to tar
    (B) tether is to horse
    (C) steer is to wheel
    (D) sink is to leak
    (E) load is to truck

60. Nimble is to acrobat as
    (A) verbose is to speaker
    (B) literate is to scholar
    (C) eloquent is to monarch
    (D) cynical is to philosopher
    (E) popular is to friend

STOP
**IF YOU FINISH BEFORE TIME IS CALLED, YOU MAY CHECK YOUR WORK ON THIS SECTION ONLY.
DO NOT TURN TO ANY OTHER SECTION IN THE TEST.**

SECTION 4
25 Questions

Following each problem in this section, there are five suggested answers. Work each problem in your head or in the blank space provided at the right of the page. Then look at the five suggested answers and decide which one is best.

Note: Figures that accompany problems in this section are drawn as accurately as possible EXCEPT when it is stated in a specific problem that its figure is not drawn to scale.

Sample Problem:

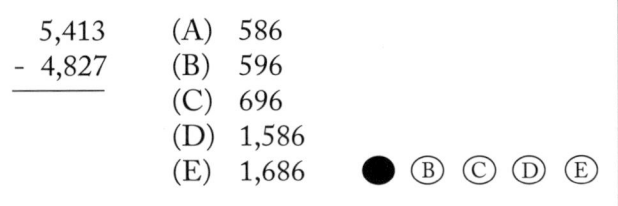

USE THIS SPACE FOR FIGURING.

1. A comic book artist can draw 2 comic book pages per day. At this rate, what is the total number of pages the artist can draw in 30 days?

   (A) 60
   (B) 45
   (C) 32
   (D) 28
   (E) 15

2. If $7 - n = 7 + n$, what is the value of n?

   (A) -7
   (B) 0
   (C) $\frac{1}{7}$
   (D) 1
   (E) 14

3. Tony and Marion together have $15. If Tony has x dollars, which of the following gives the number of dollars Marion has?

   (A) $\frac{15}{x}$
   (B) $15x$
   (C) $x - 15$
   (D) $15 + x$
   (E) $15 - x$

GO ON TO THE NEXT PAGE.

4. Compute: 3.1 + 73.48 + 0.075
   (A) 10.523
   (B) 74.54
   (C) 76.33
   (D) 76.655
   (E) 77.655

5. A sheet of 35-cent stamps has 6 rows of stamps and 4 stamps in each row. What is the cost of 2 sheets of these stamps?
   (A) $16.80
   (B) $10.40
   (C) $8.40
   (D) $7.00
   (E) $4.20

6. For the parallelogram shown, what is the value of x?
   (A) 100
   (B) 80
   (C) 60
   (D) 40
   (E) 10

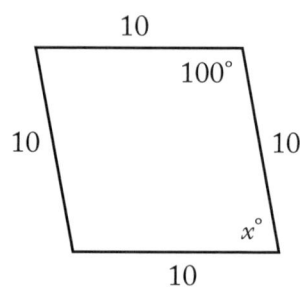

7. A mass of 400 grams is equivalent to how many kilograms?
   (A) 40
   (B) 25
   (C) 4
   (D) 2.5
   (E) 0.4

8. Each month, Dwayne reads 2 fiction books and 1 nonfiction book, and Kristina reads 1 fiction book and 2 nonfiction books. At this rate, how many more fiction books will Dwayne read than Kristina will read in one year?
   (A) 0
   (B) 1
   (C) 6
   (D) 12
   (E) 24

GO ON TO THE NEXT PAGE.

Practice Test IV: Middle Level

USE THIS SPACE FOR FIGURING.

9. Which of the following fractions is least?

   (A) $\frac{4}{7}$

   (B) $\frac{26}{51}$

   (C) $\frac{79}{160}$

   (D) $\frac{112}{224}$

   (E) $\frac{210}{410}$

10. A light bulb manufacturer expects that in each batch of 10,000 light bulbs produced, 14 will be defective. In a recent batch of 10,000 light bulbs, it was found that 29% of the expected number of defective light bulbs were defective. Of the following, which is the best estimate for the number of defective light bulbs in this batch?

    (A) 4
    (B) 6
    (C) 8
    (D) 30
    (E) 40

11. If $r = 6$, $s = 3$, and $t = 2$, what is the value of $\frac{r^2 - st}{s}$?

    (A) 2
    (B) 3
    (C) 10
    (D) 22
    (E) 34

12. The recipe for a cake that serves 6 people requires 1.25 pounds of butter. How many $\frac{1}{4}$-pound sticks of butter will be required to make enough cakes to serve 18 people?

    (A) 10
    (B) 12
    (C) 15
    (D) 20
    (E) 30

GO ON TO THE NEXT PAGE.

13. For integers n, which of the following must be divisible by 3 ?
    I. $24n - 6$
    II. $27(n - 6)$
    III. $36n + 4$

    (A) None
    (B) I and II only
    (C) I and III only
    (D) II and III only
    (E) I, II, and III

14. The figure is a cylinder sliced in half. Of the following, which is the best estimate for the volume of the figure?
    $(V = \pi r^2 h)$
    (A) 6
    (B) 12
    (C) 24
    (D) 36
    (E) 48

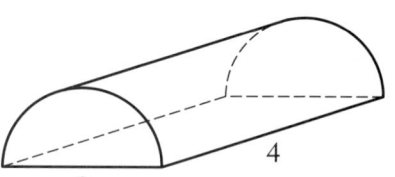

15. The first number in a sequence is 42, and each number after the first is 5 more than the preceding number. Which of the following is a number in the sequence?
    (A) 143
    (B) 158
    (C) 180
    (D) 201
    (E) 237

16. There are 20 pieces of identically wrapped candies in a box, of which 8 are chocolate, 4 are mint, 3 are licorice, and the rest are vanilla. If Mike selects a piece of candy at random, what is the probability that he will select a vanilla candy?

    (A) $\frac{1}{20}$
    (B) $\frac{1}{5}$
    (C) $\frac{1}{4}$
    (D) $\frac{1}{3}$
    (E) $\frac{3}{4}$

GO ON TO THE NEXT PAGE.

USE THIS SPACE FOR FIGURING.

17. What is 8,000 ÷ 40 ÷ 20 ÷ 10 ?
    (A)   1
    (B)   100
    (C)   400
    (D) 1,600
    (E) 4,000

18. Which of the following is true for all obtuse triangles?
    (A) The sides must be the same length.
    (B) The sides must be different lengths.
    (C) One of the interior angles must be a right angle.
    (D) Two of the interior angles must be acute angles.
    (E) All of the interior angles must be obtuse angles.

19. Calculate: 2 + 4(20 + 5)
    (A) 87
    (B) 102
    (C) 125
    (D) 150
    (E) 200

20. Which of the following will NOT produce the same result as 32,400 × 0.25 ?
    (A) $32{,}400 \times \frac{1}{4}$
    (B) $32{,}400 \div 4$
    (C) $32{,}400 \times \frac{1}{25}$
    (D) 324×25
    (E) $(32{,}400 \times 25) \div 100$

GO ON TO THE NEXT PAGE.

21. Of the following, which is the best estimate for how much greater the total dollar sales were for drinks and popcorn than the total dollar sales were for hot dogs in the graph?

    (A) $200
    (B) $250
    (C) $300
    (D) $1,050
    (E) $1,350

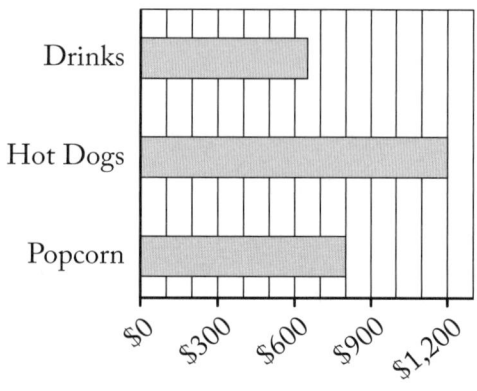

22. Of the following, which is closest to $\sqrt{50} + \sqrt{120}$?

    (A) 9
    (B) 13
    (C) 18
    (D) 85
    (E) 170

23. Square PQRS shown contains two shaded squares. If the areas of the shaded squares are 25 and 9, respectively, what is the area of the square PQRS ?

    (A) 32
    (B) 34
    (C) 61
    (D) 64
    (E) 68

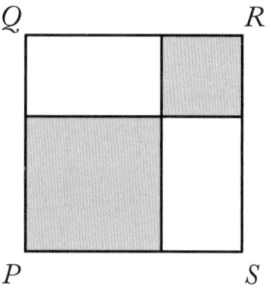

24. What is the result when $-\frac{7}{5}$ is subtracted from $\frac{11}{3}$?

   (A) $-\frac{76}{15}$

   (B) $\frac{9}{4}$

   (C) $\frac{18}{15}$

   (D) $\frac{34}{15}$

   (E) $\frac{76}{15}$

---

25. In the figure, how many non-overlapping segments equal in length to segment $\overline{OP}$ are there on segment $\overline{PQ}$?

   (A) One
   (B) Three
   (C) Four
   (D) Five
   (E) Six

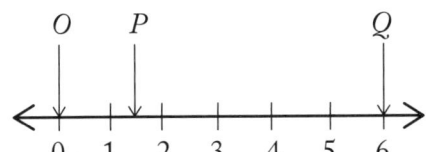

STOP
IF YOU FINISH BEFORE TIME IS CALLED, YOU MAY CHECK YOUR WORK ON THIS SECTION ONLY.
DO NOT TURN TO ANY OTHER SECTION IN THE TEST.

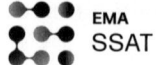

THIS PAGE INTENTIONALLY LEFT BLANK.

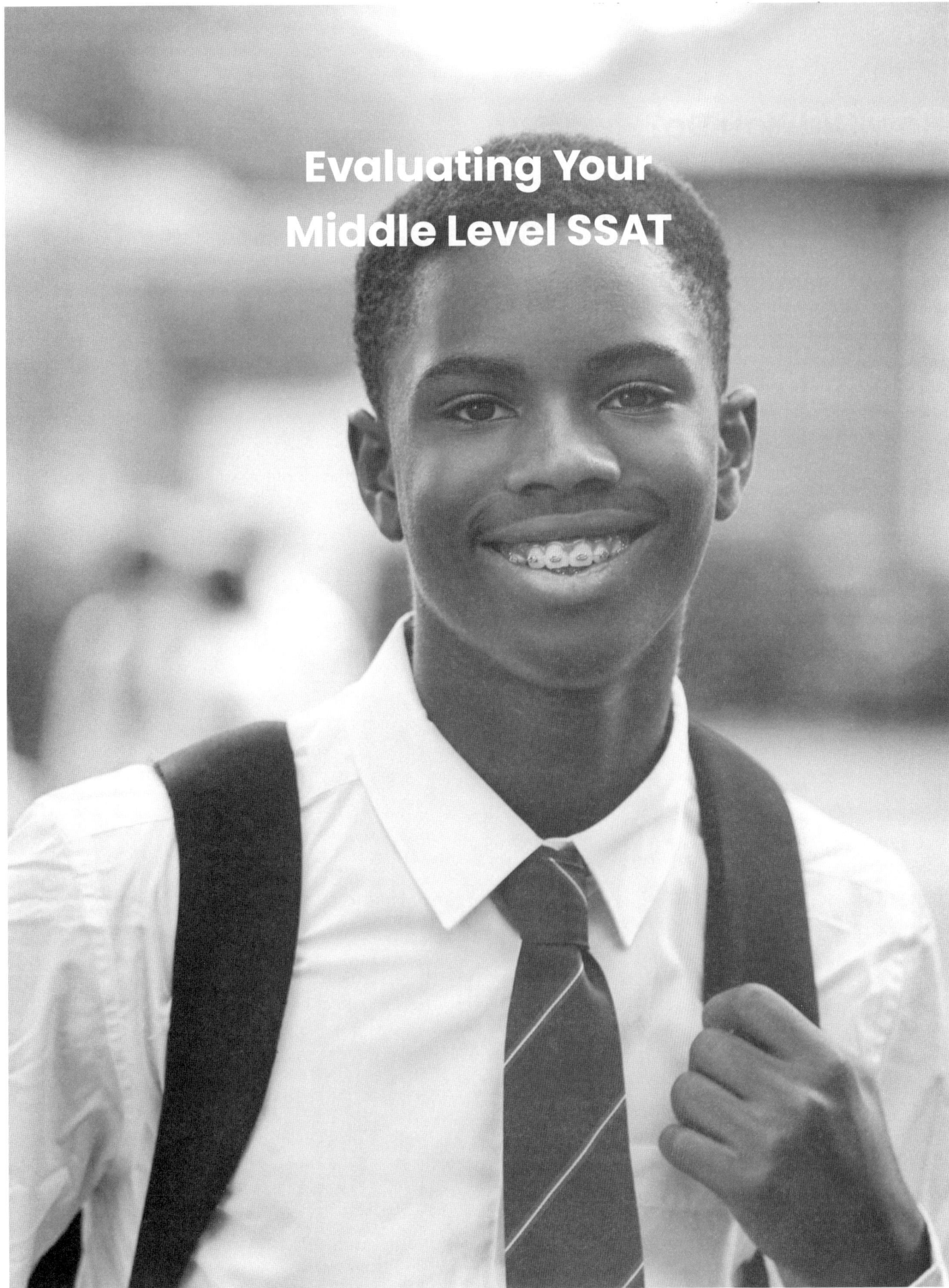
Evaluating Your Middle Level SSAT

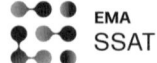

How Did You Do?

When you have completed the practice tests, give yourself a pat on the back, and then take a few moments to think about your performance.

- Did you leave many questions unanswered?
- Did you run out of time?
- Did you read the directions carefully?

Based on your understanding of how well you performed, review the particular test sections that gave you difficulty.

Scoring the Practice Tests

In order to calculate your "raw score" (right, wrong, and omitted answers) for each test section, use the answer keys on pages 218–229. *The Official Study Guide for the Middle Level SSAT* contains practice tests, not "retired" forms of the test. These tests are intended to familiarize you with the format, content, and timing of the actual test. These tests do not provide you with a score as if you were taking the actual SSAT.

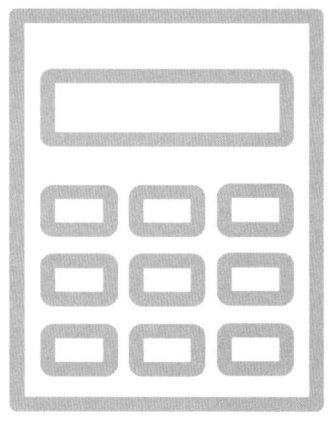
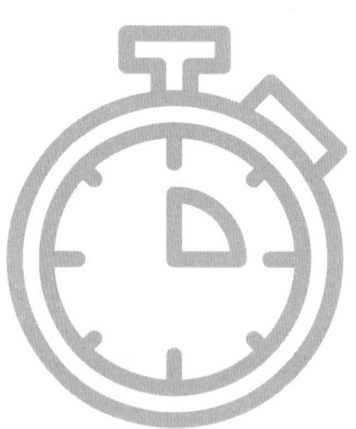

Computing Your Raw Score

1. Using the Practice Test Answer Keys found on pages 218–229, check your answer sheet against the list of correct answers.

2. Mark your answer for each test question in the "Your Answer" column. Next, give yourself a ✓ in the "C" column for each correct answer, a 0 for each wrong answer in the "W" column, and a — for each question omitted in the "O" column.

Correct Answer	Your Answer	C ✓	W 0	O —
1. A	A	✓		
2. B	C		0	
3. C				—
4. C	C	✓		
5. D	D	✓		

3. Add the total number of correct answers and enter the number in the "Total # Correct" box; add the number of 0s and enter in the "Total # Wrong" box. (It is not necessary to add the number of omits. You can use that information to go back and review those questions and to make sure that you understand all answers.)

4. Raw scores are calculated by using the following system:
   - One point is given for each correct answer.
   - No points are added or subtracted for questions omitted.
   - One fourth of a point is subtracted for each incorrect answer.

5. Divide the number of wrong answers in the "Total # Wrong" box by 4 and enter the number in the "# Wrong ÷ 4" box. For example, if you had 32 right and 19 wrong, then your raw score is 32 minus one fourth of 19, which equals 27.25 (32 - 4.75 = 27.25).

6. Round the result in box 3 to the nearest whole integer. Put the integer in Box 4. For example, round 27.25 to 27.

7. The integer in Box 4 is the raw score on the section.

8. Repeat this procedure for each simulated test section that you have taken.

Total # Correct:	1
Total # Wrong:	
# Wrong ÷ 4:	2
Box 1 - Box 2	3
Round Box 3 to nearest whole integer:	4
Raw Score:	

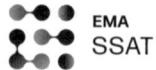

Answer Key

Middle Level Practice Test I : QUANTITATIVE (Sections 1 and 4)

For each question, mark ✓ if correct (C), **0** if wrong (W), or **−** if omitted (O).

Correct Answer	Your Answer	C ✓	W 0	O −
Section 1				
1. A	✓			
2. B	✓			
3. E	✓			
4. B	✓			
5. E	✓			
6. D	✓			
7. C				
8. B				
9. A	✓			
10. D	✓			
11. B	✓			
12. E	✓			
13. A	✓			
14. C				
15. E				
16. D				
17. D	✓			
18. E				
19. B				
20. D				
21. B	✓			
22. A				
23. D	✓			
24. A				
25. E				
Subtotal				

Correct Answer	Your Answer	C ✓	W 0	O −
Section 4				
1. E				
2. B				
3. C				
4. A				
5. A				
6. B				
7. D				
8. E				
9. B				
10. D				
11. C				
12. D				
13. C				
14. A				
15. C				
16. E				
17. B				
18. D				
19. D				
20. B				
21. C				
22. B				
23. A				
24. D				
25. B				
Subtotal				

Total # Correct:	1
Total # Wrong:	
# Wrong ÷ 4:	2
Box 1 − Box 2	3
Round Box 3 to nearest whole integer:	4

Quantitative Raw Score:
Box 4

Quantitative Estimated Scaled Score:
See Table on page 230

Answer Key

Middle Level Practice Test I : READING (Section 2)

For each question, mark ✓ if correct (C), **0** if wrong (W), or — if omitted (O).

Correct Answer	Your Answer	C ✓	W 0	O —
1. B				
2. C				
3. D				
4. E				
5. A				
6. C				
7. A				
8. B				
9. D				
10. D				
11. E				
12. E				
13. D				
14. B				
15. A				
16. C				
17. A				
18. B				
19. C				
20. D				
Subtotal				

Correct Answer	Your Answer	C ✓	W 0	O —
21. E				
22. D				
23. B				
24. A				
25. C				
26. E				
27. C				
28. D				
29. B				
30. A				
31. B				
32. B				
33. E				
34. C				
35. A				
36. C				
37. B				
38. A				
39. B				
40. D				
Subtotal				

Total # Correct:	1
Total # Wrong:	
# Wrong ÷ 4:	2
Box 1 − Box 2	3
Round Box 3 to nearest whole integer:	4

Reading Raw Score:
Box 4

Reading Estimated Scaled Score:
See Table on page 230

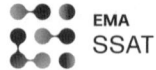

Answer Key

Middle Level Practice Test I : VERBAL (Section 3)

For each question, mark ✓ if correct (C), **0** if wrong (W), or — if omitted (O).

Correct Answer	Your Answer	C ✓	W 0	O —
1. E				
2. B				
3. A				
4. D				
5. A				
6. C				
7. A				
8. B				
9. E				
10. D				
11. C				
12. D				
13. C				
14. A				
15. E				
16. C				
17. D				
18. A				
19. D				
20. A				
21. D				
22. A				
23. C				
24. B				
25. D				
26. E				
27. A				
28. E				
29. C				
30. B				
Subtotal				

Correct Answer	Your Answer	C ✓	W 0	O —
31. B				
32. C				
33. A				
34. C				
35. B				
36. E				
37. D				
38. A				
39. B				
40. A				
41. D				
42. C				
43. E				
44. D				
45. A				
46. A				
47. E				
48. E				
49. D				
50. A				
51. D				
52. C				
53. B				
54. C				
55. E				
56. D				
57. A				
58. E				
59. B				
60. D				
Subtotal				

Total # Correct:	1
Total # Wrong:	
# Wrong ÷ 4:	2
Box 1 - Box 2	3
Round Box 3 to nearest whole integer:	4

Verbal Raw Score:
Box 4

Verbal Estimated Scaled Score:
See Table on page 230

Answer Key

Middle Level Practice Test II : QUANTITATIVE (Sections 1 and 4)

For each question, mark ✓ if correct (C), **0** if wrong (W), or — if omitted (O).

Correct Answer	Your Answer	C ✓	W 0	O —
Section 1				
1. C	C	✓		
2. B	B	✓		
3. E	E	✓		
4. A	A	✓		
5. B	B	✓		
6. D	D	✓		
7. B	B	✓		
8. C	C	✓		
9. E	E	✓		
10. D				—
11. C	C	✓		
12. B	B	✓		
13. A	A	✓		
14. D	D	✓		
15. D				—
16. E	E	✓		
17. B	B	✓		
18. E	E	✓		
19. E	E	✓		
20. A	A	✓		
21. D	A		X	
22. B	B	✓		
23. A	A	✓		
24. C	D		X	
25. A	A	✓		
Subtotal				

Correct Answer	Your Answer	C ✓	W 0	O —
Section 4				
1. C				
2. A				
3. D				
4. B				
5. C				
6. E				
7. B				
8. E				
9. D				
10. C				
11. A				
12. D				
13. D				
14. A				
15. E				
16. C				
17. E				
18. A				
19. B				
20. A				
21. D				
22. E				
23. E				
24. B				
25. C				
Subtotal				

Total # Correct:	1
Total # Wrong:	
# Wrong ÷ 4:	2
Box 1 - Box 2	3
Round Box 3 to nearest whole integer:	4

Quantitative Raw Score:
Box 4

Quantitative Estimated Scaled Score:
See Table on page 230

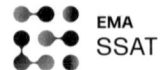

Answer Key

Middle Level Practice Test II : READING (Section 2)

For each question, mark ✓ if correct (C), **0** if wrong (W), or — if omitted (O).

Correct Answer	Your Answer	C ✓	W 0	O —
1. C				
2. D				
3. B				
4. D				
5. E				
6. C				
7. A				
8. E				
9. D				
10. C				
11. A				
12. D				
13. A				
14. B				
15. E				
16. E				
17. D				
18. B				
19. A				
20. E				
Subtotal				

Correct Answer	Your Answer	C ✓	W 0	O —
21. D				
22. E				
23. B				
24. C				
25. B				
26. B				
27. A				
28. C				
29. A				
30. E				
31. D				
32. B				
33. E				
34. D				
35. C				
36. B				
37. D				
38. C				
39. E				
40. A				
Subtotal				

Total # Correct:	1
Total # Wrong:	
# Wrong ÷ 4:	2
Box 1 - Box 2	3
Round Box 3 to nearest whole integer:	4

Reading Raw Score:
Box 4

Reading Estimated Scaled Score:
See Table on page 230

Answer Key

Middle Level Practice Test II : VERBAL (Section 3)

For each question, mark ✓ if correct (C), **0** if wrong (W), or **−** if omitted (O).

Correct Answer	Your Answer	C ✓	W 0	O −
1. B				
2. A				
3. E				
4. C				
5. B				
6. D				
7. C				
8. C				
9. E				
10. D				
11. D				
12. A				
13. D				
14. A				
15. E				
16. B				
17. D				
18. B				
19. E				
20. D				
21. A				
22. C				
23. B				
24. C				
25. B				
26. C				
27. D				
28. E				
29. B				
30. A				
Subtotal				

Correct Answer	Your Answer	C ✓	W 0	O −
31. E				
32. A				
33. E				
34. D				
35. A				
36. B				
37. D				
38. E				
39. C				
40. A				
41. D				
42. B				
43. C				
44. A				
45. C				
46. E				
47. C				
48. A				
49. C				
50. D				
51. E				
52. A				
53. E				
54. C				
55. A				
56. C				
57. B				
58. B				
59. E				
60. C				
Subtotal				

Total # Correct:	1
Total # Wrong:	
# Wrong ÷ 4:	2
Box 1 − Box 2	3
Round Box 3 to nearest whole integer:	4

Verbal Raw Score:
Box 4

Verbal Estimated Scaled Score:
See Table on page 230

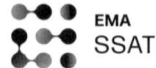

Answer Key

Middle Level Practice Test III : QUANTITATIVE (Sections 1 and 4)

For each question, mark ✓ if correct (C), **0** if wrong (W), or **−** if omitted (O).

Correct Answer	Your Answer	C ✓	W 0	O −
Section 1				
1. D				
2. A				
3. B				
4. D				
5. E				
6. C				
7. C				
8. D				
9. C				
10. B				
11. C				
12. A				
13. B				
14. D				
15. E				
16. E				
17. C				
18. E				
19. A				
20. C				
21. B				
22. B				
23. A				
24. E				
25. D				
Subtotal				

Correct Answer	Your Answer	C ✓	W 0	O −
Section 4				
1. A				
2. B				
3. A				
4. D				
5. E				
6. D				
7. E				
8. C				
9. E				
10. A				
11. B				
12. B				
13. A				
14. D				
15. D				
16. E				
17. D				
18. B				
19. C				
20. C				
21. B				
22. D				
23. C				
24. E				
25. C				
Subtotal				

Total # Correct:	1
Total # Wrong:	
# Wrong ÷ 4:	2
Box 1 − Box 2	3
Round Box 3 to nearest whole integer:	4

Quantitative Raw Score:
Box 4

Quantitative Estimated Scaled Score:
See Table on page 230

Answer Key

Middle Level Practice Test III : READING (Section 2)

For each question, mark ✓ if correct (C), **0** if wrong (W), or — if omitted (O).

Correct Answer	Your Answer	C ✓	W 0	O —
1. B				
2. C				
3. B				
4. A				
5. A				
6. E				
7. C				
8. A				
9. E				
10. B				
11. D				
12. D				
13. B				
14. E				
15. A				
16. C				
17. E				
18. D				
19. A				
20. B				
Subtotal				

Correct Answer	Your Answer	C ✓	W 0	O —
21. D				
22. C				
23. B				
24. E				
25. D				
26. E				
27. A				
28. C				
29. C				
30. B				
31. B				
32. A				
33. E				
34. D				
35. C				
36. A				
37. D				
38. C				
39. E				
40. D				
Subtotal				

Total # Correct:	1
Total # Wrong:	
# Wrong ÷ 4:	2
Box 1 - Box 2	3
Round Box 3 to nearest whole integer:	4

Reading Raw Score:
Box 4

Reading Estimated Scaled Score:
See Table on page 230

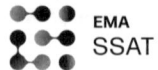

Answer Key

Middle Level Practice Test III : VERBAL (Section 3)

For each question, mark ✓ if correct (C), **0** if wrong (W), or **−** if omitted (O).

Correct Answer	Your Answer	C ✓	W 0	O −
1. D				
2. A				
3. D				
4. A				
5. C				
6. A				
7. C				
8. E				
9. B				
10. D				
11. B				
12. E				
13. B				
14. A				
15. A				
16. D				
17. B				
18. E				
19. C				
20. D				
21. A				
22. C				
23. C				
24. C				
25. B				
26. E				
27. A				
28. E				
29. B				
30. D				
Subtotal				

Correct Answer	Your Answer	C ✓	W 0	O −
31. D				
32. E				
33. D				
34. B				
35. E				
36. B				
37. C				
38. A				
39. D				
40. C				
41. E				
42. A				
43. E				
44. C				
45. B				
46. A				
47. B				
48. D				
49. E				
50. C				
51. A				
52. B				
53. D				
54. D				
55. B				
56. A				
57. C				
58. E				
59. E				
60. C				
Subtotal				

Total # Correct:		1
Total # Wrong:		
# Wrong ÷ 4:		2
Box 1 − Box 2		3
Round Box 3 to nearest whole integer:		4

Verbal Raw Score:
Box 4

Verbal Estimated Scaled Score:
See Table on page 230

Answer Key

Middle Level Practice Test IV : QUANTITATIVE (Sections 1 and 4)

For each question, mark ✓ if correct (C), **0** if wrong (W), or — if omitted (O).

Correct Answer	Your Answer	C ✓	W 0	O —
Section 1				
1. B		✓		
2. D		✓		
3. A		✓		
4. E		✓		
5. D		✓		
6. B		✓		
7. B		✓		
8. C		✓		
9. C		✓		
10. A		✓		
11. B		✓		
12. D		✓		
13. E		✓		
14. A		✓		
15. A		✓		
16. D		✓		
17. C		✓		
18. B				
19. D		✓		
20. A		✓		
21. E		✓		
22. C		✓		
23. E				
24. D		✓		
25. B		✓		
Subtotal				

Correct Answer	Your Answer	C ✓	W 0	O —
Section 4				
1. A				
2. B				
3. E				
4. D				
5. A				
6. B				
7. E				
8. D				
9. C				
10. A				
11. C				
12. C				
13. B				
14. A				
15. E				
16. C				
17. A				
18. D				
19. B				
20. C				
21. B				
22. C				
23. D				
24. E				
25. B				
Subtotal				

Total # Correct:	1
Total # Wrong:	
# Wrong ÷ 4:	2
Box 1 − Box 2	3
Round Box 3 to nearest whole integer:	4

Quantitative Raw Score:
Box 4

Quantitative Estimated Scaled Score:
See Table on page 230

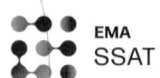

Answer Key

Middle Level Practice Test IV : READING (Section 2)

For each question, mark ✓ if correct (C), **0** if wrong (W), or **−** if omitted (O).

Correct Answer	Your Answer	C ✓	W 0	O −
1. E				
2. C				
3. B				
4. B				
5. B				
6. A				
7. D				
8. C				
9. D				
10. C				
11. E				
12. A				
13. B				
14. A				
15. B				
16. E				
17. C				
18. E				
19. E				
20. D				
Subtotal				

Correct Answer	Your Answer	C ✓	W 0	O −
21. B				
22. C				
23. B				
24. E				
25. A				
26. D				
27. C				
28. E				
29. A				
30. E				
31. D				
32. B				
33. D				
34. D				
35. E				
36. B				
37. A				
38. A				
39. E				
40. C				
Subtotal				

Total # Correct:		1
Total # Wrong:		
# Wrong ÷ 4:		2
Box 1 - Box 2		3
Round Box 3 to nearest whole integer:		4

Reading Raw Score:
Box 4

Reading Estimated Scaled Score:
See Table on page 230

Answer Key

Middle Level Practice Test IV : VERBAL (Section 3)

For each question, mark ✓ if correct (C), **0** if wrong (W), or — if omitted (O).

Correct Answer	Your Answer	C ✓	W 0	O —
1. D				
2. E				
3. C				
4. B				
5. C				
6. D				
7. E				
8. E				
9. B				
10. E				
11. A				
12. C				
13. D				
14. C				
15. A				
16. B				
17. D				
18. C				
19. C				
20. D				
21. A				
22. C				
23. E				
24. B				
25. A				
26. E				
27. C				
28. A				
29. C				
30. A				
Subtotal				

Correct Answer	Your Answer	C ✓	W 0	O —
31. B				
32. B				
33. E				
34. A				
35. D				
36. B				
37. C				
38. C				
39. A				
40. A				
41. C				
42. B				
43. A				
44. E				
45. D				
46. C				
47. C				
48. E				
49. A				
50. B				
51. C				
52. A				
53. E				
54. D				
55. E				
56. D				
57. A				
58. B				
59. B				
60. B				
Subtotal				

Total # Correct:	1
Total # Wrong:	
# Wrong ÷ 4:	2
Box 1 - Box 2	3
Round Box 3 to nearest whole integer:	4

Verbal Raw Score:
Box 4

Verbal Estimated Scaled Score:
See Table on page 230

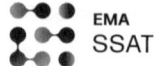

Equating Raw Scores to Scaled Scores

Scores are first calculated by awarding one point for each correct answer and subtracting one quarter of one point for each incorrect answer. These scores are called raw scores. Raw scores can vary from one edition of the test to another due to differences in difficulty among editions. Score equating is used to adjust for these differences. Even after these adjustments, no single test score provides a perfectly accurate estimate of your proficiency.

Because *The Official Study Guide for the Middle Level SSAT* contains practice tests and not "retired" forms of the test, there are no norm group data associated with these forms, and calculations of exact scaled scores or specific percentile rankings are not possible. But the following chart will give you an estimate of where your scaled scores might fall within each of the three scored sections: verbal, quantitative/math, and reading.

Table: Middle Level Estimated SSAT Scaled Scores

Raw Score	Estimated Verbal Scaled Score	Estimated Quantitative Scaled Score	Estimated Reading Scaled Score
60	710		
55	710		
50	707	710	
45	695	692	
40	677	674	710
35	656	656	701
30	635	638	671
25	617	619	641
20	596	599	614
15	575	578	587
10	551	554	557
5	528	530	524
0	506	506	497
-5	479	479	458

These are estimated scaled scores based on the raw-to-scaled conversion of many forms, and a student's score can vary when taking the test.

Notes

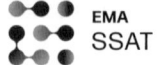

Notes

Notes

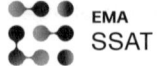

Notes

Notes

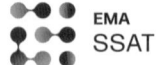

Notes

Notes

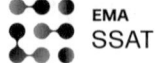

Notes

Notes

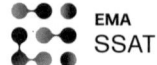

Notes

Made in the USA
Coppell, TX
06 February 2020

Appendix: Measurement Conversion Table

Volume Equivalents (Liquid)

US Standard	US Standard (Ounces)	Metric (Approximate)
2 tablespoons	1 fl. oz.	30 mL
¼ cup	2 fl. oz.	60mL
½ cup	4 fl. oz.	120mL
1 cup	8 fl. oz.	240 mL
1 and ½ cups	12 fl. oz.	355 mL
2 cups/1 pint	16 fl. oz.	475 mL
4 cups/ 1 quart	32 fl. oz.	1 L
1 gallon	128 fl. oz.	4L

Volume Equivalents (Dry)

US Standard	Metric (Approximate)
1/8 teaspoon	0.5 mL
¼ teaspoon	1 mL
½ teaspoon	2 mL
¾ teaspoon	4 mL
1 teaspoon	5 mL
1 tablespoon	15 mL
¼ cup	59 mL
1/3 cup	79 mL
½ cup	118 mL
2/3 cup	156 mL
¾ cup	177 mL
1 cup	235 mL
2 cups	475 mL
3 cups	700 mL
4 cups	1 L

Conclusion

I can't express how honored I am to think that you found my book interesting and informative enough to read it all through to the end.

I thank you again for purchasing this book and I hope that you had as much fun reading it as I had writing it.

I bid you farewell and encourage you to move forward with your amazing Keto journey with the shiny and revolutionary Ninja Foodi!

- 6 cups chicken stock
- ½ teaspoon dried basil
- 1 teaspoon salt
- 1/6 teaspoon fresh ground pepper
- 2 cups daikon noodles, spiralized

Directions

1. Set the Ninja Foodi to Saute mode and add coconut oil, allow the oil to warm up
2. Add chicken thigh and Saute for about 10 minutes
3. Take the chicken out and shred it up
4. Add carrots, onions to the pot and cook for 2 minutes
5. Add the rest of the ingredients and lock up the lid (make sure to return the chicken as well)
6. Cook for 15 minutes on HIGh pressure
7. Do a quick release carefully. Enjoy your "Faux" noodles!

Nutrition Values (Per Serving)

- Calories: 185
- Fats: 5g
- Carbs:5g
- Protein:10g

Simple Vegetable Stock

(Prepping time: 10 minutes\ Cooking time: 30 minutes |For 4 servings)

Ingredients

- 1-2 onions, chopped
- 2-3 celery ribs, chopped
- 2 carrots, chopped
- 1 leek, green parts only, rinsed and chopped
- 1-2 garlic cloves, chopped
- 3-4 sprigs parsley
- 1-2 sprigs rosemary
- 1-3 sprigs thyme
- 2 bay leaves
- 1 teaspoon black peppercorn
- 12 cups water

Directions

1. Add the listed ingredients to your Ninja Foodi
2. Lock up the lid and cook on HIGH pressure for 30 minutes
3. Release the pressure naturally
4. Strain the stock through a strainer
5. Use immediately when needed or store in fridges

Nutrition Values (Per Serving)

- Calories: 6
- Fat: 0g
- Carbohydrates: 1g
- Protein: 0g

- Calories: 275
- Fat: 23g
- Carbohydrates: 4g
- Protein: 27g

Keto Chicken Crescent Wraps
(Prepping time: 10 minutes\ Cooking time: 15 minutes |For 4 servings)

Ingredients

- 3 (10 ounces0 cans, almond flour crescent roll dough
- 6 tablespoons butter
- 2 cooked chicken breast, skinless boneless, cubed
- 3 tablespoons onion, chopped
- ¾ (8 ounces) package cream cheese
- 3 garlic cloves, peeled and minced

Directions

1. Take a skillet to place it over medium heat, add oil and let it heat up
2. Add onion and garlic ad Saute until tender
3. Add chicken, cream cheese, butter, onion garlic to food processor and blend until smooth Spread dough over a flat surface and slice into 12 equal sized rectangles
4. Spoon chicken blend at the center of each dough piece
5. Roll piece while wrapping inner filling completely
6. Place wrapped balls in Crisping basket
7. Insert basket to your ninja Foodi and lock Air Crisp Lid, Air Crisp for 15 minutes at 360 degrees F. Serve and enjoy!

Nutrition Values (Per Serving)

- Calories: 597
- Fat: 19g
- Carbohydrates: 5g
- Protein: 37g

Diced And Spiced Up Paprika Eggs
(Prepping time: 10 minutes\ Cooking time: 5 minutes |For 4 servings)

Ingredients

- ½ teaspoon paprika
- 6 whole eggs
- ¼ teaspoon salt
- Pinch of pepper
- 1 and ½ cups of water

Directions

1. Add water to Ninja Foodi. Crack an egg into a baking dish
2. Cover dish with foil and place on a rack, place the rack in Ninja Foodie
3. Lock lid and cook on HIGH pressure for 4 minutes
4. Quick release pressure. Remove loaf of eggs and finely dice
5. Stir in spices and serve. Enjoy!

Nutrition Values (Per Serving)

- Calories: 290
- Fat: 23g
- Carbohydrates: 4g
- Protein: 16g

Faux Daikon Noodles
(Prepping time: 10 minutes\ Cooking time: 15 minutes |For 6 servings)

Ingredients

- 2 tablespoons coconut oil
- 1 pound boneless and skinless chicken thigh
- 1 cup celery, diced
- 1 cup carrots, diced
- ¾ cup green onion, chopped

A Hot Buffalo Wing Platter
(Prepping time: 10 minutes\ Cooking time: 6 hours | For 4 servings)

Ingredients

- 1 bottle of (12 ounces) hot pepper sauce
- ½ cup melted ghee
- 1 tablespoons dried oregano
- 2 teaspoons garlic powder
- 1 teaspoon onion powder
- 5 pounds chicken wing sections

Directions

Take a large bowl and mix in hot sauce, ghee, garlic powder, oregano, onion powder and mix well. Add chicken wings and toss to coat. Pour mix into Ninja Foodi and cook on LOW for 6 hours. Serve and enjoy!

Nutrition Values (Per Serving)

- Calories: 529
- Fat: 4g
- Carbohydrates: 1g
- Protein: 31g

Garlic And Mushroom Crunchies
(Prepping time: 10 minutes\ Cooking time: 8 hours | For 4 servings)

Ingredients

- ¼ cup vegetable stock
- 2 tablespoons extra virgin olive oil
- 1 tablespoon Dijon mustard
- 1 teaspoon dried thyme
- 1 teaspoon of sea salt
- ½ teaspoon dried rosemary
- ¼ teaspoon fresh ground black pepper
- 2 pounds cremini mushrooms, cleaned
- 6 garlic cloves, minced
- ¼ cup fresh parsley, chopped

Directions

1. Take a small bowl and whisk in vegetable stock, mustard, olive oil, salt, thyme, pepper and rosemary. Add mushrooms, garlic and stock mix to your Ninja Foodi
2. Close lid and cook on SLOW COOK Mode (LOW) for 8 hours
3. Open the lid and stir in parsley. Serve and enjoy!

Nutrition Values (Per Serving)

- Calories: 92
- Fat: 5g
- Carbohydrates: 8g
- Protein: 4g

Delicious Cocoa Almond Bites
(Prepping time: 10 minutes\ Cooking time: 2 hours | For 6 servings)

Ingredients

- 3 cups of raw almonds
- 3 tablespoons coconut oil, melted
- Kosher salt
- ¼ cup Erythritol
- 1 tablespoon unsweetened cocoa powder
- 1 tablespoon ground cinnamon

Directions

1. Add almonds coconut oil to the Ninja Foodi and stir until coated
2. Season with salt. Mix in Erythritol, cocoa powder, cinnamon, and cover
3. Cook on SLOW COOK MODE(HIGH) for 2 hours, making sure to stir every 30 minutes
4. Transfer nuts to a large baking sheet and spread them out to cool. Serve and enjoy!

Nutrition Values (Per Serving)

- 10 ounces kale, roughly chopped
- 1 tablespoon ghee
- 1 medium onion, sliced
- 3 medium carrots, cut into half inch pieces
- 5 garlic clove, peeled and chopped
- ½ cup chicken broth
- Fresh ground pepper
- Vinegar as needed
- ½ teaspoon red pepper flakes

Directions

1. Set your pot to Saute mode and add ghee, allow the ghee to melt
2. Add chopped onion and carrots and Saute for a while
3. Add garlic and Saute for a while. Pile the kale on top
4. Pour chicken broth and season with pepper
5. Lock up the lid and cook on HIGH pressure for 8 minutes
6. Release the pressure naturally over 10 minutes. Open and give it a nice stir
7. Add vinegar and sprinkle a bit more pepper flakes. Enjoy!

Nutrition Values (Per Serving)

- Calories: 41
- Fat: 2g
- Carbohydrates: 5g
- Protein: 2g

Delicious Bacon- Wrapped Drumsticks
(Prepping time: 10 minutes\ Cooking time: 8 hours |For 6 servings)

Ingredients

- 12 chicken drumsticks
- 12 slices thin cut bacon

Directions

1. Wrap each chicken drumsticks in bacon. Place drumsticks in your Ninja Foodi
2. Place lid and cook SLOW COOK mode (LOW) for 8 hours. Serve and enjoy!

Nutrition Values (Per Serving)

- Calories: 202
- Fat: 8g
- Carbohydrates: 3g
- Protein: 30g

Stuffed Chicken Mushrooms
(Prepping time: 10 minutes\ Cooking time: 15 minutes |For 4 servings)

Ingredients

- 12 large fresh mushrooms, stems removed

Stuffing

- 1 cup chicken meat, cubed
- ½ pound, imitation crabmeat, flaked
- 2 cups butter
- Garlic powder to taste
- 2 garlic cloves, peeled and minced

Directions

1. Take a non-stick skillet and place it over medium heat, add butter and let it heat up
2. Stir in chicken and Saute for 5 minutes. Add ingredients for stuffing and cook for 5 minutes
3. Remove heat and let the chicken cool down. Divide filling into mushroom caps
4. Place stuffed mushroom caps in your Crisping basket and transfer basket to Foodi
5. Lock Crisping Lid and Air Crisp for 10 minutes at 375 degrees F. Serve and enjoy!

Nutrition Values (Per Serving)

- Calories: 385
- Fat: 36g
- Carbohydrates: 4g
- Protein: 8g

- 2 tablespoons fresh oregano, chopped

Directions

1. Add listed ingredients to your Ninja Foodi and gently stir. Lock lid and cook on SLOW COOK mode for 5-7 hours. Serve and enjoy!

Nutrition Values (Per Serving)

- Calories: 247
- Fat: 5g
- Carbohydrates: 15g
- Protein: 34g

The Kool Poblano Cheese Frittata
(Prepping time: 10 minutes\ Cooking time: 25 minutes | For 4 servings)

Ingredients

- 4 whole eggs
- 1 cup half and half
- 10 ounces canned green chilies
- ½ -1 teaspoon salt
- ½ teaspoon ground cumin
- 1 cup Mexican blend shredded cheese
- ¼ cup cilantro, chopped

Directions

1. Take a bowl and beat eggs and a half and half
2. Add diced green chilis, salt, cumin and ½ cup of shredded cheese
3. Pour the mixture into 6 inches greased metal pan and cover with foil
4. Add 2 cups of water to the Ninja Foodi. Place trivet in the pot and place the pan in the trivet
5. Lock up the lid and cook on HIGH pressure for 20 minutes
6. Release the pressure naturally over 10 minutes
7. Scatter half cup of the cheese on top of your quiche and broil for a while until the cheese has melted. Enjoy!

Nutrition Values (Per Serving)

- Calories: 257
- Fat: 19g
- Carbohydrates: 6g
- Protein:14g

The Divine Fudge Meal
(Prepping time: 10 minute + chill times\ Cooking time: 10-20 minutes | For 20 servings)

Ingredients

- ½ teaspoon organic vanilla extract
- 1 cup heavy whip cream
- 2 ounces butter, soft
- 2 ounces 70% dark chocolate, finely chopped

Directions

1. Set your Ninja Foodi to Saute mode and add vanilla, heavy cream. Saute for 5 minutes
2. Add butter and chocolate and Saute for 2 minutes. Transfer to serving the dish
3. Chill for few hours and enjoy!

Nutrition Values (Per Serving)

- Calories: 292
- Fat: 26g
- Carbohydrates: 8g
- Protein: 5g

The Original Braised Kale And Carrot Salad
(Prepping time: 5 minutes\ Cooking time: 30 minutes | For 4 servings)

Ingredients

3. Make the vinaigrette by combining the hot pepper, anchovies, olive oil, capers, pepper, salt and mix well. Quick release the pressure
4. Strain the veggies out and mix with vinaigrette and the orange slices. Enjoy!

Nutrition Values (Per Serving)

- Calories: 163
- Fats: 11g
- Carbs: 15g
- Protein: 3g

Faithful Roasted Garlic
(Prepping time: 10 minutes\ Cooking time: 20 minutes |For 4 servings)

Ingredients

- 3 large garlic bulbs
- 1 cup of water

Directions

1. Slice off ¼ of the garlic bulb from the top, keeping the bulb intact
2. Add water to your Ninja Foodi and a steamer trivet
3. Transfer garlic bulb on rack and lock lid, cook on HIGH pressure for 5-6 minutes
4. Naturally, release the pressure over 10 minutes
5. Transfer the soft garlic to grill rack in your oven and roast for 5 minutes. Serve and enjoy!

Nutrition Values (Per Serving)

- Calories: 8
- Fat: 0g
- Carbohydrates: 1.5g
- Protein: 0g

Feisty Chicken Thighs
(Prepping time: 5 minutes\ Cooking time:6-8 hours |For 6 servings)

Ingredients

- 3 pounds boneless chicken thighs, skinless
- 2 tablespoons apple cider vinegar
- ½ cup agave nectar
- 2 teaspoon garlic powder
- 2 teaspoon paprika
- 1 teaspoon chili powder
- 1 teaspoon red pepper flakes
- 1 teaspoon black pepper
- 2 teaspoon salt

Directions

1. Take a bowl and add garlic pepper, paprika, chili powder, red pepper flakes, salt, and pepper. Take another bowl and mix in agave nectar, vinegar and keep the mix on the side
2. Use the seasoning mix to properly coat the chicken thigh
3. Pour nectar, vinegar mix over chicken. Transfer the mix to Ninja Foodi
4. Lock lid and cook on SLOW COOK MODE (LOW) for 6-8 hours
5. Once done, unlock the lid. Drizzle the glaze on top and serve. Enjoy!

Nutrition Values (Per Serving)

- Calories: 234
- Fat: 15g
- Carbohydrates: 14g
- Protein: 8g

Garlic And Tomato "Herbed" Chicken Thighs
(Prepping time: 10 minutes\ Cooking time: 5-7 hours |For 4 servings)

Ingredients

- 3 pounds boneless, skinless chicken thighs
- ½ cup low-sodium chicken broth
- 2 cups cherry tomatoes, halved
- 4 garlic cloves, minced
- 2 teaspoons garlic salt
- ¼ teaspoon ground white pepper
- 2 tablespoons fresh basil, chopped

- 24 mushrooms, caps and stems diced
- 1 cup cheddar cheese, shredded
- ½ orange bell pepper, diced
- ½ onion, diced
- 4 bacon slices, diced
- ½ cup sour cream

Directions

1. Set your Ninja Foodie to Saute mode and add mushroom stems, onion, bacon, bell pepper and Saute for 5 minutes. Add 1 cup cheese, sour cream and cook for 2 minutes more
2. Stuff mushrooms with cheese and vegetable mixture and top with cheddar cheese
3. Transfer them to your Crisping Basket and lock Air Crisping lid
4. Air Crisp for 8 minutes at 350 degrees F. Serve and enjoy!

Nutrition Values (Per Serving)

- Calories: 288
- Fat: 6g
- Carbohydrates: 3g
- Protein: 25g

Tasty Brussels
(Prepping time: 10 minutes\ Cooking time: 3 minutes |For 4 servings)

Ingredients

- 1 pound Brussels sprouts
- ¼ cup pine nuts
- 1 tablespoon extra virgin olive oil
- 1 pomegranate
- ½ teaspoon salt
- 1 pepper, grated

Directions

1. Remove outer leaves and trim the stems off the washed Brussels sprouts
2. Cut the largest ones in uniform halves
3. Add 1 cup of water to the Ninja Foodi
4. Place steamer basket and add sprouts in the basket
5. Lock up the lid and cook on HIGH pressure for 3 minutes
6. Release the pressure naturally
7. Transfer the sprouts to serving dish and dress with olive oil, pepper, and salt
8. Sprinkle toasted pine nuts and pomegranate seeds! Serve warm and enjoy!

Nutrition Values (Per Serving)

- Calories: 118
- Fat: 10g
- Carbohydrates: 7g
- Protein: 3g

Visible Citrus And Cauli Salad
(Prepping time: 10 minutes\ Cooking time: 10 minutes |For 4 servings)

Ingredients

- 1 small sized cauliflower with the florets divided
- 1 Romanesco cauliflower with the florets divided
- 1 pound of broccoli florets
- 2 seedless oranges peeled up and sliced thinly

For vinaigrette ingredients

- 1 zested and squeezed orange
- 4 anchovies
- 1 hot pepper sliced up and chopped
- 1 tablespoon of capers
- 4 tablespoon of extra virgin olive oil
- Salt as needed
- Pepper as needed

Directions

1. Add broccoli, cauliflower florets to your Ninja Foodi
2. Lock up the lid and cook on HIGH pressure for 7 minutes

- ¼ teaspoon garlic powder

Directions

1. Add the above-mentioned ingredients to the Ninja Foodi
2. Lock up the lid and cook on HIGH pressure for 10 minutes
3. Release the pressure naturally
4. Spoon the mix into washed jars and cover the slices with a bit of cooking liquid
5. Add vinegar to submerge the chilly. Enjoy!

Nutrition Values (Per Serving)

- Calories: 3.1
- Fat: 0g
- Carbohydrates: 0.6g
- Protein: 0.1g

Easy To Swallow Beet Chips
(Prepping time: 10 minutes\ Cooking time: 8 hours | For 8 servings)

Ingredients

- ½ beet, peeled and cut into 1/8 inch slices

Directions

Arrange beet slices in single layer in the Cook and Crisp baske. Place the basket in the pot and close the crisping lid. Press the Dehydrate button and let it dehydrate for 8 hours at 135 degrees F. Once the dehydrating is done, remove the basket from pot and transfer slices to your Air Tight container, serve and enjoy!

Nutrition Values (Per Serving)

- Calories: 35
- Fat: 0g
- Carbohydrates: 8g
- Protein: 1g

Bacon Samba Bok Choy
(Prepping time: 10 minutes\ Cooking time:3 minutes | For 4 servings)

Ingredients

- ½ tablespoons fresh lemon juice
- 1 medium ripe avocado, peeled and pitted, chopped
- 6 organic eggs, boiled, peeled and cut half
- Salt to taste
- ½ cup fresh watercress, trimmed

Directions

1. Place a steamer basket at the bottom of your Ninja Foodi
2. Add water and put watercress on the basket, lock lid and pressure cook for 3 minutes
3. Quick release pressure. Remove egg yolk and transfer to a bowl
4. Add watercress, avocado, lemon juice, salt, and mash well
5. Place egg whites in serving the dish and fill whites with watercress, mix well and enjoy!

Nutrition Values (Per Serving)

- Calories: 132
- Fat: 10g
- Carbohydrates: 3g
- Protein: 6g

Sour Cream Mushroom Appetizer
(Prepping time: 10 minutes\ Cooking time: 20 minutes | For 6 servings)

Ingredients

Directions

5. Add zucchini in a colander and season with salt, add cream cheese and mix
6. Add oil into your Ninja Foodie's pot and add Zucchini
7. Lock Air Crisping Lid and set the temperature to 365 degrees F and timer to 10 minutes
8. Let it cook for 10 minutes and take the dish out once done, enjoy!

Nutrition Values (Per Serving)

- Calories: 374
- Fat: 36g
- Carbohydrates: 6g
- Protein: 7g

Pickled Up Green Chili
(Prepping time: 5 minutes\ Cooking time: 11 minutes |For 4 servings)

Ingredients

- 1 pound green chilies
- 1 and ½ cups apple cider vinegar
- 1 teaspoon pickling salt
- 1 and ½ teaspoon sugar
- ¼ teaspoon garlic powder

Directions

1. Add the listed ingredients to your pot. Lock up the lid and cook on HIGH pressure for 11 minutes. Release the pressure naturally
2. Spoon the mixture into jars and cover the slices with cooking liquid, making sure to completely submerge the chilies. Serve!

Nutrition Values (Per Serving)

- Calories: 3
- Fat: 0g
- Carbohydrates: 0.8g
- Protein: 0.1g

Spaghetti Squash And Chicken Parmesan
(Prepping time: 10 minutes\ Cooking time: 20 minutes |For 4 servings)

Ingredients

- 1 spaghetti squash
- 1 cup marinara sauce (Keto Friendly)
- 1 pound chicken, cooked and cubed
- 16 ounces mozzarella

Directions

1. Split up the squash in halves and remove the seeds
2. Add 1 cup of water to the Ninja Foodi and place a trivet on top
3. Add the squash halves on the trivet. Lock up the lid and cook for 20 minutes at HIGH pressure
4. Do a quick release. Remove the squashes and shred them using a fork into spaghetti portions
5. Pour sauce over the squash and give it a nice mix
6. Top them up with the cubed up chicken and top with mozzarella
7. Broil for 1-2 minutes and broil until the cheese has melted

Nutrition Values (Per Serving)

- Calories: 127
- Fats: 8g
- Carbs:11g
- Protein:5g

Spice Lover's Jar Of Chili
(Prepping time: 10 minutes\ Cooking time: 11 minutes |For 4 servings)

Ingredients

- 1 pound green chilies
- 1 and ½ cups apple cider vinegar
- 1 teaspoon pickling salt
- 1 and ½ teaspoons date paste

6. Cook in batches if needed, serve and enjoy!

Nutrition Values (Per Serving)

- Calories: 609
- Fat: 50g
- Carbohydrates: 10g
- Protein: 29g

Juicy Garlic Chicken Livers
(Prepping time: 10 minutes\ Cooking time: 8 hours |For 6 servings)

Ingredients

- 1 pound chicken livers
- 8 garlic cloves, minced
- 8 ounces cremini mushrooms, quartered
- 4 slices uncooked bacon, chopped
- 1 onion, chopped
- 1 cup bone broth
- 1 teaspoon dried thyme
- 1 teaspoon dried rosemary
- 1 teaspoon salt
- 1 teaspoon freshly ground black pepper
- ¼ cup fresh parsley, chopped

Directions

1. Add livers, bacon, garlic, mushrooms, onion, thyme, broth, rosemary to Ninja Foodi
2. Season with salt and pepper. Place lid and cook on SLOW COOK Mode (LOW) for 8 hours
3. Remove lid and stir in parsley. Serve and enjoy!

Nutrition Values (Per Serving)

- Calories: 210
- Fat: 9g
- Carbohydrates: 6g
- Protein: 24g

The Original Zucchini Gratin
(Prepping time: 10 minutes\ Cooking time: 15 minutes |For 4 servings)

Ingredients

- 2 zucchinis
- 1 tablespoon fresh parsley, chopped
- 2 tablespoons bread crumbs
- 4 tablespoons parmesan cheese, grated
- 1 tablespoon vegetable oil
- Salt and pepper to taste

Directions

1. Pre-heat your Ninja Foodi to 300 degrees F for 3 minutes
2. Slice zucchini lengthwise to get about 8 equal sizes pieces
3. Arrange pieces in your Crisping Basket (skin side down)
4. Top each with parsley, bread crumbs, cheese, oil, salt, and pepper
5. Return basket Ninja Foodi basket and cook for 15 minutes at 360 degrees F
6. Once done, serve with sauce. Enjoy!

Nutrition Values (Per Serving)

- Calories: 481
- Fat: 11g
- Carbohydrates: 10g
- Protein: 7g

Quick Bite Zucchini Fries
(Prepping time: 10 minutes\ Cooking time: 10 minutes |For 4 servings)

Ingredients

- 1-2 pounds of zucchini, sliced into 2 and ½ inch sticks
- Salt to taste
- 1 cup cream cheese
- 2 tablespoons olive oil

Egg Dredged Casserole
(Prepping time: 10 minutes\ Cooking time: 5 minutes |For 6 servings)

Ingredients

- 4 whole eggs
- 1 tablespoons milk
- 1 tomato, diced
- ½ cup spinach
- ¼ teaspoon salt
- ¼ teaspoon ground black pepper

Directions

1. Take a baking pan (small enough to fit Ninja Foodi) and grease it with butter
2. Take a medium bowl and whisk in eggs, milk, salt, pepper, add veggies to the bowl and stir
3. Pour egg mixture into the baking pan and lower the pan into the Ninja Foodi
4. Close Air Crisping lid and Air Crisp for 325 degrees for 7 minutes
5. Remove the pan from eggs and enjoy hot!

Nutrition Values (Per Serving)

- Calories: 78
- Fat: 5g
- Carbohydrates: 1g
- Protein: 7g

Excellent Bacon And Cheddar Frittata
(Prepping time: 10 minutes\ Cooking time: 10 minutes |For 6 servings)

Ingredients

- 6 whole eggs
- 2 tablespoons milk
- ½ cup bacon, cooked and chopped
- 1 cup broccoli, cooked
- ½ cup shredded cheddar cheese
- ¼ teaspoon salt
- ¼ teaspoon ground black pepper

Directions

1. Take a baking pan (small enough to fit into your Ninja Foodi) bowl, and grease it well with butter. Take a medium sized bowl and add eggs, milk, salt, pepper, bacon, broccoli, and cheese. Stir well. Pour mixture into your prepared baking pan and lower pan into your Foodi, close Air Crisping lid. Air Crisp for 7 minutes at 375 degrees F. Remove pan and enjoy!

Nutrition Values (Per Serving)

- Calories: 269
- Fat: 20g
- Carbohydrates: 3g
- Protein: 19g

Pork Packed Jalapeno
(Prepping time: 10 minutes\ Cooking time: 10 minutes |For 6 servings)

Ingredients

- 2 pounds pork sausage, ground
- 2 cups parmesan cheese, shredded
- 2 pounds large sized jalapeno peppers sliced lengthwise and seeded
- 2 (8 ounces packages), cream cheese, softened
- 2 (8 ounces) bottles, ranch dressing

Directions

1. Take a bowl and add pork sausage, cream cheese, ranch dressing and mix well
2. Slice jalapeno in half, remove seeds and clean them
3. Stuff sliced jalapeno pieces with pork mixture
4. Place peppers in crisping basket and transfer basket to your Ninja Foodi
5. Lock Air Crisping lid and cook on Air Crisp mode for 10 minutes at 350 degrees F

The Great Mediterranean Spinach
(Prepping time: 10 minutes\ Cooking time: 15 minutes |For 4 servings)

Ingredients

- 4 tablespoons butter
- 2 pounds spinach, chopped and boiled
- Salt and pepper to taste
- 2/3 cup Kalamata olives, halved and pitted
- 1 and ½ cups feta cheese, grated
- 4 teaspoons fresh lemon zest, grated

Directions

1. Take a bowl and mix in spinach, butter, salt, pepper and mix well
2. Transfer to Ninja Foodi the seasoned spinach
3. Lock Air Crisper and Air Crisp for 15 minutes at 350 degrees F. Serve and enjoy!

Nutrition Values (Per Serving)

- Calories: 247
- Fat: 13g
- Carbohydrates: 4g
- Protein: 6g

Quick Turkey Cutlets
(Prepping time: 10 minutes\ Cooking time: 22 minutes |For 4 servings)

Ingredients

- 1 teaspoon Greek seasoning
- 1 pound turkey cutlets
- 2 tablespoons olive oil
- 1 teaspoon turmeric powder
- ½ cup almond flour

Directions

1. Add Greek seasoning, turmeric powder, almond flour to a bowl
2. Dredge turkey cutlets in it and keep it on the side for 30 minutes
3. Set your Foodi to Saute mode and add oil and cutlets, Saute for 2 minutes
4. Lock lid and cook on LOW-MEDIUM pressure for 20 minutes
5. Quick release pressure. Serve and enjoy!

Nutrition Values (Per Serving)

- Calories: 233
- Fat: 19g
- Carbohydrates: 3.7g
- Protein: 36g

Veggies Dredged In Cheese
(Prepping time: 10 minutes\ Cooking time: 30 minutes |For 4 servings)

Ingredients

- 2 onions, sliced
- 2 tomatoes, sliced
- 2 zucchinis, sliced
- 2 teaspoons olive oil
- 2 cups cheddar cheese, grated
- 2 teaspoons mixed dried herbs
- Salt and pepper to taste

Directions

Arrange all the listed ingredients to your Ninja Foodi. Top with olive oil, herbs, cheddar, salt and pepper. Lock lid and Air Crisp for 30 minutes at 350 degrees F. Serve and enjoy!

Nutrition Values (Per Serving)

- Calories: 305
- Fat: 22g
- Carbohydrates: 9g
- Protein: 15g

- Calories: 132
- Fat: 10g
- Carbohydrates: 3g
- Protein: 5g

- Carbohydrates: 5g
- Protein: 16g

The Original Steamed Artichoke
(Prepping time: 5 minutes \ Cooking time: 25 minutes | For 4 servings)

Ingredients

- 2 medium sized whole artichokes
- 1 lemon wedge
- 1 cup water

Directions

1. Rinse artichokes under water and clean it, remove any damaged outer leaves
2. Take a sharp knife and trim off stem and top third of each choke
3. Rub the cut with lemon wedge to prevent browning
4. Add 1 cup water to your Foodi and place steamer basket in the pot, add artichokes to the rack
5. Lock lid and cook on HIGH pressure for 20 minutes. Release pressure naturally over 10 minutes
6. Open lid and transfer to plate. Serve and enjoy!

Nutrition Values (Per Serving)

- Calories: 564
- Fat: 40g
- Carbohydrates: 5g
- Protein: 2g

Crispy Avocado Chips
(Prepping time: 10 minutes \ Cooking time: 10 minutes | For 4 servings)

Ingredients

- 4 tablespoons butter
- 4 raw avocados, peeled and sliced into chips form
- Salt and pepper to taste

Directions

1. Season avocado slices with salt and pepper
2. Grease the pot of your Ninja Foodi with butter and add the avocado slices
3. Lock Crisping lid and cook on "Air Crisp" mode for 10 minutes at 350 degrees F
4. Remove the dish from Ninja Foodi and serve, enjoy!

Nutrition Values (Per Serving)

- Calories: 391
- Fat: 38g
- Carbohydrates: 15g
- Protein: 3.5g

The Crazy Egg-Stuffed Avocado Dish
(Prepping time: 10 minutes \ Cooking time: 5 minutes | For 6 servings)

Ingredients

- ½ tablespoon fresh lemon juice
- 1 medium ripe avocado, peeled, pitted and chopped
- 6 organic eggs, boiled, peeled and cut in half lengthwise
- Salt to taste
- ½ cup fresh watercress, trimmed

Directions

1. Place steamer basket at the bottom of your Ninja Foodie
2. Add water. Add watercress on the basket and lock lid
3. Cook on HIGH pressure for 3 minutes, quick release the pressure and drain the watercress
4. Remove egg yolks and transfer them to a bowl
5. Add watercress, avocado, lemon juice, salt into the bowl and mash with fork
6. Place egg whites in a serving bowl and fill them with the watercress and avocado dish
7. Serve and enjoy!

Nutrition Values (Per Serving)

3. Take a small bowl and add stevia, salt, pepper , pepper flakes and mix
4. Life squash out and shred using 2 forks, pour water out of pot and dry it
5. Set your pot to Saute mode and add butter, let it heat up. Add garlic, cook for 1 and ½ minutes
6. Add sage and stevia mixture, cook for 45 seconds
7. Pour the prepared sauce over spaghetti and stir. Enjoy!

Nutrition Values (Per Serving)

- Calories: 214
- Fat: 20g
- Carbohydrates: 5g
- Protein: 5g

Spicy Cauliflower Steak
(Prepping time: 5 minutes \ Cooking time: 5 minutes | For 4 servings)

Ingredients

- 1 large cauliflower head
- 2 tablespoons extra virgin olive oil
- 2 teaspoons paprika
- 2 teaspoons ground cumin
- ¾ teaspoon kosher salt
- ¼ cup fresh cilantro, chopped
- 1 lemon quartered

Directions

1. Place a steamer insert in your pot and add 1 and ½ cups water to the pot
2. Remove leaves form cauliflower and trim the core so the leaves sit flat
3. Transfer to rack. Take a small bowl and add olive oil, paprika, cumin and salt
4. Drizzle the mix over cauliflower and rub
5. Lock lid and cook on HIGH pressure for 4 minutes, quick release pressure
6. Once done, open up the lid and transfer the cooked cauliflower to a cutting board
7. Slice into 1 inch thick steaks and divide them amongst serving plates
8. Sprinkle cilantro, serve with lemon quarters and enjoy!

Nutrition Values (Per Serving)

- Calories: 268
- Fat: 23g
- Carbohydrates: 10g
- Protein: 5g

Subtle Buffalo Chicken Meatballs
(Prepping time: 10 minutes \ Cooking time: 40 minutes | For 6 servings)

Ingredients

- 1 pound chicken, ground
- 1 carrot, minced
- 2 celery stalks, minced
- ¼ cup blue cheese, crumbled
- ¼ cup buffalo sauce (check for Keto friendliness)
- 1 whole egg
- ¼ cup almond meal
- 2 tablespoons extra virgin olive oil
- ½ cup water

Directions

1. Set your Ninja to Saute mode and set it to HIGH, let it pre-heated for 5 minutes
2. Take a large mixing bowl and add chicken, carrot, celery, blue cheese, buffalo sauce, almond meal, egg. Mix and shape the mixture into 1 and ½ inch balls
3. Pour olive oil into your pot, and add the meatballs in batches, sear until all sides are browned. Keep the seared balls on the side
4. Place Cook and Crisp Basket in the pot and add water, add the seared meatballs
5. Place pressure lid and seal the pressure valves
6. Cook on HIGH pressure for 5 minutes, quick release the pressure once did
7. Close crisping lid and cook for 10 minutes at 360 degrees F
8. After 5 minutes of cooking, open the lid and lift the basket to give it a shake, lower it back and continue cooking. Enjoy once done!

Nutrition Values (Per Serving)

- Calories: 204
- Fat: 13g

3. Transfer Brussels to a plate and toss with olive oil, salt ,pepper and sprinkle of pine nuts. Enjoy!

Nutrition Values (Per Serving)
- Calories: 112
- Fat: 7g
- Carbohydrates: 4g
- Protein: 5g

Simple Mushroom Saute
(Prepping time: 10 minutes\ Cooking time: 15 minutes |For 8 servings)

Ingredients

- 1 pound white mushrooms, stems trimmed
- 2 tablespoons unsalted butter
- ½ teaspoon salt
- ¼ cup water

Directions

1. Quarter medium mushrooms and cut any large mushrooms into eight
2. Put mushrooms, butter, and salt in your Foodi's inner pot
3. Add water and lock pressure lid, making sure to seal the valve
4. Cook on HIGH pressure for 5 minutes, quick release pressure once did
5. Once done, set your pot to Saute mode on HIGH mode and bring the mix to a boil over 5 minutes until all the water evaporates
6. Once the butter/water has evaporated, stir for 1 minute until slightly browned. Enjoy!

Nutrition Values (Per Serving)

- Calories: 50
- Fat: 4g
- Carbohydrates: 2g
- Protein: 2g

Delicious Assorted Nuts
(Prepping time: 5 minutes\ Cooking time: 15 minutes |For 4 servings)

Ingredients

- 1 tablespoon butter, melted
- ½ cup raw cashew nuts
- 1 cup raw almonds
- Salt to taste

Directions

1. Add nuts to your Ninja Foodi pot
2. Lock lid and cook on "Air Crisp" mode for 10 minutes at 350 degrees F
3. Remove nuts into a bowl and add melted butter and salt. Toss well to coat
4. Return the mix to your Ninja Foodi, lock lid and bake for 5 minutes on BAKE/ROAST mode
5. Serve and enjoy!

Nutrition Values (Per Serving)

- Calories: 189
- Fat: 16g
- Carbohydrates: 7g
- Protein: 7g

Garlic And Sage Spaghetti Squash
(Prepping time: 5 minutes\ Cooking time: 17 minutes |For 4 servings)

Ingredients

- 1 spaghetti squash, halved crosswise and seeded
- 2 teaspoons stevia
- ¼ teaspoon salt
- 1/8 teaspoon black pepper
- 1/8 teaspoon crushed red pepper flakes
- 1/5 cup unsalted butter
- 2 cloves garlic, thinly sliced
- 12 fresh sage leaves

Directions

1. Place steamer insert in your Ninja Foodi. Add 1 and ½ cup water to the pot
2. Place spaghetti squash halves on steamer rack and lock lid, cook on HIGH pressure for 12 minutes. Quick release pressure

Lovely Cauliflower Soup
(Prepping time: 10 minutes\ Cooking time:301 minutes | For 5 servings)

Ingredients

- 5 slices bacon, chopped
- 1 onion, chopped
- 3 garlic cloves, minced
- 1 cauliflower head, trimmed
- 4 cups chicken broth
- 1 cup almond milk
- 1 teaspoon salt
- 1 teaspoon black pepper
- 1 and ½ cups cheddar cheese, shredded
- Sour cream and chopped fresh chives for serving

Directions

1. Set your pot to Saute mode and pre-heat it for 5 minutes on HIGH settings
2. Add bacon, onion, garlic to your pot and cook for 5 minutes. Reserve bacon for garnish
3. Add cauliflower, chicken broth to the pot and place pressure cooker lid, seal the pressure valves
4. Cook on HIGH pressure for 10 minutes, quick release the pressure once did
5. Add milk, and mash the soup reaches your desired consistency
6. Season with salt, pepper and sprinkle cheese evenly on top of the soup
7. Close crisping lid and Broil for 5 minutes
8. Once done, top with reserved crispy bacon and serve with sour cream and chives.Enjoy!

Nutrition Values (Per Serving)

- Calories: 253
- Fat: 17g
- Carbohydrates: 12g
- Protein: 13g

Elegant Broccoli Pops
(Prepping time: 60 minutes\ Cooking time: 12 minutes | For 4 servings)

Ingredients

- 1/3 cup parmesan cheese, grated
- 2 cups cheddar cheese, grated
- Salt and pepper to taste
- 3 eggs, beaten
- 3 cups broccoli florets
- 1 tablespoon olive oil

Directions

1. Add broccoli into a food processor and pulse until finely crumbed
2. Transfer broccoli to a large sized bowl and add remaining ingredients to the bowl, mix well
3. Make small balls using the mixture and let them chill for 30 minutes
4. Place balls in your Ninja Foodi pot and Air Crisping lid
5. Let it cook for 12 minutes at 365 degrees F on the "Air Crisp" mode
6. Once done, remove and enjoy!

Nutrition Values (Per Serving)

- Calories: 162
- Fat: 12g
- Carbohydrates: 2g
- Protein: 12g

Great Brussels Bite
(Prepping time: 5 minutes\ Cooking time: 3 minutes | For 4 servings)

Ingredients

- 1 pound Brussels sprouts
- ¼ cup pine nuts
- Salt and pepper to taste
- Olive oil as needed
- 1 cup water

Directions

1. Place a steamer basket in your Ninja Foodi and add Brussels to the basket
2. Add water and lock lid, cook on HIGH pressure for 3 minutes. Quick release pressure

Chapter 10: Snacks Recipes

Ultimate Creamy Zucchini Fries
(Prepping time: 10 minutes\ Cooking time: 10 minutes |For 4 servings)

Ingredients

- 1-2 pounds of zucchini, sliced into 2 and ½ inch sticks
- Salt to taste
- 1 cup cream cheese
- 2 tablespoons olive oil

Directions

1. Add zucchini in a colander and season with salt, add cream cheese and mix
2. Add oil into your Ninja Foodi's pot and add Zucchini
3. Lock Air Crisping Lid and set the temperature to 365 degrees F and timer to 10 minutes
4. Let it cook for 10 minutes and take the dish out once done, enjoy!

Nutrition Values (Per Serving)

- Calories: 374
- Fat: 36g
- Carbohydrates: 6g
- Protein: 7g

The Onion And Smoky Mushroom Medley
(Prepping time: 5 minutes\ Cooking time: 2 minutes |For 4 servings)

Ingredients

- 1 tablespoon ghee
- 1 carton (8 ounces) button mushrooms, sliced
- 1 onion, diced
- ½ teaspoon salt
- 2 tablespoon coconut aminos
- 1/8 teaspoon smoked paprika

Directions

1. Set your Ninja Foodi to Saute mode and add ghee, let it heat up
2. Add mushrooms, onion and seasoning, Saute for 5 minutes
3. Lock lid and cook on HIGH pressure for 3 minutes.Quick release pressure. Serve warm and enjoy!

Nutrition Values (Per Serving)

- Calories: 268
- Fat: 20g
- Carbohydrates: 11g
- Protein: 10g

Cool Beet Chips
(Prepping time: 10 minutes\ Cooking time: 8 hours |For 8 servings)

Ingredients

- ½ beet, peeled and cut into 1/8 inch slices

Directions

1. Arrange beet slices in single layer in the Cook and Crisp basket
2. Place the basket in the pot and close the crisping lid
3. Press the Dehydrate button and let it dehydrate for 8 hours at 135 degrees F
4. Once the dehydrating is done, remove the basket from pot and transfer slices to your Air Tight container, serve and enjoy!

Nutrition Values (Per Serving)

- Calories: 35
- Fat: 0g
- Carbohydrates: 8g
- Protein: 1g

2. Set your Ninja Foodi to Saute mode and add spinach, mushrooms
3. Whisk eggs, milk, cream cheese, herbs, and Sautéed vegetables in a bowl and mix well
4. Take a 6-inch baking pan and grease it well
5. Pour mixture and transfer to your Ninja Foodie (on a trivet)
6. Cook on HIGH pressure for 2 minutes. Quick release pressure. Serve and enjoy!

Nutrition Values (Per Serving)

- Calories: 300
- Fat: 25g

- Carbohydrates: 5g
- Protein: 14g

Ultimate Cheese Dredged Cauliflower Snack
(Prepping time: 10 minutes\ Cooking time: 30 minutes |For 4 servings)

Ingredients

- 1 tablespoon mustard
- 1 head cauliflower
- 1 teaspoon avocado mayonnaise

- ½ cup parmesan cheese, grated
- ¼ cup butter, cut into small pieces

Directions

1. Set your Ninja Foodi to Saute mode and add butter and cauliflower
2. Saute for 3 minutes. Add remaining ingredients and stir
3. Lock lid and cook on HIGH pressure for 30 minutes. Release pressure naturally over 10 minutes
4. Serve and enjoy!

Nutrition Values (Per Serving)

- Calories: 155
- Fat: 13g

- Carbohydrates: 4g
- Protein: 6g

Nutrition Values (Per Serving)

- Calories: 95
- Fat: 3.1g
- Carbohydrates: 10g
- Protein: 2g

Rise And Shine Breakfast Casserole

(Prepping time: 10 minutes \ Cooking time: 10 minutes | For 6 servings)

Ingredients

- 4 whole eggs
- 1 tablespoons milk
- 1 cup ham, cooked and chopped
- ½ cup cheddar cheese, shredded
- ¼ teaspoon salt
- ¼ teaspoon ground black pepper

Directions

1. Take a baking pan (small enough to fit into your Ninja Foodi) bowl, and grease it well with butter. Take a medium bowl and whisk in eggs, milk, salt, pepper and add ham, cheese, and stir. Pour mixture into baking pan and lower the pan into your Ninja Foodi
2. Set your Ninja Foodi Air Crisp mode and Air Crisp for 325 degrees F for 7 minutes
3. Remove pan from eggs and enjoy!

Nutrition Values (Per Serving)

- Calories: 169
- Fat: 13g
- Carbohydrates: 1g
- Protein: 12g

Cauliflower And Egg Dish

(Prepping time: 10 minutes \ Cooking time: 4 minutes | For 4 servings)

Ingredients

- 21 ounces cauliflower, separated into florets
- 1 cup red onion, chopped
- 1 cup celery, chopped
- ½ cup of water
- Salt and pepper to taste
- 2 tablespoons balsamic vinegar
- 1 teaspoon stevia
- 4 boiled eggs, chopped
- 1 cup Keto Friendly mayonnaise

Directions

1. Add water to Ninja Foodi
2. Add steamer basket and add cauliflower, lock lid and cook on High Pressure for 5 minutes
3. Quick release pressure. Transfer cauliflower to bowl and add eggs, celery, onion and toss
4. Take another bowl and mix in mayo, salt, pepper, vinegar, stevia and whisk well
5. Add a salad, toss well. Divide into salad bowls and serve. Enjoy!

Nutrition Values (Per Serving)

- Calories: 170
- Fat: 4g
- Carbohydrates: 5g
- Protein: 5g

Just A Simple Egg Frittata

(Prepping time: 10 minutes \ Cooking time: 15 minutes | For 4 servings)

Ingredients

- 5 whole eggs
- ¾ teaspoon mixed herbs
- 1 cup spinach
- ¼ cup shredded cheddar cheese
- ½ cup mushrooms
- Salt and pepper to taste
- ¾ cup half and half
- 2 tablespoons butter

Directions

1. Dice mushrooms, chop spinach finely

Nutrition Values (Per Serving)

- Calories: 111
- Fat: 6g
- Carbohydrates: 2g
- Protein: 2g

Obvious Paprika And Cabbage
(Prepping time: 10 minutes \ Cooking time: 4 minutes | For 4 servings)

Ingredients

- 1 and ½ pounds green cabbage, shredded
- Salt and pepper to taste
- 3 tablespoon ghee
- 1 cup vegetable stock
- ¼ teaspoon sweet paprika

Directions

1. Set your Ninja Foodi to Saute mode and add ghee, let it melt
2. Add cabbage, salt, pepper, and stock, stir well
3. Lock lid and cook on HIGH pressure for 7 minutes. Quick release pressure
4. Add paprika and toss well. Divide between plates and serve. Enjoy!

Nutrition Values (Per Serving)

- Calories: 170
- Fat: 4g
- Carbohydrates: 5g
- Protein: 5g

Authentic Western Omelet
(Prepping time: 5 minutes \ Cooking time: 34 minutes | For 2 servings)

Ingredients

- 3 eggs, whisked
- 3 ounces chorizo, chopped
- 1-ounces Feta cheese, crumbled
- 5 tablespoons almond milk
- ¾ teaspoon chili flakes
- ¼ teaspoon salt
- 1 green pepper, chopped

Directions

1. Add all the ingredients and mix them well. Stir it gently. Take an omelet pan and pour the mixture into it. Preheat your Ninja Foodi at "Roast/Bake" mode at 320 F.
2. Cook for 4 minutes. After that, transfer the pan with an omelet in Ninja Foodi
3. Cook for 30 minutes more at the same mode. Serve hot and enjoy!

Nutrition Values (Per Serving)

- Calories: 426
- Fat: 38.2g
- Carbohydrates: 6.8g
- Protein: 21.7g

Bowl Full Of Broccoli Salad
(Prepping time: 10 minutes \ Cooking time: 5 minutes | For 4 servings)

Ingredients

- 1 pound broccoli, cut into florets
- 2 tablespoons balsamic vinegar
- 2 garlic cloves, minced
- 1 teaspoon mustard seeds
- 1 teaspoon cumin seeds
- Salt and pepper to taste
- 1 cup cottage cheese, crumbled

Directions

4. Add 1 cup water to your Ninja Foodi. Place steamer basket
5. Place broccoli in basket and lock lid, cook on HIGH pressure for 5 minutes
6. Quick release pressure and remove lid. Toss broccoli with other ingredients and serve. Enjoy!

- Calories: 550
- Fat: 54g
- Carbohydrates: 5g
- Protein: 13g

Kale And Almonds Mix
(Prepping time: 10 minutes \ Cooking time: 4 minutes | For 4 servings)

Ingredients

- 1 cup of water
- 1 big kale bunch, chopped
- 1 tablespoon balsamic vinegar
- 1/3 cup toasted almonds
- 3 garlic cloves, minced
- 1 small yellow onion, chopped
- 2 tablespoons olive oil

Directions

1. Set your Ninja Foodi on Saute mode and add oil, let it heat up
2. Stir in onion and cook for 3 minutes. Add garlic, water, kale, and stir
3. Lock lid and cook on HIGH pressure for 4 minutes. Quick release pressure
4. Add salt, pepper, vinegar, almonds and toss well. Serve and enjoy!

Nutrition Values (Per Serving)

- Calories: 140
- Fat: 6g
- Carbohydrates: 5g
- Protein: 3g

Simple Treat Of Garlic
(Prepping time: 10 minutes \ Cooking time: 5 minutes | For 4 servings)

Ingredients

- 1 tablespoon extra-virgin olive oil
- 2 garlic cloves, minced
- 2 large-sized Belgian endive, halved lengthwise
- ½ cup apple cider vinegar
- ½ cup broth
- Salt and pepper to taste
- 1 teaspoon cayenne pepper

Directions

1. Set your Ninja Foodi to Saute mode and add oil, let the oil heat up
2. Add garlic and cook for 30 seconds unto browned
3. Add endive, vinegar, broth, salt, pepper, and cayenne
4. Lock lid and cook on LOW pressure for 2 minutes. Quick release pressure and serve. Enjoy!

Nutrition Values (Per Serving)

- Calories: 91
- Fat: 6g
- Carbohydrates: 3g
- Protein: 2g

Buttered Up Garlic And Fennel
(Prepping time: 10 minutes \ Cooking time: 5 minutes | For 4 servings)

Ingredients

- ½ stick butter
- 2 garlic cloves, sliced
- ½ teaspoon salt
- 1 and ½ pounds fennel bulbs, cut into wedges
- ¼ teaspoon ground black pepper
- ½ teaspoon cayenne
- ¼ teaspoon dried dill weed
- 1/3 cup dry white wine
- 2/3 cup stock

Directions

1. Set your Ninja Foodi to Saute mode and add butter, let it heat up
2. Add garlic and cook for 30 seconds. Add rest of the ingredients
3. Lock lid and cook on LOW pressure for 3 minutes. Remove lid and serve. Enjoy!

Directions

1. Take a medium bowl and whisk in yolks, heavy cream, cocoa powder, vanilla and stevia
2. Pour the mixture into 1 and ½ quart baking dish and place the dish in your Ninja Foodi insert
3. Add enough water to reach about halfway up the sides of baking dish
4. Lock lid and cook on HIGH pressure for 12 minutes
5. Quick release pressure once the cycle is complete
6. Remove baking dish from insert and let it cool
7. Chill the dessert in refrigerator and serve with garnish of whipped coconut cream and shaved dark chocolate. Enjoy!

Nutrition Values (Per Serving)

- Calories: 275
- Fat: 18g
- Carbohydrates: 3g
- Protein: 5g

Inspiring Cauliflower Hash Browns
(Prepping time: 10 minutes\ Cooking time: 30 minutes |For 6 servings)

Ingredients

- 6 whole eggs
- 4 cups cauliflower rice
- ¼ cup milk
- 1 onion, chopped
- 3 tablespoons butter
- 1 and ½ cups cooked ham, chopped
- ½ cup shredded cheese

Directions

1. Set your Ninja Foodi to sauté mode and add butter, let the butter heat up
2. Add onions and cook for 5 minutes until tender. Add iced cauliflower to pot and stir
3. Lock the Air Crisping lid and Air Crisp for 15 minutes, making sure to give them a turn about halfway through
4. Take a small bowl and mix in eggs and milk, pour mixture over browned cauliflower
5. Sprinkle ham over top. Press Air Crispy again and crisp for 10 minutes more
6. Sprinkle cheddar cheese on top and lock lid, let the crisp for 1 minute more until the cheese melts. Serve and enjoy!

Nutrition Values (Per Serving)

- Calories: 166
- Fat: 14g
- Carbohydrates: 3g
- Protein: 9g

Everybody's Favorite Cauliflower Patties
(Prepping time: 5 minutes \ Cooking time: 20 minutes |For 4 servings)

Ingredients

- 3 whole eggs
- 1 chili pepper, chopped
- ½ teaspoon garlic powder
- Salt and pepper to taste
- 2 cups cauliflower, chopped
- ¾ cups olive oil
- ¼ cup cheddar cheese
- ¼ cup whole mozzarella cheese

Directions

1. Cut cauliflower into small florets, remove leaves and cut out a core
2. Add 1 cup water to Ninja Food, transfer florets to steamer basket and place it on a trivet in your Ninja Foodi. Lock lid and cook on HIGH pressure for 5 minutes
3. Mash steamed cauliflower and dry them, add shredded cheese, eggs, chili, salt and pepper
4. Mix well and shape into flat patties
5. Heat up oil in your Ninja Foodi and set to Saute mode, shallow fry patties until crisp on both sides. Serve and enjoy!

Nutrition Values (Per Serving)

6. Remove ramekin and let it cool down to room temperature
7. Chill in fridge and serve topped up with whipped coconut cream. Enjoy!

Nutrition Values (Per Serving)

- Calories: 319
- Fat: 30g
- Carbohydrates: 3g
- Protein: 7g

Hearty Carrot Pumpkin Pudding

(Prepping time: 10 minutes\ Cooking time: 15 minutes |For 4 servings)

Ingredients

- 1 tablespoon extra-virgin olive oil
- 2 cups carrots, shredded
- 2 cups pureed pumpkin
- ½ sweet onion, finely chopped
- 1 cup heavy whip cream
- ½ cup cream cheese, soft
- 2 whole eggs
- 1 tablespoon granulated Erythritol
- 1 teaspoon ground nutmeg
- ½ teaspoon salt
- ¼ cup pumpkin seeds, garnish
- ¼ cup water

Directions

1. Add oil to your Ninja Foodi pot and whisk In carrots, pumpkin, onion, heavy cream, cream cheese, eggs, Erythritol, nutmeg, salt and water. Stir and lock lid
2. Cook on HIGH pressure for 10 minutes. Release pressure naturally over 10 minutes
3. Serve with a topping of pumpkin seeds. Enjoy!

Nutrition Values (Per Serving)

- Calories: 239
- Fat: 19g
- Carbohydrates: 7g
- Protein: 6g

Creative Crème Brulee

(Prepping time: 10 minutes + 3 hours chill time \ Cooking time: 15 minutes |For 4 servings)

Ingredients

- 1 cup heavy cream
- ½ tablespoons vanilla extract
- 3 egg yolks
- 1 pinch salt
- ¼ cup stevia

Directions

1. Take a bowl and mix in egg yolks, vanilla extract, salt and heavy cream
2. Mix well and beat until combined well
3. Divide the mixture between 4 greased ramekins evenly and transfer the ramekins to your Ninja Foodi. Lock lid and choose the "Bake/Roast" mode, bake for 35 minutes at 365 degrees F
4. Remove the ramekin from Ninja Foodi and wrap ramekins with plastic wrap
5. Refrigerate them to chill for about 3 hours. Serve and enjoy!

Nutrition Values (Per Serving)

- Calories: 260
- Fat: 22g
- Carbohydrates: 8g
- Protein: 5g

The Original Pot-De-Crème

(Prepping time: 15 minutes \ Cooking time: 15 minutes |For 4 servings)

Ingredients

- 6 egg yolks
- 2 cups heavy whip cream
- 1/3 cup cocoa powder
- 1 tablespoon pure vanilla extract
- ½ teaspoon liquid stevia
- Whipped coconut cream as needed for garnish
- Shaved dark chocolate, for garnish

Nutrition Values (Per Serving)

- Calories: 292
- Fat: 26g
- Carbohydrates: 8g
- Protein: 5g

Delicious Lemon Mousse

(Prepping time: 10 minutes \ Cooking time: 12 minutes | For 2 servings)

Ingredients

- 1-2 ounces cream cheese, soft
- ½ cup heavy cream
- 1/8 cup fresh lemon juice
- ½ teaspoon lemon liquid stevia
- 2 pinch salt

Directions

1. Take a bowl and mix in cream cheese, heavy cream, lemon juice, salt and stevia
2. Pour the mixture into ramekins and transfer the ramekins to your Ninja Foodi pot
3. Lock lid and select "Bake/Roast" mode and bake for 12 minutes at 350 degrees F
4. Pour the mixture into

Nutrition Values (Per Serving)

- Calories: 292
- Fat: 26g
- Carbohydrates: 8g
- Protein: 5g

The Generous Strawberry Shortcake

(Prepping time: 10 minutes \ Cooking time: 15 minutes | For 4 servings)

Ingredients

- 1 whole egg
- ½ cup almond flour
- ½ teaspoon vanilla extract
- 1 tablespoon stevia
- 1 tablespoon ghee
- 3 tablespoons strawberries, chopped
- 1 cup water
- 3 tablespoons coconut whip cream

Directions

1. Add all ingredients except whip cream to a heat resistant mug, add a cup of water to the Ninja Foodi pot. Place steaming rack in your pot and place the mug in the rack
2. Lock lid and cook on HIGH pressure for 12 minutes. Quick release pressure
3. Remove lid and remove the mug. Top with coconut whipped cream and more strawberries. Enjoy!

Nutrition Values (Per Serving)

- Calories: 275
- Fat: 18g
- Carbohydrates: 3g
- Protein: 5g

Sensational Lemon Custard

(Prepping time: 10 minutes \ Cooking time: 22 minutes | For 4 servings)

Ingredients

- 5 egg yolks
- ¼ cup fresh squeeze lemon juice
- 1 tablespoon lemon zest
- 1 teaspoon pure vanilla extract
- 1/3 teaspoon liquid stevia
- 2 cups heavy cream
- 1 cup whipped coconut cream

Directions

1. Take a medium bowl and whisk in yolks, lemon juice, zest, vanilla and liquid stevia
2. Whisk in heavy cream and divide the mix between 4 (4 ounce sized) ramekins
3. Place the provided rack at the bottom of your Ninja Foodi. Place ramekins in rack
4. Add water just enough to reach halfway up the sides of ramekins
5. Lock lid and cook on HIGH pressure for 20 minutes. Quick release pressure

Chapter 9: Dessert Recipes

The Divine Fudge Delight
(Prepping time: 20 minutes \ Cooking time: 10 minutes
\ Freeze Time: 3-5 hours | For 24 servings)

Ingredients

- ½ teaspoon organic vanilla extract
- 1 cup heavy whipping cream
- 2 ounces butter, soft
- 2 ounces 70% dark chocolate, finely chopped

Directions

1. Set your Ninja-Foodi to Saute mode with "Medium-HIGH" temperature, add vanilla and heavy cream. Saute for 5 minutes and select "LOW" temperature
2. Saute for 10 minutes more, add butter and chocolate. Saute for 2 minutes more
3. Transfer the mix to a serving dish and refrigerate for a few hours. Serve chilled and enjoy!

Nutrition Values (Per Serving)

- Calories: 292
- Fat: 26g
- Carbohydrates: 8g
- Protein: 5g

Keto-Friendly Nut Porridge
(Prepping time: 10 minutes \ Cooking time: 10 minutes | For 4 servings)

Ingredients

- 4 teaspoons coconut oil, melted
- 1 cup pecans, halved
- 2 cups water
- 2 tablespoon stevia
- 1 cup cashew nuts, raw and unsalted

Directions

1. Add cashew nuts and pecans to your food processor and pulse until chunked
2. Add nuts mixture into pot and stir in water, coconut oil and stevia
3. Set your Ninja Foodi to sauté ode and add the nut mixture. Cook for 15 minutes
4. Serve immediately and enjoy!

Nutrition Values (Per Serving)

- Calories: 260
- Fat: 22g
- Carbohydrates: 8g
- Protein: 5g

Heartfelt Vanilla Yogurt
(Prepping time: 20 minutes and 9 hours culture time \ Cooking time: 3 hours | For 4 servings)

Ingredients

- ½ cup full-fat milk
- ¼ cup yogurt started
- 1 cup heavy cream
- ½ tablespoon pure vanilla extract
- 2 teaspoons stevia

Directions

1. Pour milk in your Ninja Foodi pot, stir in heavy cream, vanilla extract and Stevia
2. Let the yogurt sit and lock lid. Cook for 3 hours on "Slow Cooker" mode
3. Take a small bowl and mix 1 cup milk with yogurt starter, add this mixture to the pot
4. Lock lid and wrap the Foodi in two small t towels
5. Let it sit for 9 hours, allowing the yogurt to culture. Refrigerate and serve. Enjoy!

4. Serve and enjoy with a sprinkle of chopped lemon grass stalks. Enjoy!

Nutrition Values (Per Serving)

- Calories: 251
- Fat: 10g

- Carbohydrates: 3g
- Protein: 34g

Gentle Salmon Stew
(Prepping time: 5 minutes\ Cooking time: 11 minutes |For 4 servings)

Ingredients

- 1 cup fish broth
- Salt and pepper to taste
- 1 medium onion, chopped

- 1-2 pounds salmon fillets, cubed
- 1 tablespoon butter

Directions

1. Add the listed ingredients to a large sized bowl and let the shrimp marinate for 30-60 minutes
2. Grease the inner pot of the Ninja Foodi with butter and transfer marinated shrimp to the pot
3. Lock the lid and select "Bake/Roast" mode and bake for 15 minutes at 355 degrees F
4. Once done, serve and enjoy!

Nutrition Values (Per Serving)

- Calories: 173
- Fat: 8g

- Carbohydrates: 0.1g
- Protein: 23g

- Carbohydrates: 12g
- Protein: 25g

Butter Dredged "Rich" Lobster

(Prepping time: 15 minutes\ Cooking time: 20 minutes | For 4 servings)

Ingredients

- 6 Lobster Tails
- 4 garlic cloves,
- ¼ cup butter

Directions

12. Preheat the Ninja Foodi to 400 degrees F at first
13. Open the lobster tails gently by using kitchen scissors
14. Remove the lobster meat gently from the shells but keep it inside the shells
15. Take a plate and place it. Add some butter in a pan and allow it melt
16. Put some garlic cloves in it and heat it over medium-low heat
17. Pour the garlic butter mixture all over the lobster tail meat
18. Let the fryer to broil the lobster at 130 degrees F
19. Remove the lobster meat from Ninja Foodi and set aside
20. Use a fork to pull out the lobster meat from the shells entirely
21. Pour some garlic butter over it if needed. Serve and enjoy!

Nutrition Values (Per Serving)

- Calories: 160
- Fat: 1g
- Carbohydrates: 1g
- Protein: 20g

The Extremely Wild Alaskan Cod

(Prepping time: 10 minutes\ Cooking time: 5-10 minutes | For 4 servings)

Ingredients

- 1 large fillet, Alaskan Cod (Frozen)
- 1 cup cherry tomatoes
- Salt and pepper to taste
- Seasoning as you need
- 2 tablespoons butter
- Olive oil as needed

Directions

7. Take an ovenproof dish small enough to fit inside your pot
8. Add tomatoes to the dish, cut large fish fillet into 2-3 serving pieces and lay them on top of tomatoes. Season with salt, pepper and your seasoning
9. Top each fillet with 1 tablespoon butter and drizzle olive oil
10. Add 1 cup of water to the pot. Place trivet to the Ninja Foodi and place dish on the trivet
11. Lock lid and cook on HIGH pressure for 9 minutes
12. Release pressure naturally over 10 minutes. Serve and enjoy!

Nutrition Values (Per Serving)

- Calories: 449
- Fat: 32g
- Carbohydrates: 11g
- Protein: 25g

Magical Shrimp Platter

(Prepping time: 10 minutes\ Cooking time: 15 minutes | For 4 servings)

Ingredients

- 2 tablespoons butter
- ½ teaspoon smoked paprika
- 1 red chili pepper, seeded and chopped
- 1 pound shrimp, peeled and deveined
- Lemongrass stalks

Directions

1. Take a bowl and mix in all ingredients except lemongrass, let the mixture marinate for 60 minutes
2. Transfer the marinated fillet to your Ninja Foodi pot
3. Close lid and set to "Bake/Roast" mode and bake for 15 minutes at 345 degrees F

- Calories: 416
- Fat: 31g
- Carbohydrates: 5g
- Protein: 26g

Almond Cod Fillets
(Prepping time: 10 minutes\ Cooking time: 5-10 minutes |For 4 servings)

Ingredients

- 1 pound frozen cod fish fillets
- 2 garlic cloves, halved
- 1 cup chicken broth
- 2 tablespoons almonds, sliced½ teaspoon paprika
- ½ cup packed parsley
- 2 tablespoons oregano

Directions

7. Take the fish out of freezer and let it defrost
8. Take a food processor and stir in garlic, oregano, parsley, paprika, 1 tablespoon almond and process. Set your Ninja Foodi to "SAUTE" mode and add olive oil, let it heat up
9. Add remaining almonds and toast, transfer to a towel. Pour broth in pot and add herb mixture
10. Cut fish into 4 pieces and place in a steamer basket, transfer steamer basket to the pot
11. Lock lid and cook on HIGH pressure for 3 minutes. Quick release pressure once done
12. Serve steamer fish by pouring over the sauce. Enjoy!

Nutrition Values (Per Serving)
- Calories: 246
- Fat: 10g
- Carbohydrates: 8g
- Protein: 15g

Simple Sweet And Sour Fish Magnifico
(Prepping time: 10 minutes\ Cooking time: 6 minutes |For 4 servings)

Ingredients

- 2 drops liquid stevia
- ¼ cup butter
- 1 pound fish chunks
- 1 tablespoon vinegar
- Salt and pepper to taste

Directions

1. Set your Ninja Foodi to Saute mode and add butter, let it melt
2. Add fish chunks and Saute for 3 minutes. Add stevia, salt and pepper, stir
3. Lock Crisping Lid and cook on "Air Crisp" mode for 3 minutes at 360 degrees F
4. Serve once done and enjoy!

Nutrition Values (Per Serving)

- Calories: 274
- Fat: 15g
- Carbohydrates: 2g
- Protein: 33g

Cod With Broccoli, Lemon And Dill Mismash
(Prepping time: 15 minutes\ Cooking time: 2-5 minutes |For 4 servings)

Ingredients

- 1 pound, 1 inch thick frozen cod fillets
- 2 cups broccoli
- 1 cup water
- Dill weed
- Lemon pepper to taste
- Dash of salt

Directions

1. Cut fish into four pieces. Season fish pieces with lemon pepper, salt, dill weed
2. Add 1 cup water to the Ninja Foodi
3. Lower down steamer basket and add fish, broccoli florets to the steamer basket
4. Lock lid and cook on LOW pressure for 2 minutes. Quick release pressure. Serve and enjoy!

Nutrition Values (Per Serving)
- Calories: 463
- Fat: 33g

6. Add sea bass, diced tomatoes, tomato paste, broth to the pot, place the lid and seal the valves
7. Cook on HIGH pressure for 5 minutes, quick release the pressure once did
8. Set your pot to Saute mode again with the temperature set at Medium-HIGH mode and add shrimp. Place lid and seal the pressure valve, cook for 4 minutes until the shrimp is opaque
9. Season with ¼ teaspoon salt and serve, enjoy!

Nutrition Values (Per Serving)

- Calories: 326
- Fat: 9g
- Carbohydrates: 10g
- Protein: 46g

The Great Lobster Bisque
(Prepping time: 10 minutes\ Cooking time: 10 minutes | For 4 servings)

Ingredients

- 2 teaspoons unsalted butter
- 1 onion, chopped
- 1 tablespoon garlic, minced
- 1 tablespoon fresh ginger, minced
- 2 cups vegetable broth
- 1 cup tomatoes, chopped
- 3 cups cauliflower, chopped
- 2 tablespoons Keto-Friendly pesto
- ½ teaspoon salt
- 1 -2 teaspoons fresh ground black pepper
- 1 pound cooked lobster meat
- 1 cup heavy whip cream

Directions

1. Pre-heat your Ninja Foodi by setting to Saute mode on HIGH settings
2. Once the inner pot is hot, add butter and let it heat up
3. Once the butter is shimmering, add onion, garlic and ginger. Saute for 2-3 minutes
4. Add broth, stir, making sure to scrape the bottom of the pan to remove any browned bits
5. Add tomatoes, cauliflower, pesto, salt and pepper
6. Lock lid and cook on HIGH pressure for 4 minutes. Release pressure naturally over 10 minutes
7. Use an immersion blender to puree the veggies in the soup
8. Turn Saute mode on and let the meat cook for a while, stir in cream and serve. Enjoy!

Nutrition Values (Per Serving)

- Calories: 441
- Fat: 30g
- Carbohydrates: 10g
- Protein: 30g

Elegant Fish Curry
(Prepping time: 5 minutes\ Cooking time: 4 minutes | For 4 servings)

Ingredients

- 2 tablespoons coconut oil
- 1 and ½ tablespoons fresh ginger, grated
- 2 teaspoons garlic, minced
- 1 tablespoon curry powder
- ½ teaspoon ground cumin
- 2 cups coconut milk
- 16 ounces firm white fish, cut into 1 inch chunks
- 1 cup kale, shredded
- 2 tablespoons cilantro, chopped

Directions

1. Pre-heat your Ninja Foodi to by selecting the Saute mode and setting the temperature to HIGH heat
2. Add coconut oil and let it heat up, add ginger and garlic and Saute for 2 minutes until light browned. Stir in curry powder, cumin, Saute for 2 minutes until fragrant
3. Stir in coconut milk, reduce heat to low and simmer for 5 minutes
4. Lock lid and cook on LOW pressure for 4 minutes. Release pressure naturally over 10 minutes
5. Stir in kale and cilantro, simmer in Saute mode for 2 minutes. Serve and enjoy!

Nutrition Values (Per Serving)

1. Set your Ninja Foodi to Saute mode and add butter and let it melt
2. Add rosemary, garlic and Saute for 1 minute. Add sea scallops, salt and pepper
3. Saute for 2 minutes more
4. Lock Crisping Lid and cook on "Air Crisp" mode for 3 minutes at 350 degrees F
5. Once done, serve and enjoy!

Nutrition Values (Per Serving)

- Calories: 279
- Fat: 16g
- Carbohydrates: 4g
- Protein: 25g

Sensational Coconut Fish Curry
(Prepping time: 10 minutes\ Cooking time: 5-10 minutes |For 4 servings)

Ingredients

- 1 and ½ pounds white fish fillets, rinsed and cut into bite sized pieces
- 1 heaping cup cherry tomatoes
- 2 green chilies, sliced into strips
- 2 garlic cloves, finely chopped
- 1 tablespoon ginger, freshly grated
- 6 curry leaves such as bay leaves
- 1 tablespoon ground coriander
- 1 tablespoon ground cumin
- ½ teaspoon ground turmeric
- 1 teaspoon chili powder
- ½ teaspoon ground fenugreek
- 2 cups coconut milk, unsweetened
- 1 teaspoon olive oil
- Salt to taste
- Lemon juice to taste

Directions

1. Set your Ninja Foodi to Saute mode and add oil and curry leaves
2. Gently fry for 1 minute, add onion, garlic, ginger and Saute until onion are tender
3. Add coriander, turmeric, chili powder, fenugreek (all ground) and Saute with onions for 1 minute
4. Deglaze pot with coconut milk, scraping browned bits
5. Add green chilies, tomatoes and fish and stir to coat
6. Lock lid and cook on HIGH pressure for 3 minutes, quick release pressure
7. Open lid and season with salt and lemon juice. Enjoy!

Nutrition Values (Per Serving)

- Calories: 276
- Fat: 21g
- Carbohydrates: 4g
- Protein: 18g

Warm Cajun Bass Stew
(Prepping time: 10 minutes\ Cooking time: 28 minutes |For 6 servings)

Ingredients

- 1 pound sea bass fillets, patted dry and cut into 2 inch chunks
- 3 tablespoons Cajun seasoning, divided
- ½ teaspoon salt
- 2 tablespoons extra virgin olive oil
- 2 yellow onion, diced
- 2 bell peppers, diced
- 4 celery stalks, diced
- 1 can (28 ounces) diced tomatoes, drained
- ¼ cup tomato paste
- 1 and ½ cups veggie broth
- 2 pounds large shrimp, peeled and deveined

Directions

1. Set your Pot to Saute mode at a temperature of Medium-HIGH heat, let it pre-heat for 5 minutes
2. Season sea bass on both sides with 1 and ½ tablespoons Cajun seasoning and ¼ teaspoon salt
3. Put 1 tablespoon oil and sea bass in your pre-heated pot
4. Saute for 4 minutes
5. Add remaining 1 tablespoon oil and onions to the pot and cook for 3 minutes, add bell peppers, celery, and 1 and ½ tablespoons Cajun seasoning to the pot. Cook for 2 minutes more

- Calories: 361
- Fat: 22g
- Carbohydrates: 11g
- Protein: 30g

The Smoked White Fish

(Prepping time: 10 minutes\ Cooking time: 2 hours | For 4 servings)

Ingredients

- 2 pounds Whitefish fillets, raw
- 1 tablespoon onion powder
- ½ teaspoon cumin
- 1 tablespoon paprika
- 1 tablespoon garlic powder
- 1 tablespoon olive oil
- Fresh lemon juice
- Fresh cilantro, chopped
- Salt and pepper to taste

Directions

1. Set up your Ninja Foodi to 200 degrees F on a low heat setting
2. Use olive oil to brush the fish fillets
3. Add cumin, garlic powder, onion powder, paprika, salt, and pepper in a bowl and mix them well
4. Rub this prepared seasoning all over the pork from all the sides
5. Spray some olive oil more on the fillets
6. Put the seasoned fillets on the rack and put it inside the Ninja Foodi at a low temperature
7. Cook for 2 hours. Garnish it with chopped cilantro and fresh lemon juice. Serve and enjoy!

Nutrition Values (Per Serving)

- Calories: 142
- Fat: 2g
- Carbohydrates: 0g
- Protein: 30g

Cool Lemon And Dill Fish Packages

(Prepping time: 10 minutes\ Cooking time: 5-10 minutes | For 4 servings)

Ingredients

- 2 tilapia cod fillets
- Salt, pepper and garlic powder to taste
- 2 sprigs fresh dill
- 4 slices lemon
- 2 tablespoons butter

Directions

8. Lay out 2 large squares of parchment paper
9. Place fillet in center of each parchment square and season with salt, pepper and garlic powder
10. On each fillet, place 1 sprig of dill, 2 lemon slices, 1 tablespoon butter
11. Place trivet at the bottom of your Ninja Foodi. Add 1 cup water into the pot
12. Close parchment paper around fillets and fold to make a nice seal
13. Place both packets in your pot. Lock lid and cook on HIGH pressure for 5 minutes
14. Quick release pressure. Serve and enjoy!

Nutrition Values (Per Serving)

- Calories: 259
- Fat: 11g
- Carbohydrates: 8g
- Protein: 20g

Heart-Throb Buttery Scallops

(Prepping time: 10 minutes\ Cooking time: 15 minutes | For 4 servings)

Ingredients

- 4 garlic cloves, minced
- 4 tablespoons fresh rosemary, chopped
- 2 pounds sea scallops
- ½ cup butter
- Salt and pepper to taste

Directions

Directions

1. Add a cup of water to your Ninja Foodi and place a steamer rack on top
2. Place the fish. Season the fish with salt and pepper and lock up the lid
3. Cook on HIGH pressure for 3 minutes. Once done, quick release the pressure
4. Remove the fish and allow it to cool
5. Break the fillets into a bowl and add egg, yellow and green onions
6. Add ½ a cup of almond meal and mix with your hand. Divide the mixture into patties
7. Take a large skillet and place it over medium heat. Add oil and cook the patties.Enjoy!

Nutrition Values (Per Serving)

- Calories: 238
- Fat: 15g
- Carbohydrates: 1g
- Protein: 23g

Small-Time Herby Cods

(Prepping time: 5 minutes\ Cooking time: 8 minutes | For 4 servings)

Ingredients

- 4 garlic cloves, minced
- 2 teaspoons coconut aminos
- ¼ cup butter
- 6 whole eggs
- 2 small onions, chopped
- 3 (4 ounces each) skinless cod fish fillets, cut into rectangular pieces
- 2 green chilies, chopped
- Salt and pepper to taste

Directions

1. Take a shallow dish and add all ingredients except cod, beat the mixture well
2. Dip each fillet into the mixture and keep it on the side
3. Transfer prepared fillets to your Ninja Foodi Crisping basket and transfer basket to Pot
4. Lock Crisping lid and cook on "Air Crisp" mode for 8 minutes at 330 degrees F. Serve and enjoy!

Nutrition Values (Per Serving)

- Calories: 409
- Fat: 25g
- Carbohydrates: 7g
- Protein: 37g

Tomato And Shrimp Medley

(Prepping time: 10 minutes\ Cooking time: 5 minutes | For 4 servings)

Ingredients

- 3 tablespoons unsalted butter
- 1 tablespoon garlic
- ½ teaspoon red pepper flakes
- 1 and ½ cup onion, chopped
- 1 can (14 and ½ ounces) tomatoes, diced
- 1 teaspoon dried oregano
- 1 teaspoon salt
- 1 pound frozen shrimp, peeled
- 1 cup crumbled feta cheese
- ½ cup black olives, sliced
- ½ cup parsley, chopped

Directions

1. Pre-heat your Ninja Foodi by setting in in the Saute mode on HIGH settings, add butter and let it melt. Add garlic, pepper flakes, cook for 1 minute
2. Add onion, tomato, oregano, salt and stir well. Add frozen shrimp
3. Lock lid and cook on HIGH pressure for 1 minute. Quick release pressure
4. Mix shrimp with tomato broth, let it cool and serve with a sprinkle of feta, olives and parsley
5. Enjoy!

Nutrition Values (Per Serving)

- Calories: 234
- Fat: 14g

- Carbohydrates: 12g
- Protein: 16g

Breathtaking Cod Fillets

(Prepping time: 10 minutes\ Cooking time: 5-10 minutes |For 4 servings)

Ingredients

- 1 pound frozen cod fish fillets
- 2 garlic cloves, halved
- 1 cup chicken broth
- ½ cup packed parsley

- 2 tablespoons oregano
- 2 tablespoons almonds, sliced½ teaspoon paprika

Directions

1. Take the fish out of the freezer and let it defrost
2. Take a food processor and stir in garlic, oregano, parsley, paprika, 1 tablespoon almond and process. Set your Ninja Foodi to "SAUTE" mode and add olive oil, let it heat up
3. Add remaining almonds and toast, transfer to a towel. Pour broth in a pot and add herb mixture
4. Cut fish into 4 pieces and place in a steamer basket, transfer steamer basket to the pot
5. Lock lid and cook on HIGH pressure for 3 minutes. Quick release pressure once has done
6. Serve steamed fish by pouring over the sauce.Enjoy!

Nutrition Values (Per Serving)

- Calories: 246
- Fat: 10g

- Carbohydrates: 8g
- Protein: 15g

Lemon And Pepper Salmon Delight

(Prepping time: 5 minutes\ Cooking time: 6 minutes |For 4 servings)

Ingredients

- ¾ cup of water
- Sprigs of parsley, basil, tarragon
- 1 pound salmon, skin on
- 3 teaspoons ghee
- ¾ teaspoon salt

- ½ teaspoon pepper
- ½ lemon, sliced
- 1 red bell pepper, julienned
- 1 carrot, julienned

Directions

1. Set your Ninja Foodi to Saute mode and add water and herbs
2. Place a steamer rack and add the salmon. Drizzle ghee on top of the salmon
3. Season with pepper and salt. Cover lemon slices on top
4. Lock up the lid and cook on HIGH pressure for 3 minutes
5. Release the pressure naturally over 10 minutes
6. Transfer the salmon to a platter. Add veggies to your pot and set the pot to Saute mode
7. Cook for 1-2 minutes. Serve the cooked vegetables with salmon. Enjoy!

Nutrition Values (Per Serving)

- Calories: 464
- Fat: 34g

- Carbohydrates: 3g
- Protein: 34g

Fresh Steamed Salmon

(Prepping time: 5 minutes\ Cooking time: 5 minutes |For 4 servings)

Ingredients

- 2 salmon fillets
- ¼ cup onion, chopped
- 2 stalks green onion stalks, chopped
- 1 whole egg

- Almond meal
- Salt and pepper to taste
- 2 tablespoons olive oil

1. Pre-heat your Ninja Foodi with the Crisping Basket inside at 350 degrees F
2. Take a bowl and mix in ranch dressing and panko
3. Beat eggs in a shallow bowl and keep it on the side
4. Dip fillets in the eggs, then in the panko mix
5. Place fillets in your Ninja Foodie's insert and transfer insert to Ninja Foodi
6. Lock Air Crisping Lid and Air Crisp for 13 minutes at 350 degrees F
7. Garnish with chilies and herbs. Enjoy!

Nutrition Values (Per Serving)

- Calories: 301
- Fat: 12g
- Carbohydrates: 1.5g
- Protein: 28g

Alaskan Cod Divine
(Prepping time: 10 minutes\ Cooking time: 5-10 minutes |For 4 servings)

Ingredients

- 1 large fillet, Alaskan Cod (Frozen)
- 1 cup cherry tomatoes
- Salt and pepper to taste
- Seasoning as you need
- 2 tablespoons butter
- Olive oil as needed

Directions

1. Take an ovenproof dish small enough to fit inside your pot
2. Add tomatoes to the dish, cut large fish fillet into 2-3 serving pieces and lay them on top of tomatoes. Season with salt, pepper, and your seasoning
3. Top each fillet with 1 tablespoon butter and drizzle olive oil
4. Add 1 cup of water to the pot.Place trivet to the Ninja Foodi and place dish on the trivet
5. Lock lid and cook on HIGH pressure for 9 minutes.Release pressure naturally over 10 minutes
6. Serve and enjoy!

Nutrition Values (Per Serving)
- Calories: 449
- Fat: 32g
- Carbohydrates: 11g
- Protein: 25g

Kale And Salmon Delight
(Prepping time: 10 minutes\ Cooking time: 5 minutes |For 4 servings)

Ingredients

- 1 lemon, juiced
- 2 salmon fillets
- ¼ cup extra virgin olive oil
- 1 teaspoon Dijon mustard
- 4 cups kale, thinly sliced, ribs removed
- 1 teaspoon salt
- 1 avocado, diced
- 1 cup pomegranate seeds
- 1 cup walnuts, toasted
- 1 cup goat parmesan cheese, shredded

Directions

1. Season salmon with salt and keep it on the side. Place a trivet in your Ninja Foodi
2. Place salmon over the trivet. Lock lid and cook on HIGH pressure for 15 minutes
3. Release pressure naturally over 10 minutes. Transfer salmon to a serving platter
4. Take a bowl and add kale, season with salt
5. Take another bowl and make the dressing by adding lemon juice, Dijon mustard, olive oil, and red wine vinegar. Season kale with dressing and add diced avocado, pomegranate seeds, walnuts and cheese. Toss and serve with the fish. Enjoy!

Nutrition Values (Per Serving)

5. Lock Air Crisping lid and cook on Air Crisp mode for 15 minutes at 360 degrees F
6. Serve and enjoy!

Nutrition Values (Per Serving)

- Calories: 554
- Fat: 24g
- Carbohydrates: 5g
- Protein: 37g

Salmon Paprika
(Prepping time: 5 minutes\ Cooking time: 7 minutes |For 4 servings)

Ingredients

- 2 wild caught salmon fillets, 1 to 1 and ½ inches thick
- 2 teaspoons avocado oil
- 2 teaspoons paprika
- Salt and pepper to taste
- Green herbs to garnish

Directions

1. Season salmon fillets with salt, pepper, paprika, and olive oil
2. Place Crisping basket in your Ninja Foodi, and pre-heat your Ninja Foodie at 390 degrees F
3. Place insert insider your Foodi and place the fillet in the insert, lock Air Crisping lid and cook for 7 minutes. Once done, serve the fish with herbs on top. Enjoy!

Nutrition Values (Per Serving)

- Calories: 249
- Fat: 11g
- Carbohydrates: 1.8g
- Protein: 35g

Heartfelt Air Fried Scampi
(Prepping time: 5 minutes\ Cooking time: 5 minutes |For 4 servings)

Ingredients

- 4 tablespoons butter
- 1 tablespoon lemon juice
- 1 tablespoon garlic, minced
- 2 teaspoons red pepper flakes
- 1 tablespoon chives, chopped
- 1 tablespoon basil leaves, minced
- 2 tablespoons chicken stock
- 1 pound defrosted shrimp

Directions

1. Set your Foodi to Saute mode and add butter, let the butter melt and add red pepper flakes and garlic, Saute for 2 minutes
2. Transfer garlic to crisping basket, add remaining ingredients (including shrimp) to the basket
3. Return basket back to the Ninja Foodi and lock the Air Crisping lid, cook for 5 minutes at 390 degrees F. Once done, serve with a garnish of fresh basil

Nutrition Values (Per Serving)

- Calories: 372
- Fat: 11g
- Carbohydrates: 0.9g
- Protein: 63g

Ranch Warm Fillets
(Prepping time: 5 minutes\ Cooking time: 13 minutes |For 4 servings)

Ingredients

- ¼ cup panko
- ½ packet ranch dressing mix powder
- 1 and ¼ tablespoons vegetable oil
- 1 egg beaten
- 2 tilapia fillets
- A garnish of herbs and chilies

Directions

Ingredients

- 1 cup crab meat, cubed
- 1 tablespoon garlic, minced
- Salt as needed
- Red chili flakes as needed
- 3 cups vegetable broth
- 1 teaspoon salt

Directions

1. Coat the crab cubes in lime juice and let them sit for a while
2. Add the all ingredients (including marinated crab meat) to your Ninja Foodi and lock lid
3. Cook on SLOW COOK MODE (MEDIUM) for 3 hours
4. Let it sit for a while
5. Unlock lid and set to Saute mode, simmer the soup for 5 minutes more on LOW
6. Stir and check to season. Enjoy!

Nutrition Values (Per Serving)

- Calories: 201
- Fat: 11g
- Carbohydrates: 12g
- Protein: 13g

The Rich Guy Lobster And Butter
(Prepping time: 15 minutes\ Cooking time: 20 minutes | For 4 servings)

Ingredients

- 6 Lobster Tails
- 4 garlic cloves,
- ¼ cup butter

Directions

1. Preheat the Ninja Foodi to 400 degrees F at first
2. Open the lobster tails gently by using kitchen scissors
3. Remove the lobster meat gently from the shells but keep it inside the shells
4. Take a plate and place it
5. Add some butter in a pan and allow it melt
6. Put some garlic cloves in it and heat it over medium-low heat
7. Pour the garlic butter mixture all over the lobster tail meat
8. Let the fryer to broil the lobster at 130 degrees F
9. Remove the lobster meat from Ninja Foodi and set aside
10. Use a fork to pull out the lobster meat from the shells entirely
11. Pour some garlic butter over it if needed. Serve and enjoy!

Nutrition Values (Per Serving)

- Calories: 160
- Fat: 1g
- Carbohydrates: 1g
- Protein: 20g

Lovely Panko Cod
(Prepping time: 5 minutes\ Cooking time: 15 minutes | For 6 servings)

Ingredients

- 2 uncooked cod fillets, 6 ounces each
- 3 teaspoons kosher salt
- ¾ cup panko bread crumbs
- 2 tablespoons butter, melted
- ¼ cup fresh parsley, minced
- 1 lemon. Zested and juiced

Directions

1. Pre-heat your Ninja Foodi at 390 degrees F and place Air Crisper basket inside
2. Season cod and salt
3. Take a bowl and add bread crumbs, parsley, lemon juice, zest, butter, and mix well
4. Coat fillets with the bread crumbs mixture and place fillets in your Air Crisping basket

- 2 tilapia cod fillets
- Salt, pepper and garlic powder to taste

- 2 sprigs fresh dill
- 4 slices lemon
- 2 tablespoons butter

Directions

1. Layout 2 large squares of parchment paper
2. Place fillet in center of each parchment square and season with salt, pepper and garlic powder
3. On each fillet, place 1 sprig of dill, 2 lemon slices, 1 tablespoon butter
4. Place trivet at the bottom of your Ninja Foodi. Add 1 cup water into the pot
5. Close parchment paper around fillets and fold to make a nice seal
6. Place both packets in your pot . Lock lid and cook on HIGH pressure for 5 minutes
7. Quick release pressure . Serve and enjoy!

Nutrition Values (Per Serving)

- Calories: 259
- Fat: 11g

- Carbohydrates: 8g
- Protein: 20g

Adventurous Sweet And Sour Fish

(Prepping time: 10 minutes\ Cooking time: 6 minutes |For 4 servings)

Ingredients

- 2 drops liquid stevia
- ¼ cup butter
- 1 pound fish chunks

- 1 tablespoon vinegar
- Salt and pepper to taste

Directions

1. Set your Ninja Foodi to Saute mode and add butter, let it melt
2. Add fish chunks and Saute for 3 minutes. Add stevia, salt, and pepper, stir
3. Lock Crisping Lid and cook on "Air Crisp" mode for 3 minutes at 360 degrees F
4. Serve once done and enjoy!

Nutrition Values (Per Serving)

- Calories: 274
- Fat: 15g

- Carbohydrates: 2g
- Protein: 33g

Garlic And Lemon Prawn Delight

(Prepping time: 5 minutes\ Cooking time: 5 minutes |For 4 servings)

Ingredients

- 2 tablespoons olive oil
- 1 pound prawns
- 2 tablespoons garlic, minced
- 2/3 cup fish stock

- 1 tablespoon butter
- 2 tablespoons lemon juice
- 1 tablespoon lemon zest
- Salt and pepper to taste

Directions

1. Set your Ninja Foodi to Saute mode and add butter and oil, let it heat up
2. Stir in remaining ingredients. Lock lid and cook on LOW pressure for 5 minutes
3. Quick release pressure. Serve and enjoy!

Nutrition Values (Per Serving)

- Calories: 236
- Fat: 12g

- Carbohydrates: 2g
- Protein: 27g

Lovely Carb Soup

(Prepping time: 5 minutes\ Cooking time: 6-7 hours |For 4 servings)

- 2 pounds sea scallops
- 12 cup butter
- Salt and pepper to taste

Directions

1. Set your Ninja Foodi to Saute mode and add butter, rosemary, and garlic
2. Saute for 1 minute. Add scallops, salt, and pepper
3. Saute for 2 minutes. Lock Crisping lid and Crisp for 3 minutes at 350 degrees F. Serve and enjoy!

Nutrition Values (Per Serving)

- Calories: 279
- Fat: 16g
- Carbohydrates: 5g
- Protein: 25g

Awesome Cherry Tomato Mackerel
(Prepping time: 5 minutes\ Cooking time: 7 minutes |For 4 servings)

Ingredients

- 4 Mackerel fillets
- ¼ teaspoon onion powder
- ¼ teaspoon lemon powder
- ¼ teaspoon garlic powder
- ½ teaspoon salt
- 2 cups cherry tomatoes
- 3 tablespoons melted butter
- 1 and ½ cups of water
- 1 tablespoon black olives

Directions

1. Grease baking dish and arrange cherry tomatoes at the bottom of the dish
2. Top with fillets sprinkle all spices. Drizzle melted butter over
3. Add water to your Ninja Foodi
4. Lower rack in Ninja Foodi and place baking dish on top of the rack
5. Lock lid and cook on LOW pressure for 7 minutes . Quick release pressure. Serve and enjoy!

Nutrition Values (Per Serving)

- Calories: 325
- Fat: 24g
- Carbohydrates: 2g
- Protein: 21g

Lovely Air Fried Scallops
(Prepping time: 5 minutes\ Cooking time: 5 minutes |For 4 servings)

Ingredients

- 12 scallops
- 3 tablespoons olive oil
- Salt and pepper to taste

Directions

1. Gently rub scallops with salt, pepper, and oil
2. Transfer to your Ninja Foodie's insert, and place the insert in your Foodi
3. Lock Air Crisping lid and cook for 4 minutes at 390 degrees F
4. Half through, make sure to give them a nice flip and keep cooking. Serve warm and enjoy!

Nutrition Values (Per Serving)

- Calories: 372
- Fat: 11g
- Carbohydrates: 0.9g
- Protein: 63g

Packets Of Lemon And Dill Cod
(Prepping time: 10 minutes\ Cooking time: 5-10 minutes |For 4 servings)

Ingredients

2. Add olive oil as well. Add garlic and cook for 1 minute
3. Add lemon juice, shrimp and cook for 1 minute
4. Stir in rest of the ingredients and lock lid, cook on LOW pressure for 5 minutes
5. Quick release pressure and serve . Enjoy!

Nutrition Values (Per Serving)

- Calories: 277
- Fat: 6g
- Carbohydrates: 5g
- Protein: 27g

Heartfelt Sesame Fish
(Prepping time: 8 minutes\ Cooking time: 8 minutes |For 4 servings)

Ingredients

- 1 and ½ pound salmon fillet
- 1 teaspoon sesame seeds
- 1 teaspoon butter, melted
- ½ teaspoon salt
- 1 tablespoon apple cider vinegar
- ¼ teaspoon rosemary, dried

Directions

1. Take apple cider vinegar and spray it to the salmon fillets
2. Then add dried rosemary, sesame seeds, butter and salt
3. Mix them well. Take butter sauce and brush the salmon properly
4. Place the salmon on the rack and lower the air fryer lid. Set the air fryer mode
5. Cook the fish for 8 minutes at 360 F.Serve hot and enjoy!

Nutrition Values (Per Serving)

- Calories: 239
- Fat: 11.2g
- Carbohydrates: 0.3g
- Protein: 33.1g

Awesome Sock-Eye Salmon
(Prepping time: 5 minutes\ Cooking time: 5 minutes |For 4 servings)

Ingredients

- 4 sockeye salmon fillets
- 1 teaspoon Dijon mustard
- ¼ teaspoon garlic, minced
- ¼ teaspoon onion powder
- ¼ teaspoon lemon pepper
- ½ teaspoon garlic powder
- ¼ teaspoon salt
- 2 tablespoons olive oil
- 1 and ½ cup of water

Directions

1. Take a bowl and add mustard, lemon juice, onion powder, lemon pepper, garlic powder, salt, olive oil. Brush spice mix over salmon
2. Add water to Instant Pot. Place rack and place salmon fillets on rack
3. Lock lid and cook on LOW pressure for 7 minutes
4. Quick release pressure .Serve and enjoy!

Nutrition Values (Per Serving)

- Calories: 353
- Fat: 25g
- Carbohydrates: 0.6g
- Protein: 40g

Buttered Up Scallops
(Prepping time: 10 minutes\ Cooking time: 5 minutes |For 4 servings)

Ingredients

- 4 garlic cloves, minced
- 4 tablespoons rosemary, chopped

Chapter 8: Seafood And Fish Recipes

Hearty Swordfish Meal
(Prepping time: 5 minutes\ Cooking time: 150 minutes |For 4 servings)

Ingredients

- 5 swordfish fillets
- ½ a cup of melted clarified butter
- 6 garlic cloves, chopped
- 1 tablespoon black pepper

Directions

1. Take a mixing bowl and add garlic, clarified butter, black pepper
2. Take a parchment paper and add the fillet. Cover and wrap the fish
3. Keep repeating until the fillets are wrapped up
4. Transfer wrapped fish to Ninja Foodi pot and lock lid
5. Allow them to cook for 2 and a ½ hour at high pressure. Release the pressure naturally
6. Serve and enjoy!

Nutrition Values (Per Serving)

- Calories: 379
- Fat: 26g
- Carbohydrates: 1g
- Protein: 34g

Gentle And Simple Fish Stew
(Prepping time: 5 minutes\ Cooking time: 20 minutes |For 4 servings)

Ingredients

- 3 cups fish stock
- 1 onion, diced
- 1 cup broccoli, chopped
- 2 cups celery stalks, chopped
- 1 and ½ cups cauliflower, diced
- 1 carrot, sliced
- 1 pound white fish fillets, chopped
- 1 cup heavy cream
- 1 bay leaf
- 2 tablespoons butter
- ¼ teaspoon pepper
- ½ teaspoon salt
- ¼ teaspoon garlic powder

Directions

1. Set your Ninja Foodi to Saute mode and add butter, let it melt
2. Add onion and carrots, cook for 3 minutes. Stir in remaining ingredients
3. Lock lid and cook on HIGH pressure for 4 minutes.Naturally, release pressure over 10 minutes
4. Discard bay leaf . Serve and enjoy!

Nutrition Values (Per Serving)

- Calories: 298
- Fat: 18g
- Carbohydrates: 6g
- Protein: 24g

Cool Shrimp Zoodles
(Prepping time: 5 minutes\ Cooking time: 3 minutes |For 4 servings)

Ingredients

- 4 cups zoodles
- 1 tablespoon basil, chopped
- 2 tablespoons Ghee
- 1 cup vegetable stock
- 2 garlic cloves, minced
- 2 tablespoons olive oil
- ½ lemon
- ½ teaspoon paprika

Directions

1. Set your Ninja Foodi to Saute mode and add ghee, let it heat up

93

13. Mix pork with cooking liquid and serve with lettuce, grated carrots, squire of lime and any other topping you desire. Enjoy!

Nutrition Values (Per Serving)

- Calories: 245
- Fat: 18g
- Carbohydrates: 4g
- Protein: 13g

Cuban And Garlic Pork Meal
(Prepping time: 10 minutes\ Cooking time: 80 minutes |For 4 servings)

Ingredients

- 3 pounds boneless pork shoulder blade roast, fat trimmed and removed
- 6 garlic cloves, minced
- 2/3 cup grapefruit juice
- ½ tablespoon fresh oregano
- ½ tablespoon cumin
- 1 lime, juiced
- 1 tablespoon salt
- 1 bay leaf
- Lime wedges as needed
- Cilantro, chopped, for garnish
- Hot sauce as needed
- Salsa as needed

Directions

1. Cut the pork chops in 4 individual pieces and add them to a bowl
2. Take a small sized blender and add garlic, grapefruit juice, lime, oregano, cumin, salt, and blend well. Pour the marinade over your pork and allow it to sit for 60 minutes
3. Transfer the mix to your Ninja Foodi and add bay leaf
4. Cover and cook on HIGH pressure for 80 minutes. Release the pressure naturally
5. Remove the pork and shred it up. Return the pork back to the Foodi and add 1 cup of liquid
6. Season with some salt and allow it warm for a while (over Saute mode)
7. Enjoy!

Nutrition Values (Per Serving)

- Calories: 213
- Fat: 9g
- Carbohydrates: 2g
- Protein: 26g

Mean Cream Mushroom Garlic Chicken
(Prepping time: 10 minutes\ Cooking time: 15 minutes |For 4 servings)

Ingredients

- 2 pounds chicken thighs
- 7 ounces Cremini mushrooms
- 2 teaspoons garlic, minced
- ½ cup chicken broth
- ½ cup whipping cream
- 1 teaspoon cayenne pepper
- 1 tablespoon lemon juice
- 1 tablespoon parsley, chopped
- 1 tablespoon olive oil
- Salt and pepper to taste

Directions

1. Trim the stems of mushrooms. Wash and rinse chicken thighs under cold water
2. Pat dry with paper towels
3. Use kitchen scissors to trim excess skin and d fat from chicken thighs
4. Season both sides with salt and pepper, keep them on the side (covered)
5. Set your Ninja Foodi to Saute mode and add olive oil, let it heat up
6. Add chicken thighs and brown both sides. Scoop out excess fat and discard
7. Add garlic, whipping cream, mushrooms, broth, salt and pepper
8. Lock lid and cook on HIGH pressure for 10 minutes. Release pressure naturally over 10 minutes
9. Open the lid and set your pot to Saute mode. Add lemon juice and parsley. Serve and enjoy!

Nutrition Values (Per Serving)

- Calories: 390
- Fat: 20g
- Carbohydrates: 2g
- Protein: 48g

1. Set your Ninja Foodi to "SAUTE" mode and add oil, let it heat up
2. Add pork, salt and pepper, brown each side for 3 minutes until both sides are slightly browned
3. Transfer them to a plate. Add water, liquid smoke to the pot and return the meat, stir
4. Lock lid and cook on HIGH pressure for 90 minutes, release pressure naturally over 10 minutes
5. Transfer meat to cutting board and shred using 2 forks, divide between serving plates and serve with the cooking liquid on top, add green beans on the side if you prefer. Enjoy!

Nutrition Values (Per Serving)

- Calories: 357
- Fat: 28g
- Carbohydrates: 2g
- Protein: 20g

Easy-Going Kid Friendly Pork Chops

(Prepping time: 15 minutes\ Cooking time: 5-10 minutes |For 4 servings)

Ingredients

- 3-4 pork chops -12 to ¾ inch thick each
- 1 egg, beaten
- 1-2 cups Almond flour as needed
- Salt and pepper to taste
- 1-2 cups almond meal
- ½ cup onions, chopped
- 2-4 garlic cloves, squashed and chopped
- 1 tablespoons butter
- 1-2 tablespoons coconut oil

Directions

1. Set your Ninja Foodi to "Saute" mode and add butter, let it heat up
2. Dredge the pork chops in beaten egg, then in flour and finally in almond meal
3. Add them to the pot and brown all sides. Add onions and cook for a minute
4. Add garlic and cook for 1 minute more
5. Transfer the browned meat, onion and garlic to a plate, make sure to keep the drippings in the pot. Add 2-3 tablespoons of water and place and place a steamer rack in your pot
6. Add browned pork chops on the steamer and lock lid
7. Cook on HIGH Pressure for 5 minutes, once done, let the pressure release naturally over 10 minutes. Remove from pot and serve. Enjoy!

Nutrition Values (Per Serving)

- Calories: 446
- Fat: 25g
- Carbohydrates: 6g
- Protein: 21g

Amazing Mexican Pulled Pork Lettuce

(Prepping time: 10 minutes\ Cooking time: 60 minutes |For 4 servings)

Ingredients

- 4 pounds pork roast
- 1 head butter lettuce, washed and dried
- 2 carrots, grated
- 2 tablespoons olive oil
- 2 lime wedges
- 1 onion, chopped
- 1 tablespoon salt
- 2-3 cups water

For Spice Mix

- 1 tablespoons unsweetened cocoa powder
- 2 teaspoons oregano
- 1 teaspoon red pepper flakes
- 1 teaspoon garlic powder
- 1 teaspoon white pepper
- 1 teaspoon cumin
- 1/8 teaspoon cayenne
- 1/8 teaspoon coriander

Directions

8. Marinate pork overnight by transferring the meat to a bowl and mixing in all of the spices
9. Set your Ninja Foodi to "SAUTE" mode and add roast, let it brown
10. Add 2-3 cups water to fully submerge the roast
11. Lock lid and cook on HIGH pressure for 55 minutes. Release pressure naturally over 10 minutes
12. Set your pot to "SAUTE" mode again and take out the meat, shred the meat and keep it on the side. Reduce the liquid by half and strain/skim any excess fat

- 2 tablespoons olive oil
- 1 tablespoon garlic, minced
- 1 tablespoon fresh ginger, minced
- 2 tablespoons coconut aminos
- 2 tablespoons black vinegar
- 1-2 teaspoons stevia
- 1-2 teaspoons salt

- ½ onion, sliced
- 1 pound pork shoulder, cut into 2 inch chunks
- 2 pepper corns, crushed
- 3 cups water
- 3-4 cups bok choy, chopped
- ¼ cup fresh cilantro, chopped

Directions

1. Pre-heat your Ninja Foodi by setting it to Saute mode on HIGH settings
2. Once the inner pot it hot enough, add oil and let heat until shimmering
3. Add garlic and ginger and Saute for 1-2 minutes
4. Add coconut aminos, vinegar, sweetener, pepper corn, salt, onion, pork, water and stir
5. Lock lid and cook on HIGH pressure for 20 minutes. Release pressure naturally over 10 minutes
6. Open lid and add bok choy, close lid and let it cook in the remaining heat for 10 minutes
7. Ladle soup into serving bowl and serve with topping of cilantro. Enjoy!

Nutrition Values (Per Serving)

- Calories: 256
- Fat: 20g

- Carbohydrates: 5g
- Protein: 14g

Healthy Cranberry Keto-Friendly BBQ Pork
(Prepping time: 10 minutes\ Cooking time: 45 minutes |For 4 servings)

Ingredients

- 3-4 pounds pork shoulder, boneless, fat trimmed

For Sauce

- 3 tablespoons liquid smoke
- 2 tablespoons tomato paste
- 2 cups fresh cranberries
- ¼ cup hot sauce (Keto-Friendly)
- 1/3 cup blackstrap molasses
- ½ cup water
- ½ cup apple cider vinegar

- 1 teaspoon salt
- 1 tablespoons adobo sauce (Keto Friendly and Sugar Free)
- 1 cup tomato puree (Keto-Friendly and Sugar Free)
- 1 chipotle pepper in adobo sauce, diced

Directions

6. Cut pork against halves/thirds and keep it on the side
7. Set your Ninja Foodi to "SAUTE" mode and let it heat up
8. Add cranberries and water to the pot
9. Let them simmer for 4-5 minutes until cranberries start to pop, add rest of the sauce ingredients and simmer for 5 minutes more. Add pork to the pot and lock lid
10. Cook on HIGH pressure for 40 minutes. Quick release pressure
11. Use fork to shred the pork and serve on your favorite greens

Nutrition Values (Per Serving)

- Calories: 250
- Fat: 17g

- Carbohydrates: 5g
- Protein: 15g

Decisive Kalua Pork
(Prepping time: 10 minutes\ Cooking time: 90 minutes |For 4 servings)

Ingredients

- 4 pounds pork shoulder, cut into half
- ½ cup water
- 2 tablespoons olive oil
- Salt and pepper to taste

- 1 tablespoon liquid smoke
- Steamer green beans for serving (optional)

Directions

11. Lock lid and cook on HIGH pressure for 40 minutes. Once done, quick release pressure
12. Slice the meat and serve with the sauce. Enjoy!

Nutrition Values (Per Serving)
- Calories: 331
- Fat: 21g
- Carbohydrates: 2g
- Protein: 19g

Deliciously Spicy Pork Salad Bowl
(Prepping time: 10 minutes\ Cooking time: 90 minutes | For 6 servings)

Ingredients

- 4 pounds pork shoulder
- Butter as needed
- 2 teaspoons salt
- 2 cups chicken stock
- 1 teaspoon smoked paprika powder
- 1 teaspoon garlic powder
- 1 teaspoon black pepper
- 1 pinch dried oregano leaves
- 4 tablespoons coconut oil
- 6 garlic cloves

Directions

8. Remove rind from pork and cut meat from bone, slice into large chunks
9. Trim fat off met. Set your Foodi to Saute mode and add oil, let it heat up
10. Once the oil is hot, layer chunks of meat in the bottom of the pot and Saute for around 30 minutes until browned
11. While the meat are being browned, peel garlic cloves and cut into small chunks
12. Once the meat is browned, transfer it to a large sized bowl
13. Add a few tablespoons of chicken stock to the pot an deglaze it, scraping off browned bits
14. Transfer browned bits to the bowl with meat chunks. Repeat if any more meat are left
15. Once done, add garlic, oregano leaves, smoked paprika,. Garlic powder, pepper and salt to the meat owl and mix it up. Add all chicken stock to pot and bring to a simmer over Saute mode
16. Once done, return seasoned meat to the pot and lock lid, cook on HIGH pressure for 45 minutes. Release pressure naturally over 10 minutes
17. Open lid and shred the meat using fork, transfer shredded meat to a bowl and pour cooking liquid through a mesh to separate fat into the bowl with shredded meat. Serve with lime and enjoy!

Nutrition Values (Per Serving)
- Calories: 307
- Fat: 23g
- Carbohydrates: 8g
- Protein: 15g

Special "Swiss" Pork chops
(Prepping time: 5 minutes\ Cooking time: 18 minutes | For 4 servings)

Ingredients

- ½ cup Swiss cheese, shredded
- 4 pork chops, bone-in
- 6 bacon strips, cut in half
- Salt and pepper to taste
- 1 tablespoon butter

Directions

1. Season pork chops with salt and pepper
2. Set your Foodi to sauté mode and add butter, let the butter heat up
3. Add pork chops and sauté for 3 minutes on each side. Add bacon strips and Swiss cheese
4. Lock lid and cook on Medium-LOW pressure for 15 minutes
5. Release pressure naturally over 10 minutes. Transfer steaks to serving platter, serve and enjoy!

Nutrition Values (Per Serving)
- Calories: 483
- Fat: 40g
- Carbohydrates: 0.7g
- Protein: 27g

Perfect Sichuan Pork Soup
(Prepping time: 10 minutes\ Cooking time: 20 minutes | For 6 servings)

Ingredients

Ingredients

- 2 pounds pork butt, chopped into 2 inch pieces
- 1 teaspoon salt
- ½ teaspoon oregano
- ½ teaspoon cumin
- 1 yellow onion, cut into half
- 6 garlic cloves, peeled and crushed
- ½ cup chicken broth

Directions

15. Insert a pan into your Ninja Foodi and add pork
16. Season with salt, cumin, oregano and mix well, making sure that the pork is well seasoned
17. Take the orange and squeeze the orange juice all over
18. Add squeezed orange to into the insert pan as well. Add garlic cloves and onions
19. Pour ½ cup chicken broth into the pan
20. Lock the lid of the Ninja Foodi, making sure that the valve is sealed well
21. Set pressure to HIGH and let it cook for 20 minutes
22. Once the timer beeps, quick release the pressure
23. Open the lid and take out orange, garlic cloves, and onions
24. Set your Nina Foodi to Sauté mode and adjust the temperature to medium-high
25. Let the liquid simmer for 10-15 minutes
26. After most of the liquid has been reduced, press stop button
27. Close the Ninja Foodi with "Air Crisp" lid. Pressure broil option and set timer to 8 minutes
28. Take the meat and put it in wraps. Garnish with cilantro and enjoy!

Nutrition Values (Per Serving)

- Calories: 355
- Fat: 13g
- Carbohydrates: 9g
- Protein: 43g

Mustard Dredged Pork Chops

(Prepping time: 10 minutes\ Cooking time: 30 minutes |For 4 servings)

Ingredients

- 2 tablespoons butter
- 2 tablespoons Dijon mustard (Keto-Friendly)
- 4 pork chops
- Salt and pepper to taste
- 1 tablespoon fresh rosemary, coarsely chopped

Directions

5. Take a bowl and add pork chops, cover with Dijon mustard and carefully sprinkle rosemary, salt and pepper. Let it marinate for 2 hours
6. Add butter and marinated pork chops to your Ninja Foodi pot
7. Lock lid and cook on Low-Medium Pressure for 30 minutes
8. Release pressure naturally over 10 minutes. Take the dish out, serve and enjoy!

Nutrition Values (Per Serving)

- Calories: 315
- Fat: 26g
- Carbohydrates: 1g
- Protein: 18g

Authentic Beginner Friendly Pork Belly

(Prepping time: 10 minutes\ Cooking time: 40 minutes |For 4 servings)

Ingredients

- 1 pound pork belly
- ½-1 cup white wine vinegar
- 1 garlic clove
- 1 tablespoon olive oil
- Salt and pepper to taste

Directions

7. Set your Ninja Foodi to "SAUTE" mode and add oil, let it heat up
8. Add pork and sear for 2-3 minutes until both sides are golden and crispy
9. Add vinegar until about a quarter inch, season with salt, pepper and garlic
10. Add garlic clove and Saute until the liquid comes to a boil

- 4 pounds pork roast
- 1 head butter lettuce, washed and dried
- 2 carrots, grated
- 2 tablespoons olive oil

For Spice Mix

- 1 tablespoon unsweetened cocoa powder
- 2 teaspoons oregano
- 1 teaspoon red pepper flakes
- 1 teaspoon garlic powder
- 2 lime wedges
- 1 onion, chopped
- 1 tablespoon salt
- 2-3 cups water
- 1 teaspoon white pepper
- 1 teaspoon cumin
- 1/8 teaspoon cayenne
- 1/8 teaspoon coriander

Directions

1. Marinate pork overnight by transferring the meat to a bowl and mixing in all of the spices
2. Set your Ninja Foodi to "SAUTE" mode and add roast, let it brown
3. Add 2-3 cups water to fully submerge the roast
4. Lock lid and cook on HIGH pressure for 55 minutes
5. Release pressure naturally over 10 minutes
6. Set your pot to "SAUTE" mode again and take out the meat, shred the meat and keep it on the side. Reduce the liquid by half and strain/skim any excess fat
7. Mix pork with cooking liquid and serve with lettuce, grated carrots, squire of lime and any other topping you desire. Enjoy!

Nutrition Values (Per Serving)

- Calories: 245
- Fat: 18g
- Carbohydrates: 4g
- Protein: 13g

Pork With Cranberries And Pecan

(Prepping time: 10 minutes\ Cooking time: 45 minutes |For 4 servings)

Ingredients

- ¼ cup of spicy brown mustard
- ½ a teaspoon of garlic powder
- ½ a teaspoon of stevia
- ½ a teaspoon of salt
- ¼ teaspoon of pepper freshly ground
- 3 and a ½ pound of pork shoulder, boneless and trimmed of excess fat
- 2 cups onion, chopped
- 1 cup of fresh cranberries
- 3 cups of cabbage, finely shredded
- ½ a cup of toasted pecans
- ½ a cup of dried cranberries

Directions

1. Take a small bowl and add mustard, stevia, garlic powder, pepper, and salt and mix them well
2. Rub the mix all over the pork
3. Add pork to the Ninja Foodi
4. Top with cranberries and onion
5. Lock up the lid and cook on HIGH pressure for 45 minutes
6. Release the pressure naturally
7. Transfer the pork to cutting board and shred using two forks
8. Strain the liquid making sure to discard the cranberries and onion
9. Pour the strained liquid over pork
10. Serve over shredded cabbage topped with pecans and cranberries
11. Enjoy!

Nutrition Values (Per Serving)

- Calories: 249
- Fats: 13g
- Carbs:7g
- Protein:25

Mesmerizing Pork Carnitas

(Prepping time: 10 minutes\ Cooking time: 25 minutes |For 4 servings)

2. Season with salt, cumin, oregano and mix well, making sure that the pork is well seasoned
3. Take the orange and squeeze the orange juice all over
4. Add squeezed orange to into the insert pan as well
5. Add garlic cloves and onions. Pour ½ cup chicken broth into the pan
6. Lock the lid of the Ninja Foodi, making sure that the valve is sealed well
7. Set pressure to HIGH and let it cook for 20 minutes
8. Once the timer beeps, quick release the pressure
9. Open the lid and take out orange, garlic cloves, and onions
10. Set your Nina Foodi to Sauté mode and adjust the temperature to medium-high
11. Let the liquid simmer for 10-15 minutes
12. After most of the liquid has been reduced, press the stop button
13. Close the Ninja Foodi with "Air Crisp" lid. Pressure broil option and set timer to 8 minutes
14. Take the meat and put it in wraps. Garnish with cilantro and enjoy!

Nutrition Values (Per Serving)

- Calories: 355
- Fat: 13g
- Carbohydrates: 9g
- Protein: 43g

Technical Keto Pork Belly

(Prepping time: 10 minutes \ Cooking time: 40 minutes | For 4 servings)

Ingredients

- 1 pound pork belly
- ½-1 cup white wine vinegar
- 1 garlic clove
- 1 tablespoon olive oil
- Salt and pepper to taste

Directions

1. Set your Ninja Foodi to "SAUTE" mode and add oil, let it heat up
2. Add pork and sear for 2-3 minutes until both sides are golden and crispy
3. Add vinegar until about a quarter inch, season with salt, pepper, and garlic
4. Add garlic clove and Saute until the liquid comes to a boil
5. Lock lid and cook on HIGH pressure for 40 minutes
6. Once done, quick release pressure. Slice the meat and serve with the sauce. Enjoy!

Nutrition Values (Per Serving)

- Calories: 331
- Fat: 21g
- Carbohydrates: 2g
- Protein: 19g

Jamaican Pork Pot

(Prepping time: 10 minutes \ Cooking time: 45 minutes | For 4 servings)

Ingredients

- ½ cup beef stock
- 1 tablespoon olive oil
- ¼ cup Jamaican jerk spice blend
- 4 ounces of pork shoulder

Directions

1. Rub roast with olive oil and spice blend
2. Set your Ninja Foodi to Saute mode and add meat, brown all sides
3. Pour beef broth. Lock lid and cook on HIGH pressure for 45 minutes
4. Quick release pressure. Shred pork and serve!

Nutrition Values (Per Serving)

- Calories: 308
- Fat: 18g
- Carbohydrates: 5g
- Protein: 31g

The Mexican Pulled Pork Ala Lettuce

(Prepping time: 10 minutes \ Cooking time: 60 minutes | For 4 servings)

Ingredients

Directions

1. Set your Ninja Foodi to Saute mode. Season the chops with pepper and salt
2. Toss your chops into your pot and cook for 4 minutes
3. Transfer the chops to a plate and repeat to cook and brown the rest
4. Pour in 1 tablespoon of butter and Toss in your carrots, dill to the cooker and let it cook for about 1 minute
5. Pour in the wine and scrape off any browned bits in your cooker while the liquid comes to a boil
6. Stir in the broth. return the chops to your pot
7. Lock up the lid and let it cook for about 18 minutes at high pressure
8. Naturally, release the pressure by keeping it aside for 8 minutes
9. Unlock and serve with some sauce poured over

Nutrition Values (Per Serving)

- Calories: 296
- Fat: 25g
- Carbohydrates: 2g
- Protein: 17g

Cranberry Pork BBQ Dish
(Prepping time: 10 minutes\ Cooking time: 45 minutes | For 4 servings)

Ingredients

- 3-4 pounds pork shoulder, boneless, fat trimmed

For Sauce

- 3 tablespoons of liquid smoke
- 2 tablespoons tomato paste
- 2 cups fresh cranberries
- ¼ cup hot sauce (Keto-Friendly)
- 1/3 cup blackstrap molasses
- ½ cup of water
- ½ cup apple cider vinegar
- 1 teaspoon salt
- 1 tablespoon adobo sauce (Keto Friendly and Sugar-Free)
- 1 cup tomato puree (Keto-Friendly and Sugar-Free)
- 1 chipotle pepper in adobo sauce, diced

Directions

1. Cut pork against halves/thirds and keep it on the side
2. Set your Ninja Foodi to "SAUTE" mode and let it heat up. Add cranberries and water to the pot
3. Let them simmer for 4-5 minutes until cranberries start to pop, add rest of the sauce ingredients and simmer for 5 minutes more. Add pork to the pot and lock lid
4. Cook on HIGH pressure for 40 minutes. Quick release pressure
5. Use a fork to shred the pork and serve on your favorite greens

Nutrition Values (Per Serving)

- Calories: 250
- Fat: 17g
- Carbohydrates: 5g
- Protein: 15g

Definitive Pork Carnita
(Prepping time: 10 minutes\ Cooking time: 25 minutes | For 4 servings)

Ingredients

- 2 pounds pork butt, chopped into 2-inch pieces
- 1 teaspoon salt
- ½ teaspoon oregano
- ½ teaspoon cumin
- 1 yellow onion, cut into half
- 6 garlic cloves, peeled and crushed
- ½ cup chicken broth

Directions

1. Insert a pan into your Ninja Foodi and add pork

Directions

1. Add the pork cubes to a pot and place it over medium heat
2. Add enough water to submerge them. Allow the water to come to a boil
3. Boil the cubes for 3 minutes and drain and rinse the cubes to remove any impurities
4. Keep them on the side. Set your Ninja Foodi to Saute mode and add maple syrup
5. Add cooked cubes and cook them for 1 minute until browned
6. After 10 minutes, add the remaining ingredients into the mix and bring the whole mixture to a boil. Lock up the lid and cook for 25 minutes at HIGH pressure
7. Allow the pressure to release naturally.
8. Open up the lid and set your Ninja Foodi to Saute mode again
9. Allow the contents to simmer for a while until the liquid has been reduced sufficiently enough to just coat the cubes. Serve with a garnish of cilantro. Enjoy!

Nutrition Values (Per Serving)

- Calories: 335
- Fats: 13g
- Carbs:16g
- Protein:31g

Cool Spicy Pork Salad Bowl

(Prepping time: 10 minutes\ Cooking time: 90 minutes |For 6 servings)

Ingredients

- 4 pounds pork shoulder butter
- 2 teaspoons salt
- 2 cups chicken stock
- 1 teaspoon smoked paprika powder
- 1 teaspoon garlic powder
- 1 teaspoon black pepper
- 1 pinch dried oregano leaves
- 4 tablespoons coconut oil
- 6 garlic cloves

Directions

1. Remove rind from pork and cut meat from the bone, slice into large chunks
2. Trim fat off met
3. Set your Foodi to Saute mode and add oil, let it heat up
4. Once the oil is hot, layer chunks of meat in the bottom of the pot and Saute for around 30 minutes until browned
5. While the meat is being browned, peel garlic cloves and cut into small chunks
6. Once the meat is browned, transfer it to a large-sized bowl
7. Add a few tablespoons of chicken stock to the pot a deglaze it, scraping off browned bits
8. Transfer browned bits to the bowl with meat chunks. Repeat if any more meat is left
9. Once done, add garlic, oregano leaves, smoked paprika, Garlic powder, pepper, and salt to the meat owl and mix it up. Add all chicken stock to the pot and bring to a simmer over Saute mode
10. Once done, return seasoned meat to the pot and lock lid, cook on HIGH pressure for 45 minutes. Release pressure naturally over 10 minutes
11. Open the lid and shred the meat using a fork, transfer shredded meat to a bowl and pour cooking liquid through a mesh to separate fat into the bowl with shredded meat
12. Serve with lime and enjoy!

Nutrition Values (Per Serving)

- Calories: 307
- Fat: 23g
- Carbohydrates: 8g
- Protein: 15g

Dill And Butter Pork Chops

(Prepping time: 10 minutes\ Cooking time: 20 minutes |For 4 servings)

Ingredients

- 2 tablespoons unsalted butter
- 4 pieces ½ inch thick pork loin chops
- ½ teaspoon salt
- ½ teaspoon pepper
- 16 baby carrots
- ½ cup white wine vinegar
- ½ cup chicken broth

4. Lock lid and cook on HIGH pressure for 1 minute. Quick release pressure
5. Arrange lettuce and green cabbage in serving bowls and add pulled pork on top
6. Top with guacamole and serve. Enjoy!

Nutrition Values (Per Serving)
- Calories: 417
- Fat: 95g
- Carbohydrates: 6g
- Protein: 75g

Awesome Sauerkraut Pork
(Prepping time: 10 minutes\ Cooking time: 35 minutes |For 4 servings)

Ingredients

- 3 pounds of pork shoulder
- Salt and pepper to taste
- 3 tablespoons butter
- 2 onions, chopped
- 3 cloves garlic, sliced
- 6 cups sauerkraut, divided
- 1 pound hot dog, sliced and cooked
- ½ pound kielbasa, sliced and cooked

Directions

1. Season pork roast with salt and pepper
2. Set your Ninja Foodi to Saute mode and add butter, let the butter melt
3. Add pork roast and brown. Pour 2 cups water, onion and garlic
4. Season with salt and pepper and lock lid. Cook on HIGH pressure for 35 minutes
5. Release pressure naturally over 10 minutes
6. Shred pork and stir in sauerkraut, hotdog, and kielbasa. Serve and enjoy!

Nutrition Values (Per Serving)
- Calories: 792
- Fat: 83g
- Carbohydrates: 14g
- Protein: 68g

Spice Lover's Jalapeno Hash
(Prepping time: 5 minutes\ Cooking time: 10 minutes |For 4 servings)

Ingredients

- 4 jalapeno peppers, chopped
- ½ cup chicken stock
- 3 ounces bacon, chopped and cooked
- 6 ounces zucchini, chopped
- 1 teaspoon ground black pepper
- 1 teaspoon butter

Directions

1. Add jalapeno peppers and zucchini into the Ninja Foodi pot
2. Put bacon, ground black pepper, butter, and chicken stock
3. Seal the lid. Set Pressure High. Cook the meat for 5 minutes
4. Then make natural pressure release for 10 minutes
5. Once cooked, let the meal chill for a few minutes. Serve with chicken stock and enjoy!

Nutrition Values (Per Serving)

- Calories: 139
- Fat: 10.3g
- Carbohydrates: 3.2g
- Protein: 8.8g

The Premium Red Pork
(Prepping time: 10 minutes\ Cooking time: 40 minutes |For 6 servings)

Ingredients

- 2 pounds of pork belly
- 2 tablespoons maple syrup
- 3 tablespoons sherry
- 1 tablespoon blackstrap molasses
- 2 tablespoons coconut amino
- 1 teaspoon salt
- 1/3 cup water
- 1 piece ginger, peeled and smashed
- Few sprigs of cilantro, garnish

Chapter 7: Pork Recipes

Spicy "Faux" Pork Belly
(Prepping time: 10 minutes\ Cooking time: 15 minutes | For 4 servings)

Ingredients

- 1 pound of pork belly, chopped
- 4 cups cauliflower, riced
- ½ a cup of bone broth
- ½ red onion, sliced
- ½ a cup of cilantro
- 2 green onion, sliced

- 1 tablespoon of lime juice
- 3 cloves garlic cloves, sliced
- 1 teaspoon turmeric
- 1 tablespoon oregano
- 1 tablespoon cumin
- ½ a teaspoon salt

Directions

1. Add all of the ingredients to your Instant Pot except ¼ cup of cilantro
2. Lock up the lid and cook on HIGH pressure for 15 minutes
3. Release the pressure naturally over 10 minutes
4. Open the lid and serve with sprinkled cilantro leaves
5. Enjoy!

Nutrition Values (Per Serving)

- Calories: 277
- Fat: 18g

- Carbohydrates: 3g
- Protein: 24g

Spiced Up Chipotle Pork Roast
(Prepping time: 5 minutes\ Cooking time:605 minutes | For 4 servings)

Ingredients

- 6 ounces bone broth
- 7 and ¼ ounces tomatoes, diced
- 2 ounces green chilies, diced
- 2 pounds pork roast

- ½ teaspoon cumin, onion powder each
- 1 teaspoon chipotle powder

Direction

1. Add listed ingredients to your Ninja Foodi. Lock lid and cook on HIGH pressure for 60 minutes
2. Release pressure naturally over 10 minutes. Serve and enjoy!

Nutrition Values (Per Serving)

- Calories: 460
- Fat: 31g

- Carbohydrates: 4g
- Protein: 40g

Happy Burrito Bowl Pork
(Prepping time: 10 minutes\ Cooking time: 5 minutes | For 4 servings)

Ingredients

- 1 and ½ tablespoons pork lard
- 1 onion, sliced
- 2 bell peppers, sliced
- 1 garlic clove, chopped
- Salt and pepper to taste
- 1 pound pulled pork

- ½ cup of chicken pork
- ½ cup chicken broth
- 6 cups lettuce, chopped
- 6 cups cabbage, chopped
- ¼ cup guacamole

Directions

1. Set your Ninja Foodi to Saute mode and add lard, let it melt and add onion and bell pepper
2. Cook for 2 minutes, stirring for 2 minutes. Add garlic, salt, and pepper
3. Stir well. Add pulled pork and chicken pork

Nutrition Values (Per Serving)
- Calories: 423
- Fat: 35g
- Carbohydrates: 4g
- Protein: 22g

Traditional Beef Sirloin Steak
(Prepping time: 5 minutes\ Cooking time: 17 minutes |For 4 servings)

Ingredients

- 3 tablespoons butter
- ½ teaspoon garlic powder
- 1-2 pounds beef sirloin steaks
- Salt and pepper to taste
- 1 garlic clove, minced

Directions

6. Set your Ninja Foodi to sauté mode and add butter, let the butter melt
7. Add beef sirloin steaks . Saute for 2 minutes on each side
8. Add garlic powder, garlic clove, salt, and pepper
9. Lock lid and cook on Medium-HIGH pressure for 15 minutes
10. Release pressure naturally over 10 minutes
11. Transfer prepare Steaks to a serving platter, enjoy!

Nutrition Values (Per Serving)
- Calories: 246
- Fat: 13g
- Carbohydrates: 2g
- Protein: 31g

Beef And Broccoli Platter
(Prepping time: 10 minutes\ Cooking time: 20 minutes |For 4 servings)

Ingredients

- 3 pounds beef chuck roast, cut into thin strips
- 1 tablespoon olive oil
- 1 yellow onion, peeled and chopped
- ½ cup beef stock
- 1 pound broccoli florets
- 2 teaspoons toasted sesame oil
- 2 tablespoons arrowroot

For Marinade

- 1 cup coconut aminos
- 1 tablespoon sesame oil
- 2 tablespoons fish sauce
- 5 garlic cloves, peeled and minced
- 3 red peppers, dried and crushed
- ½ teaspoon Chinese five spice powder
- Toasted sesame seeds, for serving

Directions

8. Take a bowl and mix in coconut aminos, fish sauce, 1 tablespoon sesame oil, garlic, five spice powder, crushed red pepper and stir
9. Add beef strips to the bowl and toss to coat. Keep it on the side for 10 minutes
10. Set your Ninja Foodi to "Saute" mode and add oil, let it heat up, add onion and stir cook for 4 minutes. Add beef and marinade, stir cook for 2 minutes. Add stock and stir
11. Lock the pressure lid of Ninja Foodi and cook on HIGH pressure for 5 minutes
12. Release pressure naturally over 10 minutes
13. Mix arrowroot with ¼ cup liquid from the pot and gently pour the mixture back to the pot and stir
14. Place a steamer basket in the pot and add broccoli to the steamer rack, lock lid and cook on HIGH pressure for 3 minutes more, quick release pressure
15. Divide the dish between plates and serve with broccoli, toasted sesame seeds and enjoy!

Nutrition Values (Per Serving)
- Calories: 433
- Fat: 27g
- Carbohydrates: 8g
- Protein: 20g

1. Set your Ninja Foodi to Saute mode add beef, brown the beef
2. Add onion and garlic
3. Add parmesan, ricotta, egg in a small dish and keep it on the side
4. Add sauce to browned meat, reserve half for later
5. Sprinkle mozzarella and half of ricotta cheese to the browned meat
6. Top with remaining meat sauce
7. For the final layer, add more mozzarella cheese and remaining ricotta
8. Stir well . Cover with foil transfer to Ninja Foodi
9. Lock lid and cook on HIGH pressure for 8-10 minutes
10. Quick release pressure. Drizzle parmesan cheese on top. Enjoy!

Nutrition Values (Per Serving)

- Calories: 365
- Fats: 25g
- Carbs: 6g
- Protein: 25g

The Wisdom Worthy Corned Beef
(Prepping time: 10 minutes\ Cooking time: 60 minutes | For 4 servings)

Ingredients

- 4 pounds beef brisket
- 2 garlic cloves, peeled and minced
- 2 yellow onions, peeled and sliced
- 11 ounces celery, thinly sliced
- 1 tablespoon dried dill
- 3 bay leaves
- 4 cinnamon sticks, cut into halves
- Salt and pepper to taste
- 17 ounces of water

Directions

7. Take a bowl and add beef, add water and cover, let it soak for 2-3 hours
8. Drain and transfer to the Ninja Foodi
9. Add celery, onions, garlic, bay leaves, dill, cinnamon, dill, salt, pepper and rest of the water to the Ninja Foodi
10. Stir and combine it well. Lock lid and cook on HIGH pressure for 50 minutes
11. Release pressure naturally over 10 minutes
12. Transfer meat to cutting board and slice, divide amongst plates and pour the cooking liquid (alongside veggies) over the servings. Enjoy!

Nutrition Values (Per Serving)

- Calories: 289
- Fat: 21g
- Carbohydrates: 14g
- Protein: 9g

Hearty Korean Ribs
(Prepping time: 10 minutes\ Cooking time: 45 minutes | For 6 servings)

Ingredients

- 1 teaspoon olive oil
- 2 green onions, cut into 1-inch length
- 3 garlic cloves, smashed
- 3 quarter sized ginger slices
- 4 pounds beef short ribs, 3 inches thick, cut into 3 rib portions
- ½ cup of water
- ½ cup coconut aminos
- ¼ cup dry white wine
- 2 teaspoons sesame oil
- Mince green onions for serving

Directions

6. Set your Ninja Foodi to "SAUTE" mode and add oil, let it shimmer
7. Add green onions, garlic, ginger, Saute for 1 minute
8. Add short ribs, water, amines, wine, sesame oil, and stir until the ribs are coated well
9. Lock lid and cook on HIGH pressure for 45 minutes . Release pressure naturally over 10 minutes
10. Remove short ribs from pot and serve with the cooking liquid. Enjoy!

- Calories: 303
- Fats: 21g
- Carbs: 4g
- Protein: 21g

Hybrid Beef Prime Roast
(Prepping time: 10 minutes\ Cooking time: 45 minutes | For 4 servings)

Ingredients

- 2 pounds chuck roast
- 1 tablespoon olive oil
- 1 teaspoon salt
- 1 teaspoon ground black pepper
- 1 teaspoon onion powder
- 1 teaspoon garlic powder
- 4 cups beef stock

Directions

1. Place roast in Ninja Food pot and season it well with salt and pepper
2. Add oil and set the pot to Saute mode, sear each side of roast for 3 minutes until slightly browned . Add beef broth, onion powder, garlic powder, and stir
3. Lock lid and cook on HIGH pressure for 40 minutes
4. Once the timer goes off, naturally release pressure over 10 minutes
5. Open the lid and serve hot. Enjoy!

Nutrition Values (Per Serving)

- Calories: 308
- Fat: 22g
- Carbohydrates: 2g
- Protein: 24g

The Epic Carne Guisada
(Prepping time: 10 minutes\ Cooking time: 45 minutes | For 4 servings)

Ingredients

- 3 pounds beef stew
- 3 tablespoon seasoned salt
- 1 tablespoon oregano chili powder
- 1 tablespoon organic cumin
- 1 pinch crushed red pepper
- 2 tablespoons olive oil
- ½ medium lime, juiced
- 1 cup beef bone broth
- 3 ounces tomato paste
- 1 large onion, sliced

Directions

1. Trim the beef stew as needed into small bite-sized portions
2. Toss the beef stew pieces with dry seasoning
3. Set your Ninja Foodi to Saute mode and add oil, allow the oil to heat up
4. Add seasoned beef pieces and brown them
5. Combine the browned beef pieces with rest of the ingredients
6. Lock up the lid and cook on HIGH pressure for 3 minutes. Release the pressure naturally . Enjoy!

Nutrition Values (Per Serving)

- Protein: 33g
- Carbs: 11g
- Fats: 12g
- Calories: 274

No-Noodle Pure Lasagna
(Prepping time: 10 minutes\ Cooking time: 10-15 minutes | For 4 servings)

Ingredients

- 2 small onions
- 2 garlic cloves, minced
- 1 pound ground beef
- 1 large egg
- 1 and ½ cups ricotta cheese
- ½ cup parmesan cheese
- 1 jar (25 ounces0 marinara sauce
- 8 ounces mozzarella cheese, sliced

Directions

- 1 teaspoon ground cumin
- 1-2 bay leaves
- 2 tablespoons green olives, capers
- 2 tablespoons brine
- 3 tablespoons water

Directions

1. Set your Ninja Foodi to Saute mode and add meat, salt, and pepper, slightly brown
2. Add garlic, tomato, onion, cilantro and Saute for 1 minute
3. Add olives, brine, leaf, cumin, and mix. Pour in sauce, water, and stir
4. Lock lid and cook on HIGH pressure for 15 minutes. Quick release pressure

Nutrition Values (Per Serving)

- Calories: 207
- Fats: 8g
- Carbs: 4g
- Protein: 25g

Simple/Aromatic Meatballs
(Prepping time: 8 minutes\ Cooking time: 11 minutes |For 4 servings)

Ingredients

- 2 cups ground beef
- 1 egg, beaten
- 1 teaspoon Taco seasoning
- 1 tablespoon sugar-free marinara sauce
- 1 teaspoon garlic, minced
- ½ teaspoon salt

Directions

1. Take a big mixing bowl and place all the ingredients into the bowl
2. Add all the ingredients into the bowl. Mix together all the ingredients by using a spoon or fingertips. Then make the small size meatballs and put them in a layer in the air fryer rack
3. Lower the air fryer lid. Cook the meatballs for 11 minutes at 350 F. Serve immediately and enjoy!

Nutrition Values (Per Serving)

- Calories: 205
- Fat: 12.2g
- Carbohydrates: 2.2g
- Protein: 19.4g

Generous Shepherd's Pie
(Prepping time: 10 minutes\ Cooking time: 10-15 minutes |For 4 servings)

Ingredients

- 2 cups of water
- 4 tablespoons butter
- 4 ounces cream cheese
- 1 cup mozzarella
- 1 whole egg
- Salt and pepper to taste
- 1 tablespoon garlic powder
- 2-3 pounds ground beef
- 1 cup frozen carrots
- 8 ounces mushrooms, sliced
- 1 cup beef broth

Directions

1. Add water to Ninja Foodi, arrange cauliflower on top, lock lid and cook for 5 minutes on HIGH pressure
2. Quick release and transfer to a blender, add cream cheese, butter, mozzarella cheese, egg, pepper, and salt. Blend well. Drain water from Ninja Foodi and add beef
3. Add carrots, garlic powder, broth and pepper, and salt
4. Add in cauliflower mix and lock lid, cook for 10 minutes on HIGH pressure
5. Release pressure naturally over 10 minutes. Serve and enjoy!

Nutrition Values (Per Serving)

Nutrition Values (Per Serving)
- Calories: 433
- Fat: 27g
- Carbohydrates: 8g
- Protein: 20g

The Juicy Beef Chili
(Prepping time: 10 minutes \ Cooking time: 40 minutes |For 4 servings)

Ingredients

- 1 and ½ pounds ground beef
- 1 sweet onion, peeled and chopped
- Salt and pepper to taste
- 28 ounces canned tomatoes, diced
- 17 ounces beef stock
- 6 garlic clove, peeled and chopped
- 7 jalapeno peppers, diced
- 2 tablespoons olive oil
- 4 carrots, peeled and chopped
- 3 tablespoons chili powder
- 1 bay leaf
- 1 teaspoon chili powder

Directions

1. Set your Ninja Foodi to "Saute" mode and add half of oil, let it heat up
2. Add beef and stir brown for 8 minutes, transfer to a bowl
3. Add remaining oil to the pot and let it heat up, add carrots, onion, jalapenos, garlic and stir Saute for 4 minutes. Add tomatoes and stir
4. Add bay leaf, stock, chili powder, chili powder, salt, pepper and beef, stir and lock lid
5. Cook on HIGH pressure for 25 minutes. Release pressure naturally over 10 minutes
6. Stir the chili and serve. Enjoy!

Nutrition Values (Per Serving)
- Calories: 448
- Fat: 22g
- Carbohydrates: 7g
- Protein: 15g

Generous Ground Beef Stew
(Prepping time: 5 minutes \ Cooking time: 5 minutes |For 4 servings)

Ingredients

- 1 tablespoon olive oil
- 1 and ½ pounds lean ground beef
- 1 large yellow onion, chopped
- 1 teaspoon ground cinnamon
- 1 teaspoon ground cumin
- ½ teaspoon dried sage
- ½ teaspoon dried oregano
- ½ teaspoon salt
- ½ teaspoon pepper
- 2 tablespoons almond meal
- 2 and ½ cups beef broth
- 2 teaspoons stevia

Directions

1. Set your Ninja Foodi to Saute mode and add oil, let it heat up
2. Add ground beef and stir for about 5 minutes until browned
3. Add onion, and cook for 3 minutes more
4. Stir in cinnamon, cumin, sage, oregano, salt, pepper and cook for 1 minute
5. Stir in almond meal and cook for 1 minute more. Stir in broth
6. Lock lid and cook on HIGH pressure for 5 minutes, release pressure naturally over 10 minutes
7. Stir well until loosely covered, serve and enjoy!

Nutrition Values (Per Serving)
- Calories: 480
- Fat: 23g
- Carbohydrates: 12g
- Protein: 20g

Quick Picadillo Dish
(Prepping time: 10 minutes \ Cooking time: 15-20 minutes |For 4 servings)

Ingredients

- ½ pound lean ground beef
- 2 garlic cloves, minced
- ½ large onion, chopped
- 1 teaspoon salt
- 1 tomato, chopped
- ½ red bell pepper, chopped
- 1 tablespoon cilantro
- ½ can (4 ounces) tomato sauce

Directions

1. Set your Ninja Foodi to Saute mode and add sesame oil, garlic, ginger, red pepper flakes and Saute for 1 minute. Deglaze pot with vinegar and mix in coconut aminos and beef stock
2. Add ribs to the pot and coat them well. Lock lid and cook on HIGH pressure for 60 minutes
3. Release pressure naturally over 10 minutes. Remove the ribs and keep them on the side
4. Take small bowl and mix in arrowroot and water, stir and mix in the liquid into the pot, set the pot to Saute mode and cook until the liquid reaches your desired consistency
5. Put the ribs under a broiler to brown them slightly (also possible to do this in the Ninja Foodi using the Air Crisping lid). Serve ribs with the cooking liquid. Enjoy!

Nutrition Values (Per Serving)

- Calories: 307
- Fat: 10g
- Carbohydrates: 5g
- Protein: 32g

Everyday Lamb Roast

(Prepping time: 10 minutes\ Cooking time: 60 minutes |For 6 servings)

Ingredients

- 2 pounds lamb roasted wegmans
- 1 cup onion soup
- 1 cup beef broth
- Salt and pepper to taste

Directions

4. Transfer lamb roast to your Ninja Foodi pot. Add onion soup, beef broth, salt and pepper
5. Lock lid and cook on Medium-HIGH pressure for 55 minutes
6. Release pressure naturally over 10 minutes. Transfer to serving bowl, serve and enjoy!

Nutrition Values (Per Serving)

- Calories: 349
- Fat: 18g
- Carbohydrates: 2.9g
- Protein: 39g

The Gentle Beef And Broccoli Dish

(Prepping time: 10 minutes\ Cooking time: 20 minutes |For 4 servings)

Ingredients

- 3 pounds beef chuck roast, cut into thin strips
- 1 tablespoon olive oil
- 1 yellow onion, peeled and chopped
-
- ½ cup beef stock
- 1 pound broccoli florets
- 2 teaspoons toasted sesame oil
- 2 tablespoons arrowroot

For Marinade

- 1 cup coconut aminos
- 1 tablespoon sesame oil
- 2 tablespoons fish sauce
- 5 garlic cloves, peeled and minced
- 3 red peppers, dried and crushed
- ½ teaspoon Chinese five spice powder
- Toasted sesame seeds, for serving

Directions

1. Take a bowl and mix in coconut aminos, fish sauce, 1 tablespoon sesame oil, garlic, five spice powder, crushed red pepper and stir. Add beef strips to the bowl and toss to coat
2. Keep it on the side for 10 minutes
3. Set your Ninja Foodi to "Saute" mode and add oil, let it heat up, add onion and stir cook for 4 minutes. Add beef and marinade, stir cook for 2 minutes. Add stock and stir
4. Lock the pressure lid of Ninja Foodi and cook on HIGH pressure for 5 minutes
5. Release pressure naturally over 10 minutes
6. Mix arrowroot with ¼ cup liquid from the pot and gently pour the mixture back to the pot and stir. Place a steamer basket in the pot and add broccoli to the steamer rack, lock lid and cook on HIGH pressure for 3 minutes more, quick release pressure
7. Divide the dish between plates and serve with broccoli, toasted sesame seeds and enjoy!

4. Add carrots, and cabbage to the pot, lock lid again and cook on HIGH pressure for 5 minutes more. Quick release pressure. Transfer veggies to the plate with corned beef
5. Pass the gravy through a gravy strainer over the beef and serve. Enjoy!

<u>Nutrition Values (Per Serving)</u>
- Calories: 531
- Fat: 45g
- Carbohydrates: 9g
- Protein: 25g

Crazy Greek Lamb Gyros
(Prepping time: 10 minutes\ Cooking time: 25 minutes |For 8 servings)

<u>Ingredients</u>

- 8 garlic cloves
- 1 and ½ teaspoon salt
- 2 teaspoons dried oregano
- 1 and ½ cups water
- 2 pounds lamb meat, ground
- 2 teaspoons rosemary
- ½ teaspoon pepper
- 1 small onion, chopped
- 2 teaspoons ground marjoram

<u>Directions</u>

1. Add onions, garlic, marjoram, rosemary, salt and pepper to a food processor
2. Process until combined well, add round lamb meat and process again
3. Press meat mixture gently into a loaf pan. Transfer the pan to your Ninja Foodi pot
4. Lock lid and select "Bake/Roast" mode. Bake for 25 minutes at 375 degrees F
5. Transfer to serving dish and enjoy!

<u>Nutrition Values (Per Serving)</u>
- Calories: 242
- Fat: 15g
- Carbohydrates: 2.4g
- Protein: 21g

The Ultimate One-Pot Beef Roast
(Prepping time: 10 minutes\ Cooking time: 40 minutes |For 4 servings)

<u>Ingredients</u>

- 2-3 pounds beef, chuck roast
- 4 carrots, chopped
- 3 garlic cloves,
- 2 tablespoons olive oil
- 2 tablespoons Italian seasoning
- 2 stalks celery, chopped
- 1 onion, chopped
- 1 cup beef broth
- 1 cup dry red wine

<u>Directions</u>

1. Set your Ninja Foodi to "Saute" mode and add oil, let it heat up
2. Add roast beef to the pot and cook each side for 1-2 minute until browned
3. Transfer browned beef to plate. Add celery, carrot to the pot and top with garlic and onion
4. Add beef broth and wine to the pot, put roast on top of vegies
5. Spread seasoning on top and lock lid, Cook on HIGH pressure for 35 minutes
6. Release pressure naturally over 10 minutes. Serve and enjoy!

<u>Nutrition Values (Per Serving)</u>
- Calories: 299
- Fat: 21g
- Carbohydrates: 3g
- Protein: 14g

Easy To Swallow Beef Ribs
(Prepping time: 10 minutes\ Cooking time: 60 minutes |For 6 servings)

<u>Ingredients</u>

- 1 tablespoon sesame oil
- 2 garlic cloves, peeled and smashed
- 1 Knob fresh ginger, peeled and finely chopped
- 1 pinch red pepper flakes
- ¼ cup white wine vinegar
- 2/3 cup coconut aminos
- 2/3 cup beef stock
- 4 pounds beef ribs, chopped in half
- 2 tablespoons arrowroot
- 1-2 tablespoons water

- ½ yellow onion, chopped
- 1 tablespoon olive oil
- 2 garlic cloves, minced
- 1 jalapeno pepper, chopped
- 1 cup cherry tomatoes, quartered

- 1 teaspoon fresh lemon juice
- 1-2 pounds grass fed ground beef
- 1-2 pounds fresh collard greens, trimmed and chopped

Spices

- 1 teaspoon cumin, ground
- ½ teaspoon ginger, ground
- 1 teaspoon coriander, ground
- ½ teaspoon fennel seeds, ground

- ½ teaspoon cinnamon, ground
- Salt and pepper to taste
- ½ teaspoon turmeric, ground

Directions

1. Set your Ninja Foodi to sauté mode and add garlic, onions
2. sauté for 3 minutes. Add jalapeno pepper, beef and spices
3. Lock lid and cook on Medium-HIGH pressure for 15 minutes
4. Release pressure naturally over 10 minutes, open lid
5. Add tomatoes, collard greens and sauté for 3 minutes
6. Stir in lemon juice, salt and pepper. Stir well
7. Once the dish is ready, transfer the dish to your serving bowl and enjoy!

Nutrition Values (Per Serving)

- Calories: 409
- Fat: 16g

- Carbohydrates: 5g
- Protein: 56g

Fresh Korean Braised Ribs
(Prepping time: 10 minutes\ Cooking time: 45 minutes |For 6 servings)

Ingredients

- 1 teaspoon olive oil
- 2 green onions, cut into 1 inch length
- 3 garlic cloves, smashed
- 3 quarter sized ginger slices
- 4 pounds beef short ribs, 3 inches thick, cut into 3 rib portions

- ½ cup water
- ½ cup coconut aminos
- ¼ cup dry white wine
- 2 teaspoons sesame oil
- Mince green onions for serving

Directions

1. Set your Ninja Foodi to "SAUTE" mode and add oil, let it shimmer
2. Add green onions, garlic, ginger, Saute for 1 minute
3. Add short ribs, water, aminos, wine, sesame oil and stir until the ribs are coated well
4. Lock lid and cook on HIGH pressure for 45 minutes. Release pressure naturally over 10 minutes
5. Remove short ribs from pot and serve with the cooking liquid. Enjoy!

Nutrition Values (Per Serving)

- Calories: 423
- Fat: 35g

- Carbohydrates: 4g
- Protein: 22g

The Classical Corned Beef And Cabbage
(Prepping time: 15 minutes\ Cooking time: 90 minutes |For 4 servings)

Ingredients

- 3 pounds cabbage, cut into eight wedges
- 1 onion, quartered
- 1 celery stalk, quartered

- 1 corned beef spice packet
- 4 cups water
- 1 pound carrots ,peeled and cut to 2 and ½ inch length

Directions

1. Rinse beef thoroughly and add to Ninja Foodi
2. Add onion and celery to the pot. Add water and lock lid
3. Cook on HIGH pressure for 90 minutes, quick release pressure. Transfer beef to a plate

Directions

1. Set your Ninja Foodi to "Saute" mode and add oil, let it heat up
2. Add onions, garlic, stir cook for 4 minutes
3. Add mustard, stir and cook for 1 minute
4. Add beef and stir until all sides are browned
5. Add curry powder, salt and pepper, stir cook for 2 minutes
6. Add coconut milk and tomato sauce, stir and cove
7. Lock lid and cook on HIGH pressure for 10 minutes
8. Release pressure naturally over 10 minutes. Serve and enjoy!

Nutrition Values (Per Serving)

- Calories: 275
- Fat: 12g
- Carbohydrates: 12g
- Protein: 27g

Mesmerizing Beef Sirloin Steak

(Prepping time: 5 minutes\ Cooking time: 17 minutes |For 4 servings)

Ingredients

- 3 tablespoons butter
- ½ teaspoon garlic powder
- 1-2 pounds beef sirloin steaks
- Salt and pepper to taste
- 1 garlic clove, minced

Directions

1. Set your Ninja Foodi to sauté mode and add butter, let the butter melt
2. Add beef sirloin steaks. Saute for 2 minutes on each side
3. Add garlic powder, garlic clove, salt and pepper
4. Lock lid and cook on Medium-HIGH pressure for 15 minutes
5. Release pressure naturally over 10 minutes. Transfer prepare Steaks to serving platter, enjoy!

Nutrition Values (Per Serving)

- Calories: 246
- Fat: 13g
- Carbohydrates: 2g
- Protein: 31g

Epic Beef Sausage Soup

(Prepping time: 10 minutes\ Cooking time: 30 minutes |For 6 servings)

Ingredients

- 1 tablespoon extra virgin olive oil
- 6 cups beef broth
- 1 pound organic beef sausage, cooked and sliced
- 2 cups sauerkraut
- 2 celery stalks, chopped
- 1 sweet onion, chopped
- 2 teaspoons garlic, minced
- 2 tablespoons butter
- 1 tablespoon hot mustard
- ½ teaspoon caraway seeds
- ½ cup sour cream
- 2 tablespoons fresh parsley, chopped

Directions

1. Grease the inner pot of your Ninja Foodi with olive oil
2. Add broth, sausage, sauerkraut, celery, onion, garlic, butter, mustard, caraway seeds in the pot
3. Lock lid and cook on HIGH pressure for 30 minutes. Quick release pressure
4. Remove lid and stir in sour cream. Serve with a topping of parsley. Enjoy!

Nutrition Values (Per Serving)

- Calories: 165
- Fat: 4g
- Carbohydrates: 14g
- Protein: 11g

The Indian Beef Delight

(Prepping time: 15 minutes\ Cooking time: 20 minutes |For 4 servings)

Ingredients

Chapter 6: Beef and Lamb Recipes

Warm And Beefy Meat Loaf

(Prepping time: 10 minutes\ Cooking time: 1 hour 10 minutes |For 6 servings)

Ingredients

- ½ cup onion, chopped
- 2 garlic cloves, minced
- ¼ cup sugar free ketchup
- 1 pound grass fed-lean ground beef
- ½ cup green bell pepper, seeded and chopped
- 1 cup cheddar cheese, grated
- 2 organic eggs, beaten
- 1 teaspoon dried thyme, crushed
- 3 cups fresh spinach, chopped
- 6 cups mozzarella cheese, freshly grated
- Black pepper to taste

Directions

1. Take a bowl and add all of the listed ingredients except cheese and spinach
2. Place a wax paper on a smooth surface and arrange the meat over it
3. Top with spinach, cheese and roll the paper around the paper to form a nice meat loaf
4. Remove wax paper and transfer loaf to your Ninja Foodi
5. Lock lid and select "Bake/Roast" mode, setting the timer to 70 minutes and temperature to 380 degrees F. Let it bake and take the dish out once done. Serve and enjoy!

Nutrition Values (Per Serving)

- Calories: 409
- Fat: 16g
- Carbohydrates: 5g
- Protein: 56g

Wise Corned Beef

(Prepping time: 10 minutes\ Cooking time: 60 minutes |For 4 servings)

Ingredients

- 4 pounds beef brisket
- 2 garlic cloves, peeled and minced
- 2 yellow onions, peeled and sliced
- 11 ounces celery, thinly sliced
- 1 tablespoon dried dill
- 3 bay leaves
- 4 cinnamon sticks, cut into halves
- Salt and pepper to taste
- 17 ounces water

Directions

1. Take a bowl and add beef, add water and cover, let it soak for 2-3 hours
2. Drain and transfer to the Ninja Foodi
3. Add celery, onions, garlic, bay leaves, dill, cinnamon, dill, salt, pepper and rest of the water to the Ninja Foodi. Stir and combine it well
4. Lock lid and cook on HIGH pressure for 50 minutes
5. Release pressure naturally over 10 minutes
6. Transfer meat to cutting board and slice, divide amongst plates and pour the cooking liquid (alongside veggies) over the servings. Enjoy!

Nutrition Values (Per Serving)

- Calories: 289
- Fat: 21g
- Carbohydrates: 14g
- Protein: 9g

Elegant Beef Curry

(Prepping time: 10 minutes\ Cooking time: 20 minutes |For 4 servings)

Ingredients

- 2 pounds beef steak, cubed
- 2 tablespoons extra virgin olive oil
- 1 tablespoon Dijon mustard
- 2 and ½ tablespoons curry powder
- 2 yellow onions, peeled and chopped
- 2 garlic cloves, peeled and minced
- 10 ounces canned coconut milk
- 2 tablespoons tomato sauce
- Salt and pepper to taste

- ¼ teaspoon ground black pepper
- ¼ teaspoon cayenne pepper
- 4 large skinless turkey thighs

Directions

1. Gently lay the garlic and onions into the bottom of your Ninja Foodi
2. Pour in some wine with a sprinkle of salt, cayenne pepper, and black pepper.
3. Add turkey thighs and cover it up. Let it cook SLOW COOKER MODE (low) for about 8 hours.
4. Remove the turkey from the crock pot and clean up the flesh from the bones.
5. Keep the lid open and keep cooking until the liquid has completely evaporated, making sure to stir from time to time. Return the turkey to the pot.
6. Nestle the turkey into the mix. Serve hot. Enjoy!

Nutrition Values (Per Serving)

- Calories: 845
- Fat: 41g
- Carbohydrates: 7g
- Protein: 45g

Awesome Ligurian Chicken
(Prepping time: 10 minutes\ Cooking time: 15 minutes |For 4 servings)

Ingredients

- 2 garlic cloves, chopped
- 3 sprigs fresh rosemary
- 2 sprigs fresh sage
- ½ bunch parsley
- 3 lemon, juiced
- 4 tablespoons extra virgin olive oil
- 1 teaspoon salt
- ¼ teaspoon pepper
- 1 and ½ cup of water
- 1 whole chicken, cut into parts
- 3 and ½ ounces black gourmet salt-cured olives
- 1 fresh lemon

Directions

1. Take a bowl and add chopped up garlic, parsley, sage, and rosemary
2. Pour lemon juice, olive oil to a bowl and season with salt and pepper
3. Remove the chicken skin and from the chicken pieces and carefully transfer them to a dish
4. Pour the marinade on top of the chicken pieces and allow them to chill for 2-4 hours
5. Set your Ninja Foodi to Saute mode and add olive oil, allow it to heat up
6. Add chicken and browned on all sides
7. Measure out the marinade and add to the pot (it should cover the chicken, add a bit of water if needed). Lock up the lid and cook on HIGH pressure for 10 minutes
8. Release the pressure naturally. The chicken out and transfer to a platter
9. Cover with a foil and allow them to cool. Set your pot in Saute mode and reduce the liquid to ¼
10. Add the chicken pieces again to the pot and allow them to warm
11. Sprinkle a bit of olive, lemon slices, and rosemary. Enjoy!

Nutrition Values (Per Serving)
- Calories: 303
- Fats: 20g
- Carbs: 10g
- Protein: 12g

(Prepping time: 10 minutes\ Cooking time: 10 minutes |For 4 servings)

Ingredients

- 1 tablespoon rice vinegar
- 1 tablespoon Truvia
- 1 tablespoon garlic, minced
- 1 tablespoon fresh ginger, minced
- 1 tablespoon sesame oil
- 2 tablespoons soy sauce
- 1 and ½ pound boneless, skinless chicken thigh, cut into large pieces

Directions

1. Take a heatproof bowl and add soy sauce, ginger, sesame oil, garlic, Truvia and vinegar
2. Stir well to coat it. Cover bowl with foil. Add 2 cups of water to Ninja Foodie's inner pot
3. Place a trivet and place the bowl with chicken on the trivet
4. Lock lid and cook for 10 minutes on HIGH pressure. Release pressure naturally over 10 minutes
5. Remove chicken and shred it, mix it back into the bowl. Serve and enjoy!

Nutrition Values (Per Serving)

- Calories: 118
- Fats: 10g
- Carbs: 7g
- Protein: 3g

Chicken Korma
(Prepping time: 10 minutes\ Cooking time: 20 minutes |For 6 servings)

Ingredients

- 1 pound of chicken

For Sauce

- 1 ounce of cashews
- 1 small chopped onion
- ½ a cup of diced tomatoes
- ½ of green Serrano pepper
- 5 cloves of garlic
- 1 teaspoon of minced ginger
- 1 teaspoon of turmeric
- 1 teaspoon of Garam masala
- 1 teaspoon of cumin-coriander powder
- ½ a teaspoon of cayenne pepper
- ½ a cup of water

For topping

- 1 teaspoon of Garam masala
- ½ a cup of coconut milk
- ¼ cup of chopped cilantro

Directions

1. Add the sauce ingredients to a blender and blend them well
2. Pour the sauce to your Ninja Foodi. Place the chicken on top
3. Lock up the lid and cook on HIGH pressure for 10 minutes
4. Release the pressure naturally. Take the chicken out and cut into bite-sized portions
5. Add coconut milk, Garam masala to the pot
6. Transfer the chicken back and garnish with cilantro. Enjoy!

Nutrition Values (Per Serving)

- Calories: 388
- Fats: 14g
- Carbs: 16g
- Protein: 48g

Turkey With Garlic Sauce
(Prepping time: 10 minutes\ Cooking time: 8 hours |For 6 servings)

Ingredients

- 5 large onions, thinly sliced
- 4 garlic cloves, minced
- ¼ cup white wine vinegar
- ½ teaspoon salt

Directions

1. Add chicken breast to the Ninja Foodi
2. Add ghee, salt, diced garlic and lock up the lid
3. Cook on HIGH pressure for 35 minutes

4. Release the pressure naturally and open the lid
5. Serve with extra ghee

Nutrition Values (Per Serving)

- Protein: 47g
- Carbs: 3g
- Fats: 21g
- Calories: 404

Creamy Chicken Curry

(Prepping time: 10 minutes\ Cooking time: 10 hours |For 4 servings)

Ingredients

- 10 bone-in chicken thighs, skinless
- 1 cup sour cream
- 2 tablespoons. Curry powder
- 1 onion, chopped
- 1 jar (16 ounces) chunky salsa sauce

Directions

1. Add chicken thigh to your Ninja Foodi
2. Add onions, salsa, curry powder over chicken, stir and place the lid
3. Cook SLOW COOK MODE (LOW) for 10 hours. Open lid and transfer chicken to a serving platter
4. Pour sour cream into the sauce (cooking liquid) in the Ninja Foodi
5. Stir well and pour the sauce over chicken. Serve!

Nutrition Values (Per Serving)

- Calories: 400
- Fat: 20g
- Carbohydrates: 17g
- Protein: 39g

Lemon And Artichoke Medley

(Prepping time: 10 minutes\ Cooking time: 8 hours |For 6 servings)

Ingredients

- 1 pound boneless and skinless chicken breast
- 1 pound boneless and skinless chicken thigh
- 14 ounces (can) artichoke hearts, packed in water and drained
- 1 onion, diced
- 2 carrots, diced
- 3 garlic cloves, minced
- 1 bay leaf
- ½ teaspoon pepper
- 3 cups turnips, peeled and cubed
- 6 cups chicken broth
- 14 cup fresh lemon juice
- ¼ cup parsley, chopped

Directions

1. Add the above mentioned ingredients to your Ninja Foodi except for lemon juice and parsley
2. Cook on Slow Cooker (LOW) for 8 hours. Remove the chicken and shred it up
3. Return it back to the Ninja Foodi. Season with some pepper and salt!
4. Stir in parsley and lemon juice and serve!

Nutrition Values (Per Serving)

- Calories: 400
- Fat: 10g
- Carbohydrates: 12g
- Protein: 3g

Awesome Sesame Ginger Chicken

- 1 teaspoon of salt
- ½ a cup of water

Whole Spices

- 4 pieces of Red Chili Whole Kashmiri
- 1 teaspoon of black peppercorns
- 1 teaspoon of cumin seeds
- 2 teaspoon of coriander seeds
- 5 pieces of Green coriander
- 1 stick of cinnamon
- 4 pieces of cloves
- 1 tablespoon of cloves
- 1 tablespoon of poppy seeds
- 1 teaspoon of fennel seeds

Directions

1. Set your Ninja Foodi to Saute mode and add whole spices and cook them until dry roasted (for about 30 seconds)
2. Add garlic, ginger, grated coconut and Saute for 30 seconds more
3. Transfer the mixture to a blender and Grind until you have a paste. This is your Chettinad Spice Mix. Clean the Ninja Foodi and set your pot to Saute mode again
4. Add oil and allow it to heat it up. Add bay leaf and curry leaves, Saute for 30 seconds
5. Add diced up onions and Saute for about 30 seconds
6. Add diced up onion and Saute for 3 minutes
7. Add tomatoes, salt and ground spices and Saute for 2 minutes (including the previous blend)
8. Add chicken pieces and Saute for 3 minutes more
9. Add water and lock up the lid, cook for 5 minutes at HIGH pressure
10. Once done, do a quick release and enjoy with a garnish of cilantro. Enjoy!

Nutrition Values (Per Serving)

- Calories: 198
- Fat: 6g
- Carbohydrates: 8g
- Protein: 28g

Hawaiian Pinna Colada Chicken Meal
(Prepping time: 10 minutes\ Cooking time: 15 minutes |For 4 servings)

Ingredients

- 2 pounds organic chicken thigh
- 1 cup fresh pineapple chunks
- ½ cup coconut cream
- 1 teaspoon cinnamon
- 1/8 teaspoon salt
- 2 tablespoons coconut aminos
- ½ cup green onion, chopped
- Arrowroot flout

Directions

1. Add all of the ingredients to your Ninja Foodi except green onion
2. Lock up the lid and cook for 15 minutes at HIGH pressure
3. Once done, allow the pressure to release naturally. Open up the lid and stir well
4. Take a bowl and mix arrowroot flour and a tablespoon of water to make a slurry
5. Add the slurry to your pot and mix well to make a thick mixture
6. Set your pot to Saute mode and wait until the sauce is just thick enough
7. Garnish with some green onion and enjoy!

Nutrition Values (Per Serving)

- Calories: 358
- Fat: 20g
- Carbohydrates: 8g
- Protein: 12g

Garlic And Butter Chicken Dish
(Prepping time: 10 minutes\ Cooking time: 35 minutes |For 4 servings)

Ingredients

- 4 pieces of chicken breasts, chopped up
- ¼ cup of turmeric ghee/ normal ghee
- 1 teaspoon of salt
- 10 cloves of garlic, peeled and diced up

Nutrition Values (Per Serving)

- Calories: 340
- Fat: 19g
- Carbohydrates: 4g
- Protein: 36g

Lemongrass And Tamarind Chicken
(Prepping time: 10 minutes \ Cooking time: 4 hours | For 4 servings)

Ingredients

- 3 chicken thighs
- 1 ounce strips fresh turmeric
- 2 shallots, quartered
- Handful of mustard
- 1 stalk lemongrass, bruised and bundled up
- 2 cups chicken stock
- 1 banana pepper
- 4 tablespoons olive oil
- 2 tablespoons tamarind paste
- 2 Roma tomatoes, quartered
- 1 radish, peeled and chopped
- Fish sauce to taste
- Salt and pepper to taste

Directions

1. Add listed ingredients to your Ninja Foodi
2. Stir well and lock lid, cook on HIGH pressure for 10 minutes
3. Quick release pressure. Top with fresh cilantro. Serve and enjoy!

Nutrition Values (Per Serving)

- Calories: 445
- Fat: 32g
- Carbohydrates: 28g
- Protein: 28g

Fluffy Whole Chicken Dish
(Prepping time: 10 minutes\ Cooking time: 8 hours | For 4 servings)

Ingredients

- 1 cup mozzarella cheese
- 4 whole garlic cloves, peeled
- 1 whole chicken (2 pounds), cleaned and pat dried
- Salt and pepper to taste
- 2 tablespoons fresh lemon juice

Directions

1. Stuff chicken cavity with garlic cloves and mozzarella cheese
2. Season chicken generously with salt and pepper
3. Transfer chicken to Ninja Foodi and drizzle lemon juice
4. Lock lid and set to Slow Cooker mode, let it cook on LOW for 8 hours
5. Once done, serve and enjoy!

Nutrition Values (Per Serving)

- Calories: 309
- Fat: 12g
- Carbohydrates: 1.6g
- Protein: 45g

Sensible Chettinad Chicken
(Prepping time: 10 minutes\ Cooking time: 15 minutes | For 4 servings)

Ingredients

- 1 pound of boneless chicken thigh cut up into pieces
- 1 tablespoon of Ghee
- 1 bay leaf
- 5 curry leaves
- 1 inch Ginger piece
- 5 cloves of Garlic
- ¼ cup of grated coconut (fresh)
- 1 large onion, diced
- 2 medium tomatoes, diced

Ingredients

- 1-ounce shallot, minced
- 1 ounces ginger, sliced
- 2 medium banana peppers,
- 1 cup of coconut milk
- 1 cup chicken stock
- Juice of 1 lime, and zest
- 2 tablespoons fish sauce
- 3 pieces of 1/3 pounds each chicken breasts, meat

Directions

1. Add listed ingredients to your Ninja Foodi
2. Stir well and lock lid, cook on HIGH pressure for 10 minutes
3. Quick release pressure. Top with fresh cilantro. Serve and enjoy!

Nutrition Values (Per Serving)

- Calories: 425
- Fat: 33g
- Carbohydrates: 9g
- Protein: 24g

Hot And Spicy Paprika Chicken

(Prepping time: 10 minutes\ Cooking time: 20-25 minutes | For 4 servings)

Ingredients

- 4 piece (4 ounces each) chicken breast, skin on
- Salt and pepper to taste
- ½ cup sweet onion, chopped
- ½ cup heavy whip cream
- 2 teaspoons smoked paprika
- ½ cup sour cream
- 2 tablespoons fresh parsley, chopped

Directions

1. Season chicken with salt and pepper
2. Set your Foodi to Saute mode and add oil, let it heat up
3. Add chicken and sear both sides until nicely browned. Should take around 15 minutes
4. Remove chicken and transfer to a plate
5. Take a skillet and place it over medium heat, add onion and Sauté for 4 minutes
6. Stir in cream, paprika, bring the liquid to simmer. Return chicken to skillet and warm
7. Transfer the whole mixture to your Foodi and lock lid, cook on HIGH pressure for 5 minutes
8. Release pressure naturally over 10 minutes. Stir in cream, serve and enjoy!

Nutrition Values (Per Serving)

- Calories: 389
- Fat: 30g
- Carbohydrates: 4g
- Protein: 25g

Inspiring Turkey Cutlets

(Prepping time: 10 minutes\ Cooking time: 20-25 minutes | For 4 servings)

Ingredients

- 1 teaspoon Greek seasoning
- 1 pound turkey cutlets
- 2 tablespoons olive oil
- 1 teaspoon turmeric powder
- ½ cup almond flour

Directions

1. Take a bowl and add Greek seasoning, turmeric powder, almond flour, and mix
2. Dredge turkey cutlets in a bowl and let them sit for 30 minutes
3. Set Ninja Foodi to Sauté mode and add oil, let it heat up. Add cutlets and Sauté for 2 minutes
4. Lock lid and cook on LOW- MEDIUM pressure for 20 minutes
5. Release pressure naturally over 10 minutes. Take it out and serve, enjoy!

1. Add all ingredients to Ninja Foodi. Stir and lock lid, cook on HIGH pressure for 10 minutes
2. Release pressure naturally over 10 minutes. Serve and enjoy!

Nutrition Values (Per Serving)

- Calories: 204
- Fat: 14g
- Carbohydrates: 4g
- Protein: 14g

Taiwanese Chicken Delight
(Prepping time: 5 minutes\ Cooking time: 10 minutes |For 4 servings)

Ingredients

- 6 dried red chilis
- ¼ cup sesame oil
- 2 tablespoons ginger
- ¼ cup garlic, minced
- ¼ cup red wine vinegar
- ¼ cup coconut aminos
- Salt as needed
- 1.2 teaspoon xanthan gum (for the finish)
- ¼ cup Thai basil, chopped

Directions

1. Set your Ninja Foodi to Saute mode and add ginger, chilis, garlic and Saute for 2 minutes
2. Add remaining ingredients. Lock lid and cook on HIGH pressure for 10 minutes
3. Quick release pressure. Serve and enjoy!

Nutrition Values (Per Serving)

- Calories: 307
- Fat: 15g
- Carbohydrates: 7g
- Protein: 31g

Cabbage And Chicken Meatballs
(Prepping time: 10 minutes + 30 minutes\ Cooking time: 4-6 minutes |For 4 servings)

Ingredients

- 1 pound ground chicken
- ¼ cup heavy whip cream
- 2 teaspoons salt
- ½ teaspoon ground caraway seeds
- 1 and ½ teaspoons fresh ground black pepper, divided
- 1/4 teaspoon ground allspice
- 4-6 cups green cabbage, thickly chopped
- ½ cup almond milk
- 2 tablespoons unsalted butter

Directions

1. Transfer meat to a bowl and add cream, 1 teaspoon salt, caraway, ½ teaspoon pepper, allspice and mix it well. Let the mixture chill for 30 minutes
2. Once the mixture is ready, use your hands to scoop the mixture into meatballs
3. Add half of your balls to Ninja Foodi pot and cover with half of the cabbage
4. Add remaining balls and cover with rest of the cabbage
5. Add milk, pats of butter, season with salt and pepper
6. Lock lid and cook on HIGH pressure for 4 minutes. Quick release pressure
7. Unlock lid and serve. Enjoy!

Nutrition Values (Per Serving)

- Calories: 294
- Fat: 26g
- Carbohydrates: 4g
- Protein: 12g

Poached Chicken With Coconut Lime Cream Sauce
(Prepping time: 5 minutes \ Cooking time: 10 minutes |For 4 servings)

7. Once done, serve and enjoy!

Nutrition Values (Per Serving)

- Calories: 467
- Fat: 24g
- Carbohydrates: 1.7g
- Protein: 56g

Sensational Lime And Chicken Chili

(Prepping time: 10 minutes\ Cooking time: 23 minutes |For 6 servings)

Ingredients

- ¼ cup cooking wine (Keto-Friendly)
- ½ cup organic chicken broth
- 1 onion, diced
- 1 teaspoon salt
- ½ teaspoon paprika
- 5 garlic cloves, minced
- 1 tablespoon lime juice
- ¼ cup butter
- 2 pounds chicken thighs
- 1 teaspoon dried parsley
- 3 green chilies, chopped

Directions

1. Set your Ninja-Foodi to Sauté mode and add onion and garlic
2. Sauté for 3 minutes, add remaining ingredients
3. Lock lid and cook on Medium-HIGH pressure for 20 minutes
4. Release pressure naturally over 10 minutes. Serve and enjoy!

Nutrition Values (Per Serving)

- Calories: 282
- Fat: 15g
- Carbohydrates: 6g
- Protein: 27g

Funky-Garlic And turkey Breasts

(Prepping time: 10 minutes\ Cooking time: 17 minutes |For 4 servings)

Ingredients

- ½ teaspoon garlic powder
- 4 tablespoons butter
- ¼ teaspoon dried oregano
- 1 pound turkey breasts, boneless
- 1 teaspoon pepper
- ½ teaspoon salt
- ¼ teaspoon dried basil

Directions

1. Season turkey on both sides generously with garlic, dried oregano, dried basil, salt and pepper
2. Set your Ninja Foodi to sauté mode and add butter, let the butter melt
3. Add turkey breasts and sauté for 2 minutes on each side
4. Lock the lid and select the "Bake/Roast" setting, bake for 15 minutes at 355 degrees F
5. Serve and enjoy once done!

Nutrition Values (Per Serving)

- Calories: 223
- Fat: 13g
- Carbohydrates: 5g
- Protein: 19g

Mexico's Favorite Chicken Soup

(Prepping time: 5 minutes\ Cooking time: 20 minutes |For 4 servings)

Ingredients

- 2 cups chicken, shredded
- 4 tablespoons olive oil
- ½ cup cilantro, chopped
- 8 cups chicken broth
- 1/3 cup salsa
- 1 teaspoon onion powder
- ½ cup scallions, chopped
- 4 ounces green chilies, chopped
- ½ teaspoon habanero, minced
- 1 cup celery root, chopped
- 1 teaspoon cumin
- 1 teaspoon garlic powder
- Salt and pepper to taste

Directions

- Calories: 340
- Fat: 19g
- Carbohydrates: 3.7g
- Protein: 36g

Pulled Up Keto Friendly Chicken Tortilla's
(Prepping time: 15 minutes\ Cooking time: 15 minutes | For 4 servings)

Ingredients

- 1 tablespoon avocado oil
- 1 pound pastured organic boneless chicken breasts
- ½ cup orange juice
- 2 teaspoons gluten-free Worcestershire sauce
- 1 teaspoon garlic powder
- 1 teaspoon salt
- ½ teaspoon chili powder
- ½ teaspoon paprika

Directions

1. Set your Ninja Foodi to Sauté mode and add oil, let the oil heat up
2. Add chicken on top, take a bowl and add remaining ingredients mix well
3. Pour the mixture over chicken. Lock lid and cook on HIGH pressure for 15 minutes
4. Release pressure naturally over 10 minutes
5. Shred the chicken and serve over salad green shell such as cabbage or lettuce. Enjoy!

Nutrition Values (Per Serving)
- Calories: 338
- Fat: 23g
- Carbohydrates: 10g
- Protein: 23g

Fully-Stuffed Whole Chicken
(Prepping time: 10 minutes\ Cooking time: 8 hours | For 6 servings)

Ingredients

- 1 cup mozzarella cheese
- 4 whole garlic cloves, peeled
- 1 whole chicken (2 pounds), cleaned and pat dried
- Salt and pepper as needed
- 2 tablespoons fresh lemon juice

Directions

1. Stuff the chicken cavity with garlic cloves and mozzarella cheese
2. Season chicken generously with salt and pepper
3. Transfer chicken to your Ninja Foodi and drizzle lemon juice
4. Lock lid and set to "Slow Cooker" mode, let it cook on LOW for 8 hours
5. Once doe, serve and enjoy!

Nutrition Values (Per Serving)
- Calories: 309
- Fat: 12g
- Carbohydrates: 1.6g
- Protein: 45g

Ham-Stuffed Generous Turkey Rolls
(Prepping time: 10 minutes\ Cooking time: 20 minutes | For 8 servings)

Ingredients

- 4 tablespoons fresh sage leaves
- 8 ham slices
- 8 (6 ounces each) turkey cutlets
- Salt and pepper to taste
- 2 tablespoons butter, melted

Directions

1. Season turkey cutlets with salt and pepper
2. Roll turkey cutlets and wrap each of them with ham slices tightly
3. Coat each roll with butter and gently place sage leaves evenly over each cutlet
4. Transfer them to your Ninja Foodi
5. Lock lid and select the "Bake/Roast" mode, bake for 10 minutes a 360 degrees F
6. Open the lid and gently give it a flip, lock lid again and bake for 10 minutes more

Ingredients

- 4 pieces (4 ounces each) chicken breast, skin on
- Salt and pepper as needed
- 1 tablespoon olive oil
- ½ cup sweet onion, chopped
- ½ cup heavy whip cream
- 2 teaspoons smoked paprika
- ½ cup sour cream
- 2 tablespoons fresh parsley, chopped

Directions

1. Lightly season the chicken with salt and pepper
2. Set your Ninja Foodi to Sauté mode and add oil, let the oil heat up
3. Add chicken and sear both sides until properly browned, should take about 15 minutes
4. Remove chicken and transfer them to a plate
5. Take a skillet and place it over medium heat, add onion and Saute for 4 minutes until tender
6. Stir in cream, paprika and bring the liquid simmer
7. Return chicken to the skillet and alongside any juices
8. Transfer the whole mixture to your Ninja Foodi and lock lid, cook on HIGH pressure for 5 minutes
9. Release pressure naturally over 10 minutes. Stir in sour cream, serve and enjoy!

Nutrition Values (Per Serving)

- Calories: 389
- Fat: 30g
- Carbohydrates: 4g
- Protein: 25g

Elegant Chicken Stock
(Prepping time: 10 minutes\ Cooking time: 2hours | For 4 servings)

Ingredients

- 2 pounds meaty chicken bones
- ¼ teaspoon salt
- 3 and ½ cups water

Directions

1. Place chicken parts in Foodi and season with salt
2. Add water, place the pressure cooker lid and seal the valve, cook on HIGH pressure for 90 minutes. Release the pressure naturally over 10 minutes
3. Line a colander with cheesecloth and place it over a large bowl, pour chicken parts and stock into the colander and strain out the chicken and bones
4. Let the stock cool and let it peel off any layer of fat that might accumulate on the surface
5. Use as needed!

Nutrition Values (Per Serving)

- Calories: 51
- Fat: 3g
- Carbohydrates: 1g
- Protein: 6g

Hot Turkey Cutlets
(Prepping time: 10 minutes\ Cooking time: 15 minutes | For 4 servings)

Ingredients

- 1 teaspoon Greek seasoning
- 1 pound turkey cutlets
- 2 tablespoons olive oil
- 1 teaspoon turmeric powder
- ½ cup almond flour

Directions

1. Take a bowl and add Greek seasoning, turmeric powder, almond flour and mix well
2. Dredge turkey cutlets in the bowl and let it sit for 30 minutes
3. Set your Ninja Foodi to Sauté mode and add oil, let it heat up
4. Add cutlets and Sauté for 2 minutes. Lock lid and cook on Low-Medium Pressure for 20 minutes
5. Release pressure naturally over 10 minutes. Take the dish out, serve and enjoy!

Nutrition Values (Per Serving)

11. Close with crisping lid and select Bake/Roast, adjust the temperature to 375 degrees F, cook for 12 minutes
12. Once done, open lid and transfer chicken to the platter, add heavy cream and stir into the sauce. stir in sauce, season with salt and pepper. Pour sauce and vegetables around chicken, serve and enjoy!

Nutrition Values (Per Serving)
- Calories: 268
- Fat: 20g
- Carbohydrates: 7g
- Protein: 19g

Lemon And Butter Chicken Extravagant
(Prepping time: 10 minutes\ Cooking time: 10 minutes | For 4 servings)

Ingredients

- 4 bone-in, skin on chicken thighs
- salt and pepper as needed
- 2 tablespoons butter, divided
- 2 teaspoons garlic, minced
- 1/2 cup herbed chicken stock
- 1/2 cup heavy whip cream
- 1/2 a lemon, juiced

Directions

1. Season chicken thighs with salt and pepper
2. Set your Ninja Foodi to Sauté mode and add oil, let it heat up
3. Add chicken thighs and saute both sides until golden, total for 6 minutes
4. Remove thighs to a plater and keep it on the side. Add garlic and cook for 2 minutes
5. Whisk in chicken stock, heavy cream, lemon juice and stir, bring the sauce to simmer and reintroduce the chicken
6. Lock lid and cook for 10 minutes on HIGH pressure
7. Release pressure naturally over 10 minutes. Serve warm and enjoy!

Nutrition Values (Per Serving)
- Calories: 294
- Fat: 26g
- Carbohydrates: 4g
- Protein: 12g

Creative Cabbage And Chicken Meatball
(Prepping time: 15 minutes\ Cooking time: 4 minutes | For 4 servings)

Ingredients

- 1 pound ground chicken
- 1/4 cup heavy whip cream
- 2 teaspoon salt
- 1/2 teaspoon ground caraway seeds
- 1 and 1/2 teaspoons fresh ground black pepper, divided
- 1/4 teaspoon ground allspice
- 4-6 cups green cabbage, thickly chopped
- 1/2 cup almond milk
- 2 tablespoons unsalted butter

Directions

1. Transfer meat to a bowl
2. Add cream, 1 teaspoon salt, caraway, 1/2 teaspoon pepper, allspice and mix well
3. Refrigerate the mixture for 30 minutes
4. Once the mixture is cool, use your hands to scoop the mixture into meatballs
5. Place half of the balls to your Ninja Foodi pot and cover with half of cabbage
6. Add remaining balls and cover with remaining cabbage
7. Add milk, pats of butter and sprinkle 1 teaspoon salt, 1 teaspoon pepper
8. Lock lid and cook on HIGH pressure for 4 minutes. Quick release pressure
9. Unlock lid and serve. Enjoy!

Nutrition Values (Per Serving)
- Calories: 338
- Fat: 23g
- Carbohydrates: 7g
- Protein: 23g

Spicy Hot Paprika Chicken
(Prepping time: 10 minutes\ Cooking time: 5 minutes | For 4 servings)

Chapter 5: Chicken And Poultry Recipes

Juicy Sesame Garlic Chicken Wings
(Prepping time: 10 minutes\ Cooking time: 25 minutes /For 4 servings)

Ingredients

- 24 chicken wing segments
- 2 tablespoons toasted sesame oil
- 2 tablespoons Asian-Chile-Garlic sauce
- 2 tablespoons stevia
- 2 garlic cloves, minced
- 1 tablespoon toasted sesame seeds

Directions

1. Add 1 cup water to Foodi's inner pot, place reversible rack in the pot in lower portions, place chicken wings in the rack. Place lid into place and seal the valve
2. Select pressure mode to HIGH and cook for 10 minutes
3. Make the glaze by taking a large bowl and whisking in sesame oil, Chile-Garlic sauce, honey and garlic. Once the chicken is cooked, quick release the pressure and remove pressure lid
4. Remove rack from the pot and empty remaining water. Return inner pot to the base
5. Cover with crisping lid and select Air Crisp mode, adjust the temperature to 375 degrees F, pre-heat for 3 minutes. While the Foodi pre-heats, add wings to the sauce and toss well to coat it
6. Transfer wings to the basket, leaving any excess sauce in the bowl
7. Place the basket in Foodi and close with Crisping mode, select Air Crisp mode and let it cook for 8 minutes, gently toss the wings and let it cook for 8 minutes more
8. Once done, drizzle any sauce and sprinkle sesame seeds. Enjoy!

Nutrition Values (Per Serving)

- Calories: 440
- Fat: 32g
- Carbohydrates: 12g
- Protein: 28g

Perfectly Braised Chicken Thigh With Chokeful Of Mushrooms
(Prepping time: 10 minutes\ Cooking time: 30 minutes /For 4 servings)

Ingredients

- 4 chicken thigh, bone in- skin on
- 1 teaspoon salt
- 1 tablespoon olive oil
- ½ small onion, sliced
- ½ cup white wine vinegar
- ½ cup chicken stock
- 1 cup frozen artichoke hearts, thawed and drained
- 1 bay leaf
- Fresh ground black pepper
- ¼ cup heavy cream

Directions

1. Set your Foodi to Sauté mode and set it to Medium-HIGH, pre-heat for 5 minutes
2. Pour olive oil and wait until it shimmers
3. Add chicken thighs, skin side-side down, cook for 4-5 minutes
4. Turn and sear the other side for 1 minute. Remove from pot
5. Add onion, sprinkle with remaining salt, cook for 2 minutes more until tender
6. Add wine and bring to a boil. Cook for 2-3 minutes, until reduced by half
7. Add chicken stock, artichoke hearts, bay leaf, thyme, several grinds of pepper, stir well
8. Place chicken thigh back to the pot (skin side up), lock pressure lid into place and seal the valve
9. Select pressure mode to HIGH and cook for 5 minutes. Once done, quick release pressure
10. use tongs to transfer chicken to Reversible Rack in the upper position, add mushrooms to sauce and stir. Set rack in the pot

- 1 large head cauliflower
- 2 tablespoon extra-virgin olive oil
- 2 teaspoon paprika
- 2 teaspoon ground cumin
- ¾ teaspoon kosher salt
- 1 cup fresh cilantro, chopped
- 1 lemon, quartered

Directions

1. Place the steamer rack into your Ninja Foodi. Add 1 and a ½ cups of water
2. Remove the leaves from the cauliflower and trim the core to ensure that it is able to sit flat
3. Carefully place it on the steam rack. Take a small bowl and add olive oil, cumin, paprika, salt
4. Drizzle the mixture over the cauliflower
5. Lock up the lid and cook on HIGH pressure for 4 minutes
6. Quick release the pressure. Lift the cauliflower to a cutting board and slice into 1-inch steaks
7. Divide the mixture among serving plates and sprinkle with cilantro. Serve and enjoy!

Nutrition Values (Per Serving)

- Calories: 283
- Fats: 19g
- Carbs: 18g
- Protein: 10g

Authentic Indian Palak Paneer

(Prepping time: 10 minutes\ Cooking time: 5 minutes |For 4 servings)

Ingredients

- 2 teaspoons olive oil
- 5 garlic cloves, chopped
- 1 tablespoon fresh ginger, chopped
- 1 large yellow onion, chopped
- ½ jalapeno chile, chopped
- 1 pound fresh spinach
- 2 tomatoes, chopped
- 2 teaspoons ground cumin
- ½ teaspoon cayenne
- 2 teaspoons Garam masala
- 1 teaspoon ground turmeric
- 1 teaspoon salt
- ½ cup of water
- 1 and ½ cup paneer cubes
- ½ cup heavy whip cream

Directions

7. Pre-heat your Ninja Foodi using Saute mode on HIGH heat, once the pot is hot, add oil and let it shimmer. Add garlic, ginger and chile, Saute for 2-3 minutes
8. Add onion, spinach, tomatoes, cumin, cayenne, garam masala, turmeric, salt, and water
9. Lock lid and cook on HIGH pressure for 2 minutes. Release pressure naturally over 10 minutes
10. Use an immersion blender to puree the mixture to your desired consistency
11. Gently stir in paneer and top with a drizzle of cream. Enjoy!

Nutrition Values (Per Serving)

- Calories: 185
- Fat: 14g
- Carbohydrates: 7g
- Protein: 7g

3. Serve with topping of dill, enjoy

Nutrition Values (Per Serving)

- Calories: 207
- Fat: 16g
- Carbohydrates: 5g
- Protein: 8g

Quick Red Cabbage
(Prepping time: 10 minutes\ Cooking time: 10 minutes | For 6 servings)

Ingredients

- 6 cups red cabbage, chopped
- 1 tablespoon apple cider vinegar
- ½ cup Keto-Friendly applesauce
- 1 cup of water
- 3 garlic cloves, minced
- 1 small onion, chopped
- 1 tablespoon olive oil
- Salt and pepper to taste

Directions

1. Add olive oil to Ninja Foodi
2. Set it to Saute mode and let it heat up, add onion and garlic and Saute for 2 minutes
3. Add remaining ingredients and stir. Lock lid and cook on HIGH pressure for 10 minutes
4. Quick release pressure. Stir well and serve. Enjoy!

Nutrition Values (Per Serving)

- Calories: 81
- Fat: 6g
- Carbohydrates: 4g
- Protein: 2g

Simple Rice Cauliflower
(Prepping time: 10 minutes\ Cooking time: 15 minutes | For 4 servings)

Ingredients

- 1 large cauliflower head
- 2 tablespoons olive oil
- ¼ teaspoon salt
- ½ teaspoon dried parsley
- ½ teaspoon cumin
- ¼ teaspoon turmeric
- ¼ teaspoon paprika
- Fresh cilantro
- Lime wedges

Directions

1. Wash the cauliflower well and trim the leaves
2. Place a steamer rack on top of the pot and transfer the florets to the rack
3. Add 1 cup of water into the Ninja Foodi.Lock up the lid and cook on HIGH pressure for 1 minute
4. Once done, do a quick release.Transfer the flower to a serving platter
5. Set your pot to Saute mode and add oil, allow the oil to heat up
6. Add flowers back to the pot and cook, making sure to break them using a potato masher
7. Add spices and season with a bit of salt. Give a nice stir and squeeze a bit of lime
8. Serve and enjoy!

Nutrition Values (Per Serving)

- Calories: 169
- Fat: 14g
- Carbohydrates: 8g
- Protein: 3g

Very Spicy Cauliflower Steak
(Prepping time: 10 minutes\ Cooking time: 4 minutes | For 6 servings)

Ingredients

- Calories: 349
- Fat: 27g
- Carbohydrates: 3.2g
- Protein: 23g

Running Away Broccoli Casserole
(Prepping time: 10 minutes \ Cooking time: 7 minutes | For 4 servings)

Ingredients

- 1 tablespoon extra-virgin olive oil
- 1 pound broccoli, cut into florets
- 1 pound cauliflower, cut into florets
- ¼ cup almond flour
- 2 cups of coconut milk
- ½ teaspoon ground nutmeg
- Pinch of pepper
- 1 and ½ cup shredded Gouda cheese, divided

Directions

6. Pre-heat your Ninja Foodi by setting it to Saute mode
7. Add olive oil and let it heat up, add broccoli and cauliflower
8. Take a medium bowl stir in almond flour, coconut milk, nutmeg, pepper, 1 cup cheese and add the mixture to your Ninja Foodi. Top with ½ cup cheese and lock lid, cook on HIGH pressure for 5 minutes. Release pressure naturally over 10 minutes . Serve and enjoy!

Nutrition Values (Per Serving)

- Calories: 373
- Fat: 32g
- Carbohydrates: 6g
- Protein: 16g

Spaghetti Squash Fancy Noodles
(Prepping time: 10 minutes \ Cooking time: 7 minutes | For 6 servings)

Ingredients

- 2 pound of spaghetti squash
- 1 cup of water

Directions

1. Take a paring knife and cut the spaghetti squash in half
2. Take a largely sized spoon and scoop out the center seeds and discard the gunk
3. Place the Ninja Foodi steamer insert inside the inner pot of your Ninja Foodi. Add 1 cup of water
4. Add the half-cut squashes to the steamer insert, making sure that the cut part if facing up
5. Lock up the lid and cook on HIGH pressure for 7 minutes
6. Once done, perform a quick release. Take the squash out and fork out the strings
7. Serve with sauce or your favorite topping!

Nutrition Values (Per Serving)

- Calories: 45
- Fats: 5g
- Carbs:7g
- Protein:3g

Dill And Garlic Fiesta Platter
(Prepping time: 10 minutes \ Cooking time: 10-15 minutes | For 6 servings)

Ingredients

- 3 cups carrots, chopped
- 1 tablespoon melted butter
- ½ teaspoon garlic salt
- 1 tablespoon fresh dill, minced
- 1 cup of water

Directions

1. Add listed ingredients to Ninja Foodi. Stir and lock lid, cook on HIGH pressure for 10 minutes
2. Release pressure naturally over 10 minutes. Quick release pressure

- 1 green apple chopped
- 1 peeled and chopped butternut squash
- 1 teaspoon salt
- 2 cups of water
- ¼ cup of finely chopped parsley
- Black pepper

Directions

1. Prepare the ingredients accordingly and keep them on the side
2. Set your Ninja Foodie to Saute mode and add onions, cook for minutes
3. Add just a splash of water . Add garlic, carrot, ginger, apple, squash, and salt
4. Give it a nice stir. Add water and lock up the lid
5. Cook on HIGH pressure for 5 minutes. Naturally, release the pressure
6. Allow it to cool for 15 minutes
7. Blend the soup in batches, or you may use an immersion blender as well to blend in the pot until it is creamy. Add parsley and season with some black pepper. Serve and enjoy!

Nutrition Values (Per Serving)

- Protein: 3g
- Carbs: 14g
- Fats: 5g
- Calories: 116

Hearty Cheesy Cauliflower
(Prepping time: 10 minutes\ Cooking time: 35 minutes |For 6 servings)

Ingredients

- 1 tablespoon Keto-Friendly mustard
- 1 head cauliflower
- 1 teaspoon avocado mayonnaise
- ½ cup parmesan cheese, grated
- ¼ cup butter, cut into small pieces

Directions

1. Set your Ninja Foodi to Saute mode and add butter, let it melt
2. Add cauliflower and Saute for 3 minutes
3. Add rest of the ingredients and lock lid, cook on HIGH pressure for 30 minutes
4. Release pressure naturally over 10 minutes. Serve and enjoy!

Nutrition Values (Per Serving)

- Calories: 155
- Fat: 13g
- Carbohydrates: 2g
- Protein: 7g

Mesmerizing Spinach Quiche
(Prepping time: 10 minutes\ Cooking time: 33 minutes |For 4 servings)

Ingredients

- 1 tablespoon butter, melted
- 1 pack (10 ounces) frozen spinach, thawed
- 5 organic eggs, beaten
- Salt and pepper to taste
- 3 cups Monterey Jack Cheese, shredded

Directions

7. Set your Ninja Foodi to Saute mode and let it heat up, add butter and let the butter melt
8. Add spinach and Saute for 3 minutes, transfer the Sautéed spinach to a bowl
9. Add eggs, cheese, salt, and pepper to a bowl and mix it well
10. Transfer the mixture to greased quiche molds and transfer the mold to your Foodi
11. Close the lid and choose the "Bake/Roast" mode and let it cook for 30 minutes at 360 degrees F. Once done, open lid and transfer the dish out
12. Cut into wedges and serve. Enjoy!

Nutrition Values (Per Serving)

Complete Cauliflower Zoodles
(Prepping time: 10 minutes\ Cooking time: 8 minutes | For 6 servings)

Ingredients

- 2 tablespoons butter
- 2 cloves garlic
- 7-8 cauliflower florets
- 1 cup vegetable broth

Garnish

- Chopped sun-dried tomatoes
- Balsamic vinegar

- 2 teaspoons salt
- 2 cups spinach, coarsely chopped
- 2 green onions, chopped
- 1 pound of zoodles (Spiralized Zucchini)

- Gorgonzola cheese

Directions

1. Set your Ninja Foodi to Saute mode and add butter, allow the butter to melt
2. Add garlic cloves and Saute for 2 minutes
3. Add cauliflower, broth, salt and lock up the lid and cook on HIGH pressure for 6 minutes
4. Prepare the zoodles. Perform a naturally release over 10 minutes
5. Use an immersion blender to blend the mixture in the pot to a puree
6. Pour the sauce over the zoodles
7. Serve with a garnish of cheese, sun-dried tomatoes and a drizzle of balsamic vinegar. Enjoy!

Nutrition Values (Per Serving)

- Calories: 78
- Fats: 5g

- Carbs 0.6g
- Protein:8g

Simple Mushroom Hats And Eggs
(Prepping time: 10 minutes\ Cooking time: 9 minutes | For 1 serving)

Ingredients

- 4 ounces mushroom hats
- 1 teaspoon butter, melted
- 4 quail eggs

- ½ teaspoon ground black pepper
- ¼ teaspoon salt

Directions

1. Spread the mushroom hats with the butter inside. Then beat the eggs into mushroom hats
2. Sprinkle with salt and ground black pepper. Transfer the mushroom hats on the rack
3. Lower the air fryer lid. Cook the meat for 7 minutes at 365 F
4. Check the mushroom, if it is not cooked fully then cook them for 2 minutes more
5. Serve and enjoy!

Nutrition Values (Per Serving)

- Calories: 118
- Fat: 8.2g
- Carbohydrates: 4.6g
- Protein: 8.4g

Ginger And Butternut Bisque Yum
(Prepping time: 10 minutes\ Cooking time: 8 minutes | For 6 servings)

Ingredients

- 1 cup of diced yellow onion
- 4 minced cloves of garlic

- 2 teaspoon of peeled and chopped ginger
- 1 cup of chopped carrot

- ½ cup dark leaf kale, chopped
- 1 tablespoon lemon juice
- ½ cup spinach, chopped
- ½ teaspoon salt
- 2 garlic cloves
- ½ teaspoon pepper
- 6 whole eggs
- 3 teaspoons coconut oil

Directions

1. Set your Ninja Foodi to Saute mode and add coconut oil, add garlic, cook until fragrant
2. Add chopped cauliflower and cook for 5 minutes
3. Stir in all ingredients except eggs, cook for 2 minutes
4. Stir in eggs, lock lid and cook for 2 minutes on HIGH pressure. Quick release pressure.Enjoy!

Nutrition Values (Per Serving)

- Calories: 480
- Fat: 35g
- Carbohydrates: 8g
- Protein: 22g

Thyme And Carrot Dish With Dill
(Prepping time: 5 minutes\ Cooking time: 5 minutes |For 4 servings)

Ingredients

- ½ cup of water
- 1 pound baby carrots
- 3 tablespoons stevia
- 1 tablespoon thyme, chopped
- 1 tablespoon dill, chopped
- Salt and pepper to taste
- 2 tablespoons ghee

Direction

1. Add trivet to your Ninja Foodi, add carrots and add water
2. Lock lid and cook on HIGH pressure for 3 minutes. Quick release pressure
3. Drain and transfer to a bowl. Set your Ninja Foodi to Saute mode and add ghee, let it melt
4. Add stevia, thyme dill, and carrots. Stir well for a few minutes. Serve and enjoy!

Nutrition Values (Per Serving)

- Calories: 162
- Fat: 4g
- Carbohydrates: 8g
- Protein: 3g

Creative Coconut Cabbage
(Prepping time: 10 minutes \ Cooking time: 7 minutes |For 4 servings)

Ingredients

- 2 tablespoons lemon juice
- 1/3 medium carrot, sliced
- ½ ounces, yellow onion, sliced
- 1/2 cup cabbage, shredded
- 1 teaspoon turmeric powder
- 1 ounce dry coconut
- ½ tablespoon mustard powder
- ½ teaspoon mild curry powder
- 1 large garlic cloves, diced
- 1 and ½ teaspoons salt
- 1/3 cup water
- 3 tablespoons olive oil
- 3 large whole eggs
- 3 large egg yolks

Directions

1. Set your Ninja Foodi to Saute mode and add oil, stir in onions, salt and cook for 4 minutes
2. Stir in spices, garlic and Saute for 30 seconds
3. Stir in rest of the ingredients, lock lid and cook on HIGH pressure for 3 minutes
4. Naturally, release pressure over 10 minutes. Serve and enjoy!

Nutrition Values (Per Serving)

- Calories: 400
- Fat: 34g
- Carbohydrates: 10g
- Protein: 14g

- 2 cups radishes, quartered
- ½ cup chicken stock
- Salt and pepper to taste
- 2 tablespoons melted ghee
- 1 tablespoon chives, chopped
- 1 tablespoon lemon zest, grated

Direction

1. Add radishes, stock, salt, pepper, zest to your Ninja Foodi and stir
2. Lock lid and cook on HIGH pressure for 7 minutes
3. Quick release pressure. Add melted ghee, toss well. Sprinkle chives and enjoy!

Nutrition Values (Per Serving)

- Calories: 102
- Fat: 4g
- Carbohydrates: 6g
- Protein: 5g

Garlic And Swiss Chard Garlic
(Prepping time: 10 minutes \ Cooking time: 4 minutes / For 4 servings)

Ingredients

- 2 tablespoons ghee
- 3 tablespoons lemon juice
- ½ cup chicken stock
- 4 bacon slices, chopped
- 1 bunch Swiss chard, chopped
- ½ teaspoon garlic paste
- Salt and pepper to taste

Directions

1. Set your Ninja Foodi to Saute mode and add bacon, stir well and cook for a few minutes
2. Add ghee, lemon juice, garlic paste, and stir. Add Swiss chard, salt, pepper, and stock
3. Lock lid and cook on HIGH pressure for 3 minutes. Quick release pressure and serve. Enjoy!

Nutrition Values (Per Serving)

- Calories: 160
- Fat: 8g
- Carbohydrates: 6g
- Protein: 4g

Healthy Rosemary And Celery Dish
(Prepping time: 10 minutes \ Cooking time: 5 minutes / For 4 servings)

Ingredients

- 1 pound celery, cubed
- 1 cup of water
- 2 garlic cloves, minced
- Salt and pepper
- ¼ teaspoon dry rosemary
- 1 tablespoon olive oil

Direction

1. Add water to your Ninja Foodi and place steamer basket
2. Add celery cubs to basket and lock lid, cook on HIGH pressure for 4 minutes
3. Quick release pressure. Take a bowl and add mix in oil, garlic, and rosemary. Whisk well
4. Add steamed celery to the bowl and toss well, spread on a lined baking sheet
5. Broil for 3 minutes using the Air Crisping lid at 250 degrees F. Serve and enjoy!

Nutrition Values (Per Serving)

- Calories: 100
- Fat: 3g
- Carbohydrates: 8g
- Protein: 3g

Awesome Veggie Hash
(Prepping time: 10 minutes \ Cooking time: 15 minutes / For 4 servings)

Ingredients

- 1 cups cauliflower, chopped
- 1 teaspoon mustard

- Calories: 274
- Fat: 18g
- Carbohydrates: 6g
- Protein: 10g

Awesome Butternut Squash Soup
(Prepping time: 10 minutes\ Cooking time: 16 minutes | For 4 servings)

Ingredients

- 1 and ½ pounds butternut squash, baked, peeled and cubed
- ½ cup green onions, chopped
- 3 tablespoons butter
- ½ cup carrots, peeled and chopped
- ½ cup celery, chopped
- 29 ounces vegetable stock
- 1 garlic clove, peeled and minced
- ½ teaspoon Italian seasoning
- 15 ounces canned tomatoes, diced
- Salt and pepper to taste
- 1/8 teaspoon red pepper flakes
- 1/8 teaspoon nutmeg, grated
- 1 and ½ cup half and half

Directions

1. Set your Ninja Foodi to "Saute" mode and add butter, let it melt
2. Add celery, carrots, onion and stir cook for 3 minutes
3. Add garlic, stir cook for 1 minute
4. Add squash, tomatoes, stock, Italian seasoning, salt, pepper, pepper flakes and nutmeg, stir
5. Lock lid and cook on HIGH pressure for 10 minutes. Release pressure naturally over 10 minutes
6. Use an immersion blender to puree the mix
7. Set the food to Saute mode on LOW and add half and half, stir cook for 1-2 minutes until thickened. Divide and serve with a sprinkle of green onions on top. Enjoy!

Nutrition Values (Per Serving)
- Calories: 250
- Fat: 22g
- Carbohydrates: 8g
- Protein: 3g

Comfortable Mushroom Soup
(Prepping time: 10 minutes\ Cooking time: 10 minutes | For 6 servings)

Ingredients

- 1 small onion, diced
- 8 ounces white button mushrooms, chopped
- 8 ounces portabella mushrooms
- 2 garlic cloves, minced

Cashew Cream

- 1/3 cup of raw cashew
- ¼ cup dry white wine vinegar
- 2 and ½ cup mushroom stock
- 2 teaspoons salt
- 1 teaspoon fresh thyme
- ¼ teaspoon black pepper

- ½ a cup of mushroom stock

Directions

1. Add onion, mushroom to the pot and set your Ninja Foodi to Saute mode
2. Cook for 8 minutes and stir from time to time
3. Add garlic and Saute for 2 minutes more. Add wine and Saute until evaporated
4. Add thyme, pepper, salt, Mushroom stock, and stir
5. Lock up the lid and cook on HIGH pressure for 5 minutes
6. Perform quick release. Transfer cashew and water to the blender and blend well
7. Remove lid and transfer mix to the blender. Blend until smooth. Server and enjoy!

Nutrition Values (Per Serving)

- Calories: 193
- Fats: 12g
- Carbs:15g
- Protein: 5

Chives And Radishes Platter
(Prepping time: 10 minutes\ Cooking time: 7 minutes | For 4 servings)

Ingredients

(Prepping time: 10 minutes\ Cooking time: 6 minutes |For 4 servings)

Ingredients

- 4 tablespoons butter, melted
- Salt and pepper to taste
- 2 pounds broccoli florets
- 1 cup whipping cream

Directions

6. Place a steamer basket in your Ninja Foodi (bottom part) and add water
7. Place florets on top of the basket and lock lid. Cook on HIGH pressure for 5 minutes
8. Quick release pressure. Transfer florets from the steamer basket to the pot
9. Add salt, pepper, butter and stir
10. Lock crisping lid and cook on Air Crisp mode for 360 degrees F. Serve and enjoy!

Nutrition Values (Per Serving)

- Calories: 178
- Fat: 14g
- Carbohydrates: 8g
- Protein: 5g

Offbeat Cauliflower And Cheddar Soup
(Prepping time: 10 minutes\ Cooking time: 5 minutes |For 8 servings)

Ingredients

- ¼ cup butter
- ½ sweet onion, chopped
- 1 head cauliflower, chopped
- 4 cups herbed vegetable stock
- ½ teaspoon ground nutmeg
- 1 cup heavy whip cream
- Salt and pepper as needed
- 1 cup cheddar cheese, shredded

Directions

1. Set your Ninja Foodi to sauté mode and add butter , let it heat up and melt
2. Add onion and Cauliflower, Saute for 10 minutes until tender and lightly browned
3. Add vegetable stock and nutmeg, bring to a boil
4. Lock lid and cook on HIGH pressure for 5 minutes, quick release pressure once done
5. Remove pot and from Foodi and stir in heavy cream, puree using immersion blender
6. Season with more salt and pepper and serve with a topping of cheddar. Enjoy!

Nutrition Values (Per Serving)

- Calories: 227
- Fat: 21g
- Carbohydrates: 4g
- Protein: 8g

Powerful Medi-Cheese Spinach
(Prepping time: 5 minutes\ Cooking time: 15 minutes |For 4 servings)

Ingredients

- 4 tablespoons butter
- 2 pounds spinach, chopped and boiled
- Salt and pepper to taste
- 2/3 cup Kalamata olives, halved and pitted
- 1 and ½ cups feta cheese, grated
- 4 teaspoons fresh lemon zest, grated

Directions

1. Take a bowl and mix spinach, butter, salt, pepper and transfer the mixture to your Crisping Basket of the Ninja Foodi. Transfer basket to your Foodi and lock Crisping lid
2. Cook for 15 minutes on Air Crisp mode on 340 degrees F
3. Serve by stirring in olives, lemon zest and feta. Enjoy!

Nutrition Values (Per Serving)

3. Open lid and add more broth, set your pot to Saute mode and adjust heat to HIGH
4. Add yellow squash, parsley and remaining 1 tablespoon garlic
5. Let it cook for 2-3 minutes until the squash is soft
6. Stir in cream and sprinkle parmesan. Serve and enjoy!

Nutrition Values (Per Serving)

- Calories: 210
- Fat: 14g
- Carbohydrates: 10g
- Protein: 10g

Delicious Mushroom Stroganoff
(Prepping time: 5 minutes\ Cooking time: 10 minutes |For 6 servings)

Ingredients

- ¼ cup unsalted butter, cubed
- 1 pound cremini mushrooms, halved
- 1 large onion, halved
- 4 garlic cloves, minced
- 2 cups vegetable broth
- ½ teaspoon salt
- ¼ teaspoon fresh black pepper
- 1 and ½ cups sour cream
- ¼ cup fresh flat-leaf parsley, chopped
- 1 cup grated parmesan cheese

Directions

1. Add butter, mushrooms, onion, garlic, vegetable broth, salt, pepper and paprika
2. Gently stir and lock lid. Cook on HIGH pressure for 5 minutes
3. Release pressure naturally over 10 minutes
4. Serve by stirring in sour cream and with a garnish of parsley and parmesan cheese. Enjoy!

Nutrition Values (Per Serving)

- Calories: 453
- Fat: 37g
- Carbohydrates: 11g
- Protein: 19g

Everyday Use Veggie-Stock
(Prepping time: 10 minutes\ Cooking time: 100 minutes |For 1 quart)

Ingredients

- 1 onion, quartered
- 2 large carrots, peeled and cut into 1 inch pieces
- 1 tablespoon olive oil
- 12 ounces mushrooms, sliced
- ¼ teaspoon salt
- 3 and ½ cups water

Directions

1. Take cook and crisp basket out of the inner pot, close crisping lid and let it pre-heat for 3 minutes at 400 degrees F on Bake/Roast settings
2. While the pot heats up, add onion, carrot chunks in the Cook and Crisp basket and drizzle vegetable oil, toss well
3. Place basket back into the inner pot, close crisping lid and cook for 15 minutes at 400 degrees F on Bake/Roast mode. Make sure to shake the basket halfway through
4. Remove basket from pot and add onions, carrots, mushrooms, water and season with salt
5. Lock pressure lid and seal the valves, cook on HIGH pressure for 60 minutes
6. Release the pressure naturally over 10 minutes
7. Line a colander with cheesecloth and place it over a large bowl, pour vegetables and stock into the colander. Strain the stock and discard veggies. Enjoy and use as needed!

Nutrition Values (Per Serving)

- Calories: 45
- Fat: 4g
- Carbohydrates: 3g
- Protein: 0g

Groovy Broccoli Florets

1. Add the pot to your Ninja Foodi and add water
2. Add steamer basket on top and add cauliflower pieces
3. Lock lid and cook on HIGH pressure for 5 minutes
4. Quick release pressure. Open lid and use an immersion blender to mash the cauliflower
5. Blend until you have your desired consistency and enjoy!

Nutrition Values (Per Serving)

- Calories: 124
- Fat: 10g
- Carbohydrates: 5g
- Protein: 5g

Beets And Greens With Cool Horseradish Sauce
(Prepping time: 5 minutes\ Cooking time: 10-15 minutes |For 4 servings)

Ingredients

- 2 large beets with greens, scrubbed and root ends trimmed
- 1 cup water, for steaming
- 2 tablespoons sour cream
- 1 tablespoon almond milk
- 1 teaspoon prepared horseradish
- ¼ teaspoon lemon zest
- 1/8 teaspoon salt
- 2 teaspoon unsalted butter
- 1 tablespoon minced fresh chives

Directions

1. Trim off beet greens and keep them on the side
2. Add water to the Ninja Foodi and place steamer basket, place beets in steamer basket
3. Lock lid and cook on HIGH pressure for 10 minutes, release pressure naturally over 10 minutes
4. While the beets are being cooked, wash greens and slice them into ½ inch thick ribbons
5. Take a bowl and whisk in sour cream, horseradish, lemon zest, 1/16 teaspoon of salt
6. Once the cooking is done, remove lid and remove beets, let them cool
7. Use a pairing knife to peel them and slice them into large bite-sized pieces
8. Remove steamer from the Ninja Foodi and pour out water
9. Set your Foodi to "Saute" mode and add butter, let it melt
10. Once the butter stops foaming, add beet greens sprinkle remaining 1/6 teaspoon salt and cook for 3-4 minutes. Return beets to the Foodi and heat for 1-2 minutes, stirring
11. Transfer beets and greens to platter and drizzle sour cream mixture
12. Sprinkle chives and serve. Enjoy!

Nutrition Values (Per Serving)

- Calories: 70
- Fat: 4g
- Carbohydrates: 9g
- Protein: 2g

Summertime Veggie Soup
(Prepping time: 10 minutes\ Cooking time: 3 minutes |For 6 servings)

Ingredients

- 3 cups leeks, sliced
- 6 cups rainbow chard, stems and leaves, chopped
- 1 cup celery, chopped
- 2 tablespoons garlic, minced
- 1 teaspoon dried oregano
- 1 teaspoon salt
- 2 teaspoons fresh ground black pepper
- 3 cups chicken broth
- 2 cups yellow summer squash, sliced into 1/ inch slices
- ¼ cup fresh parsley, chopped
- ¾ cup heavy whip cream
- 4-6 tablespoons parmesan cheese, grated

Directions

1. Add leeks, chard, celery, 1 tablespoon garlic, oregano, salt, pepper and broth to your Ninja Foodi
2. Lock lid and cook on HIGH pressure for 3 minutes. Quick release pressure

4. Release pressure naturally over 10 minutes
5. Use an immersion blender to puree the mixture to your desired consistency
6. Gently stir in paneer and top with a drizzle of cream. Enjoy!

Nutrition Values (Per Serving)

- Calories: 185
- Fat: 14g
- Carbohydrates: 7g
- Protein: 7g

Astounding Caramelized Onions
(Prepping time: 10 minutes\ Cooking time: 45 minutes |For 4 servings)

Ingredients

- 2 tablespoons unsalted butter
- 3 large onions, sliced
- 2 tablespoons water
- 1 teaspoon salt

Directions

1. Set your pot to Saute mode and adjust the heat to Medium, pre-heat the inner pot for 5 minutes
2. Add butter and let it melt, add onions, water , salt, and stir well
3. Lock pressure lid into place, making sure that the pressure valve is locked
4. Cook on HIGH pressure for 30 minutes. Quick release the pressure once done
5. Remove the lid and set the pot to Saute mode, let it sear in the Medium-HIGH mode for about 15 minutes until the liquid is almost gone. Enjoy!

Nutrition Values (Per Serving)

- Calories: 110
- Fat: 6g
- Carbohydrates: 10g
- Protein: 2g

Special Lunch-Worthy Green Beans
(Prepping time: 5 minutes\ Cooking time: 10 minutes |For 4 servings)

Ingredients

- 2-3 pounds fresh green beans
- 2 tablespoons butter
- 1 garlic clove, minced
- Salt and pepper to taste
- 1 and ½ cups water

Directions

1. Add all listed ingredients to your Ninja Foodi pot
2. Lock lid and cook on HIGH pressure for 5 minutes
3. Release pressure quickly and serve. Enjoy!

Nutrition Values (Per Serving)

- Calories: 87
- Fat: 6g
- Carbohydrates: 7g
- Protein: 3g

Healthy Cauliflower Mash
(Prepping time: 10 minutes\ Cooking time: 5 minutes |For 4 servings)

Ingredients

- 1 tablespoon butter, soft
- ½ cup feta cheese
- Salt and pepper to taste
- 1 large head cauliflower, chopped into large pieces
- 1 garlic cloves, minced
- 2 teaspoons fresh chives, minced

Directions

Chapter 4: Vegetarian And Vegan Recipes

Cheese Dredged Cauliflower Delight
(Prepping time: 5 minutes\ Cooking time: 30 minutes |For 6 servings)

Ingredients

- 1 tablespoon Keto-Friendly mustard
- 1 head cauliflower
- 1 teaspoon avocado mayonnaise
- ½ cup parmesan cheese, grated
- ¼ cup butter, cut into small pieces

Directions

1. Set your Ninja Foodi to Saute mode and add butter, let it melt
2. Add cauliflower and Saute for 3 minutes. Add remaining ingredients and lock lid
3. Cook on PRESSURE mode for 30 minutes on HIGH pressure
4. Release pressure natural over 10 minutes. Serve and enjoy!

Nutrition Values (Per Serving)

- Calories: 155
- Fat: 13g
- Carbohydrates: 2g
- Protein: 7g

Garlic And Dill Carrot Fiesta
(Prepping time: 5 minutes\ Cooking time: 12 minutes |For 4 servings)

Ingredients

- 3 cups carrots, chopped
- 1 tablespoon melted butter
- ½ teaspoon garlic sea salt
- 1 tablespoon fresh dill, minced
- 1 cup water

Directions

1. Add listed ingredients to Ninja Foodi. Stir and lock lid, cook on HIGH pressure for 10 minutes
2. Release pressure naturally over 10 minutes. Quick release pressure and remove lid
3. Serve with a topping of dill, enjoy!

Nutrition Values (Per Serving)

- Calories: 207
- Fat: 16g
- Carbohydrates: 5g
- Protein: 8g

Cool Indian Palak Paneer
(Prepping time: 10 minutes\ Cooking time: 5 minutes |For 4 servings)

Ingredients

- 2 teaspoons olive oil
- 5 garlic cloves, chopped
- 1 tablespoon fresh ginger, chopped
- 1 large yellow onion, chopped
- ½ jalapeno chile, chopped
- 1 pound fresh spinach
- 2 tomatoes, chopped
- 2 teaspoons ground cumin
- ½ teaspoon cayenne
- 2 teaspoons Garam masala
- 1 teaspoon ground turmeric
- 1 teaspoon salt
- ½ cup water
- 1 and ½ cup paneer cubes
- ½ cup heavy whip cream

Directions

1. Pre-heat your Ninja Foodi using Saute mode on HIGH heat, once the pot is hot, add oil and let it shimmer. Add garlic, ginger and chile, Saute for 2-3 minutes
2. Add onion, spinach, tomatoes, cumin, cayenne, garam masala, turmeric, salt and water
3. Lock lid and cook on HIGH pressure for 2 minutes

- 2 tablespoons butter
- 2 tablespoons Dijon mustard (Keto-Friendly)
- 4 pork chops
- Salt and pepper to taste
- 1 tablespoon fresh rosemary, coarsely chopped

Directions

1. Take a bowl and add pork chops, cover with Dijon mustard and carefully sprinkle rosemary, salt, and pepper. Let it marinate for 2 hours
2. Add butter and marinated pork chops to your Ninja Foodi pot
3. Lock lid and cook on Low-Medium Pressure for 30 minutes
4. Release pressure naturally over 10 minutes. Take the dish out, serve and enjoy!

Nutrition Values (Per Serving)
- Calories: 315
- Fat: 26g
- Carbohydrates: 1g
- Protein: 18g

Creative And Easy Lamb Roast
(Prepping time: 10 minutes\ Cooking time: 60 minutes |For 6 servings)

Ingredients

- 2 pounds lamb roast
- 1 cup onion soup
- 1 cup beef broth
- Salt and pepper to taste

Directions

1. Transfer lamb roast to your Ninja Foodi pot. Add onion soup, beef broth, salt, and pepper
2. Lock lid and cook on Medium-HIGH pressure for 55 minutes
3. Release pressure naturally over 10 minutes. Transfer to serving bowl, serve and enjoy!

Nutrition Values (Per Serving)
- Calories: 349
- Fat: 18g
- Carbohydrates: 2.9g
- Protein: 39g

Crispy Tofu And Mushrooms
(Prepping time: 10 minutes\ Cooking time: 10 minutes |For 2 servings)

Ingredients

- 8 tablespoons parmesan cheese, shredded
- 2 cups fresh mushrooms, chopped
- 2 blocks tofu, pressed and cubed
- Salt and pepper to taste
- 8 tablespoons butter

Directions

1. Take a bowl and mix in tofu, salt, and pepper
2. Set your Ninja Foodi to Saute mode and add seasoned tofu, Saute for 5 minutes
3. Add mushroom, cheese and Saute for 3 minutes. Lock crisping lid and Air Crisp for 3 minutes at 350 degrees F. Transfer to serving plate and enjoy!

Nutrition Values (Per Serving)
- Calories: 211
- Fat: 18g
- Carbohydrates: 2g
- Protein: 11g

- 1 tablespoon of agave nectar
- ¼ teaspoon of sea salt
- 1 cup of water

Directions

1. Clean and peel your carrots properly. Roughly chop up them into small pieces
2. Add 1 cup of water to your Pot
3. Place the carrots in a steamer basket and place the basket in the Ninja Foodi
4. Lock up the lid and cook on HIGH pressure for 4 minutes. Perform a quick release
5. Transfer the carrots to a deep bowl and use an immersion blender to blend the carrots
6. Add butter, nectar, salt, and puree. Taste the puree and season more if needed. Enjoy!

Nutrition Values (Per Serving)

- Calories: 143
- Fat: 9g
- Carbohydrates: 16g
- Protein: 2g

Simple Broccoli Florets
(Prepping time: 10 minutes\ Cooking time: 6 minutes |For 4 servings)

Ingredients

- 4 tablespoons butter, melted
- Salt and pepper to taste
- 2 pounds broccoli florets
- 1 cup whipping cream

Directions

1. Place a steamer basket in your Ninja Foodi (bottom part) and add water
2. Place florets on top of the basket and lock lid
3. Cook on HIGH pressure for 5 minutes. Quick release pressure
4. Transfer florets from the steamer basket to the pot. Add salt, pepper, butter, and stir
5. Lock crisping lid and cook on Air Crisp mode for 360 degrees F. Serve and enjoy!

Nutrition Values (Per Serving)

- Calories: 178
- Fat: 14g
- Carbohydrates: 8g
- Protein: 5g

Awesome Magical 5 Ingredient Shrimp
(Prepping time: 10 minutes\ Cooking time: 15 minutes |For 4 servings)

Ingredients

- 2 tablespoons butter
- ½ teaspoon smoked paprika
- 1 pound shrimps, peeled and deveined
- Lemongrass stalks
- 1 red chili pepper, seeded and chopped

Directions

1. Take a bowl and mix all of the ingredients well, except lemongrass and marinate for 1 hour
2. Transfer to Ninja Foodi and lock lid, BAKE/ROAST for 15 minutes at 345 degrees F
3. Once done, serve and enjoy!

Nutrition Values (Per Serving)

- Calories: 251
- Fat: 10g
- Carbohydrates: 3g
- Protein: 34g

Romantic Mustard Pork
(Prepping time: 10 minutes\ Cooking time: 30 minutes |For 4 servings)

Ingredients

- 4 tablespoons butter
- Salt and pepper to taste
- 2 pounds broccoli florets
- 1 cup whip cream

Directions

1. Arrange basket in the bottom of your Ninja Foodi and add water
2. Place florets on top of the basket. Lock lid and cook on HIGH pressure for 5 minutes
3. Quick release pressure and transfer florets to the pot itself
4. Season with salt, pepper and add butter
5. Lock crisping lid and Air Crisp on 360 degrees F 3 minutes
6. Transfer to a serving plate. Serve and enjoy!

Nutrition Values (Per Serving)

- Calories: 178
- Fat: 4g
- Carbohydrates: 8g
- Protein: 6g

The Epic Fried Eggs
(Prepping time: 5 minutes\ Cooking time: 10 minutes |For 2 servings)

Ingredients

- 4 eggs
- ¼ teaspoon ground black pepper
- 1 teaspoon butter, melted
- ¾ teaspoon salt

Directions

1. Take a small egg pan and brush it with butter. Beat the eggs in the pan
2. Sprinkle with the ground black pepper and salt. Transfer the egg pan in the pot
3. Lower the air fryer lid. Cook the meat for 10 minutes at 350 F. Serve immediately and enjoy!

Nutrition Values (Per Serving)

- Calories: 143
- Fat: 10.2g
- Carbohydrates: 0.9g
- Protein: 11.4g

Gentle Keto Butter Fish
(Prepping time: 10 minutes\ Cooking time: 30 minutes |For 6 servings)

Ingredients

- 1 pound salmon fillets
- 2 tablespoons ginger/garlic paste
- 3 green chilies, chopped
- Salt and pepper to taste
- ¾ cup butter

Directions

7. Season salmon fillets with ginger, garlic paste, salt, pepper
8. Place salmon fillets to Ninja Foodi and top with green chilies and butter
9. Lock lid and BAKE/ROAST for 30 minutes at 360 degrees F
10. Bake for 30 minutes and enjoy!

Nutrition Values (Per Serving)

- Calories: 507
- Fat: 45g
- Carbohydrates: 3g
- Protein: 22g

Sensational Carrot Puree
(Prepping time: 10 minutes \ Cooking time: 4 minutes |For 4 servings)

Ingredients

- 1 and a ½ pound carrots, chopped
- 1 tablespoon of butter at room temperature

Ingredients

- 4 chicken breasts, skinless
- 1 and ¼ cup of water

Direction

1. Add water to Ninja Foodi . Add frozen chicken and lock lid. Cook on HIGH pressure for 10 minutes. Quick release pressure. Open the lid and use just as you want it.

Nutrition Values (Per Serving)

- Calories: 128
- Fat: 2g
- Carbohydrates: 0g
- Protein: 23g

Italian Dark Kale Crisps
(Prepping time: 5 minutes\ Cooking time: 10 minutes | For 4 servings)

Ingredients

- 2 cups kale, Italian dark-leaf
- 1 teaspoon yeast
- 2 tablespoons coconut oil
- ½ teaspoon chili flakes
- ¼ teaspoon salt

Directions

1. Take a bowl and tear the kale roughly and place it into the bowl
2. Sprinkle the kale with coconut oil, yeast, chili flakes and salt
3. Mix up the kale well till it becomes consistent
4. Insert the air fryer basket and in the Ninja Foodi and then transfer the kale
5. Air fryer the meal for 10 minutes. Serve and enjoy!

Nutrition Values (Per Serving)

- Calories: 78
- Fat: 6.9g
- Carbohydrates: 3.3g
- Protein: 11.4g

Quick Ginger And Sesame Chicken
(Prepping time: 5 minutes\ Cooking time: 10 minutes | For 4 servings)

Ingredients

- 1 and ½ pounds chicken thighs, no skin
- 2 tablespoons coconut aminos
- 1 tablespoon agave
- 1 tablespoon ginger, minced
- 1 tablespoon garlic-sesame oil
- 1 tablespoon rice vinegar
- Red onion, sliced for salad
- Carrots julienned for salad
- Cucumbers julienned for salad

Direction

1. Slice thigh into large chunks and add rest of the ingredients to a heat-safe dish
2. Place foil over the bowl. Add 2 cups water to Ninja Foodi
3. Place steamer rack in Ninja Foodi and place the bowl over the rack
4. Lock lid and cook on HIGH pressure for 10 minutes. Naturally, release pressure over 10 minutes
5. Shred meat and serve with a tossing of the salad. Enjoy!

Nutrition Values (Per Serving)

- Calories: 286
- Fat: 21g
- Carbohydrates: 3g
- Protein: 21g

Butter Melted Broccoli Florets
(Prepping time: 10 minutes\ Cooking time: 8 minutes | For 4 servings)

Ingredients

The Coolest New York Strip Steak

(Prepping time: 10 minutes \ Cooking time: 9 minutes | For 4 servings)

Ingredients

- 24 ounces NY strip steak
- ½ teaspoon ground black pepper
- 1 teaspoon salt

Directions

1. Add steaks on a metal trivet and place trivet on your Ninja Foodi
2. Season with salt and pepper
3. Add 1 cup water to the pot (below steaks). Lock lid and cook on HIGH pressure for 1 minute
4. Quick release pressure.
5. Place Air Crisp lid and Air Crisp for 8 minutes for a medium-steak. Remove from pot and enjoy!

Nutrition Values (Per Serving)

- Calories: 503
- Fat: 46g
- Carbohydrates: 1g
- Protein: 46g

French Onion Pork Chops

(Prepping time: 5 minutes \ Cooking time: 20 minutes | For 4 servings)

Ingredients

- 4 pork chops
- 10 ounces French Onion Soup
- ½ cup sour cream
- 10 ounces chicken broth

Directions

1. Add pork chops to your Ninja Foodi. Add broth. Lock lid and cook on HIGH pressure for 12 minutes. Release pressure naturally over 10 minutes.
2. Whisk sour cream and French Onion Soup and pour mixture over pork.
3. Set your Ninja Foodi to Saute mode and cook for 6-8 minutes more. Serve and enjoy!

Nutrition Values (Per Serving)

- Calories: 365
- Fat: 26g
- Carbohydrates: 7g
- Protein: 21g

Hearty Apple Infused Water

(Prepping time: 10 minutes \ Cooking time: 4 minutes | For 4 servings)

Ingredients

- 1 whole apple, chopped
- 5 sticks of cinnamon

Directions

1. Place the above-mentioned ingredients to a mesh steamer basket
2. Place the basket in your pot. Add water to barely cover the content.
3. Lock up the lid and cook on HIGH pressure for 5 minutes
4. Once the cooking is done, quick release the pressure
5. Remove the steamer basket and discard the cooked produce
6. Allow the flavored water to cool and chill. Serve!

Nutrition Values (Per Serving)

- Calories: 194
- Fat: 0g
- Carbohydrates: 12g
- Protein: 0g

Simple And Easy Chicken Breast

(Prepping time: 5 minutes \ Cooking time: 10 minutes | For 4 servings)

2. Season with salt and pepper according to your taste
3. Set the Ninja to Medium Pressure mode and let it cook for about 10 minutes, covered, making sure to keep stirring the broccoli from time to time
4. Take a medium sized bowl and add crack in the eggs, beat the eggs gently
5. Pour milk into the eggs and give it a nice stir
6. Add the egg mixture into the Ninja (over broccoli) and gently stir, cook for 2 minutes (uncovered)
7. Once the egg has settled in, add cheese and sprinkle red pepper, black pepper, and salt
8. Enjoy with bacon strips if you prefer!

Nutrition Values (Per Serving)

- Calories: 184
- Fat: 12g
- Carbohydrates: 5g
- Protein: 12g

Original Onion And Scrambled Tofu
(Prepping time: 8 minutes\ Cooking time: 12 minutes | For 4 servings)

Ingredients

- 4 tablespoons butter
- 2 tofu blocks, pressed and cubed in to 1 inch pieces
- Salt and pepper to taste
- 1 cup cheddar cheese, grated
- 2 medium onions, sliced

Directions

1. Take a bowl and add tofu, season with salt and pepper
2. Set your Foodi to Saute mode and add butter , let it melt
3. Add onions and Saute for 3 minutes. Add seasoned tofu and cook for 2 minutes more
4. Add cheddar and gently stir
5. Lock the lid and bring down the Air Crisp mode, let the dish cook on "Air Crisp" mode for 3 minutes at 340 degrees F. Once done, take the dish out, serve and enjoy!

Nutrition Values (Per Serving)

- Calories: 184
- Fat: 12g
- Carbohydrates: 5g
- Protein: 12g

The Early Morning Ballet Of Ham And Spinach
(Prepping time: 5 minutes\ Cooking time: 30 minutes | For 6 servings)

Ingredients

- 3 pounds fresh baby spinach
- ½ cup cream
- 28 ounces ham, sliced
- 4 tablespoons butter, melted
- Salt and pepper to taste

Directions

1. Set your Ninja Foodi to Saute mode and add butter, let it melt
2. Add spinach and Saute for 3 minutes. Top with cream, ham slices, salt and pepper
3. Lock the Air Fryer lid and let it Bake/Roast for 8 minutes at 360 degrees F
4. Remove the dish from the Foodi and serve. Enjoy!

Nutrition Values (Per Serving)

- Calories: 188
- Fat: 12g
- Carbohydrates: 5g
- Protein: 14g

4. Take a small saucepan and place it over low heat, add butter, flour and stir until the mixture foams and turns into a golden beige, this is your blond roux
5. Remove from heat. Release pressure naturally over 10 minutes
6. Open lid and add roux, salt and pepper to the soup
7. Use an immersion blender to puree the soup
8. Taste and season accordingly, swirl in cream and enjoy!

Nutrition Values (Per Serving)

- Calories: 192
- Fat: 14g
- Carbohydrates: 8g
- Protein: 6g

Good-Day Pumpkin Puree
(Prepping time: 10 minutes\ Cooking time: 13-15 minutes | For 2 servings)

Ingredients

- 2 pounds small sized pumpkin, halved and seeded
- ½ cup water
- Salt and pepper to taste

Directions

1. Add water to your Ninja Foodi, place steamer rack in the pot
2. Add pumpkin halves to the rack and lock lid, cook on HIGH pressure for 13-15 minutes
3. Once done, quick release pressure and let the pumpkin cool
4. Once done, scoop out flesh into a bowl
5. Blend using an immersion blender and season with salt and pepper. Serve and enjoy!

Nutrition Values (Per Serving)

- Calories: 112
- Fat: 2g
- Carbohydrates: 7g
- Protein: 2g

Amazing Bacon And Veggie Delight
(Prepping time: 5 minutes\ Cooking time: 25 minutes | For 4 servings)

Ingredients

- 1 green bell pepper, chopped
- 4 bacon slices
- ½ cup parmesan cheese
- 1 tablespoon avocado mayonnaise (Keto Friendly)
- 2 scallions, chopped

Directions

1. Arrange your bacon slices in your Ninja Foodi pot and top them up with avocado mayo, scallions, bell peppers, parmesan cheese
2. Close lid and select the Bake/Roast mode, set timer to 25 minutes and temperature to 365 degrees F. Let it bake and remove the dish after 25 minutes. Serve and enjoy!

Nutrition Values (Per Serving)

- Calories: 197
- Fat: 13g
- Carbohydrates: 5g
- Protein: 14g

Hearty Broccoli And Scrambled Cheese Breakfast
(Prepping time: 10 minutes\ Cooking time: 5 minutes | For 4 servings)

Ingredients

- 1 pack, 12 ounces frozen broccoli florets
- 2 tablespoons butter
- salt and pepper as needed
- 8 whole eggs
- 2 tablespoons milk
- ¾ cup white cheddar cheese, shredded
- Crushed red pepper, as needed

Directions

1. Add butter and broccoli to your Ninja Foodi

Ingredients

- 1 tablespoon butter, melted
- 1 pack (10 ounces) frozen spinach, thawed
- 5 organic eggs, beaten
- Salt and pepper to taste
- 3 cups Monterey Jack Cheese, shredded

Directions

1. Set your Ninja Foodi to Saute mode and let it heat up, add butter and let the butter melt
2. Add spinach and Saute for 3 minutes, transfer the Sautéed spinach to a bowl
3. Add eggs, cheese, salt and pepper to a bowl and mix it well
4. Transfer the mixture to greased quiche molds and transfer the mold to your Foodi
5. Close lid and choose the "Bake/Roast" mode and let it cook for 30 minutes at 360 degrees F
6. Once done, open lid and transfer the dish out. Cut into wedges and serve. Enjoy!

Nutrition Values (Per Serving)

- Calories: 349
- Fat: 27g
- Carbohydrates: 3.2g
- Protein: 23g

Breakfast Broccoli Casserole
(Prepping time: 10 minutes\ Cooking time: 7 minutes |For 4 servings)

Ingredients

- 1 tablespoon extra-virgin olive oil
- 1 pound broccoli, cut into florets
- 1 pound cauliflower, cut into florets
- ¼ cup almond flour
- 2 cups coconut milk
- ½ teaspoon ground nutmeg
- Pinch of pepper
- 1 and ½ cup shredded Gouda cheese, divided

Directions

1. Pre-heat your Ninja Foodi by setting it to Saute mode
2. Add olive oil and let it heat up, add broccoli and cauliflower
3. Take a medium bowl stir in almond flour, coconut milk, nutmeg, pepper, 1 cup cheese and add the mixture to your Ninja Foodi
4. Top with ½ cup cheese and lock lid, cook on HIGH pressure for 5 minutes
5. Release pressure naturally over 10 minutes. Serve and enjoy!

Nutrition Values (Per Serving)

- Calories: 373
- Fat: 32g
- Carbohydrates: 6g
- Protein: 16g

Creamy Early Morning Asparagus Soup
(Prepping time: 10 minutes\ Cooking time: 5-10 minutes |For 4 servings)

Ingredients

- 1 tablespoon olive oil
- 3 green onions, sliced crosswise into ¼ inch pieces
- 1 pound asparagus, tough ends removed, cut into 1 inch pieces
- 4 cups vegetable stock
- 1 tablespoon unsalted butter
- 1 tablespoon almond flour
- 2 teaspoon salt
- 1 teaspoon white pepper
- ½ cup heavy cream

Directions

1. Set your Ninja Foodi to "Saute" mode and add oil, let it heat up
2. Add green onions and Saute for a few minutes, add asparagus and stock
3. Lock lid and cook on HIGH pressure for 5 minutes

Chapter 3: Breakfast Recipes

The Early Morning Veggie Hash Brown
(Prepping time: 10 minutes\ Cooking time: 20 minutes | For 3 servings)

Ingredients

- 1 tablespoon unsalted butter
- ½ teaspoon dried thyme, crushed
- ½ cup cauliflower florets, boiled and chopped
- ½ small on ion, chopped
- ½ cup water
- Salt and pepper to taste
- ½ pound turkey meat, chopped
- ¼ cup heavy cream

Directions

1. Set your Ninja Foodi to Saute mode and let it heat up, add butter and let the butter melt
2. Add onion and Saute for 3 minutes. Add chopped cauliflowers. Saute for 2 minutes longer
3. Add turkey and water
4. Close Pressure lid and set your Ninja Foodi to HIGH pressure mode, cook for 10 minutes
5. Quick release the pressure
6. Set the Ninja Foodie to BROIL mode (lid open) and add heavy cream, close the lid and let it Broil for 2 minutes. Serve and enjoy!

Nutrition Values (Per Serving)

- Calories: 151
- Fat: 11g
- Carbohydrates: 0.7g
- Protein: 11g

Sicilian Cauliflower Roast Crunch
(Prepping time: 10 minutes\ Cooking time: 10 minutes | For 4 servings)

Ingredients

- 1 medium cauliflower head, leaves removed
- ¼ cup olive oil
- 1 teaspoon red pepper, crushed
- ½ cup water
- 2 tablespoons capers, rinsed and minced
- ½ cup parmesan cheese, grated
- 1 tablespoon fresh parsley, chopped

Directions

1. Prepare the Ninja Foodi by adding water and place the cook and crisp basket inside the pot
2. Cut an "X" on the head of cauliflower by using a knife and slice it about halfway down
3. Take a basket and transfer the cauliflower in it
4. Then put on the pressure lid and seal it and set it on low pressure for 3 minutes
5. Add olive oil, capers, garlic, and crushed red pepper into it and mix them well
6. Once the cauliflower is cooked, do a quick release and remove the lid
7. Pour in the oil and spice mixture on the cauliflower
8. Spread equally on the surface then sprinkle some Parmesan cheese from the top
9. Close the pot with crisping lid. Set it on Air Crisp mode to 390 degrees F for 10 minutes
10. Once done, remove the cauliflower flower the Ninja Foodi transfer it into a serving plate
11. Cut it up into pieces and transfer them to serving plates
12. Sprinkle fresh parsley from the top. Serve and enjoy!

Nutrition Values (Per Serving)

- Calories: 119
- Fat: 10g
- Carbohydrates: 5g
- Protein: 2.2g

Heartfelt Spinach Quiche
(Prepping time: 10 minutes\ Cooking time: 33 minutes | For 4 servings)

Diet Soda

Diet soda claims to not contain sugars or carbs; it contains artificial sweeteners equally as detrimental as regular sugar. Artificial sweeteners enhance your carbohydrate intake and prevent you from reaching the metabolic state of ketosis.

Alcohol

Most alcohol beverages consist of none, or low carbs, but can still be bad for a keto lifestyle. Alcohol prevents the fat burning process or dramatically slows it down, because your body will need to process the alcohol first before the fat. To be successful with this diet, limit your alcohol intake.

Processed Foods

Avoid processed or packaged foods. Such foods are packed with artificial additives that can stray you from ketosis. Instead of choosing the processed foods, pick organic and real ingredients.
This is all you need to know about the ketogenic diet. Opinions differ between some individuals and sources, but you get the concept. The ketogenic diet and instant pot have plenty lot in common. It can be used together make fast, tasty, and healthy dishes that will improve your life. Since the keto diet asks you to avoid greasy foods, the instant pot helps by softening up foods using pressure and heat. With that being said, let's use the instant pot to prepare ketogenic meals for better health.

Best nuts and seeds for this diet include walnuts, almonds, and macadamias. They are low in calories and can help you control your carbohydrate count. You can also use products such as almond flour as an alternative to regular flour.

Fruits

You can eat fruits on the keto diet but keep in moderation. Some fruits retract you from reaching ketosis. Berries though, are the most advantageous as they are packed with nutrition and hold a low level in sugar.

What Foods Should not be on Your Plate?

To reach ketosis successfully, do your best to prevent and rid your body of foods that will hold you back from your goal. Most foods to avoid are high in carbohydrates and do not allow your body to burn fat for energy. Here is a general list of the types of foods to avoid:

Root Vegetables

Vegetables that grow and get pulled from the ground are high in carbohydrates and take you away from ketosis. Such vegetables include potatoes, beets, radishes, carrots, onions, and parsnips.

Sweet Fruits

While following the ketogenic diet you should avoid most fruits. Fruits contain fructose (similar to glucose), and is bad for reaching ketosis. Not only avoid fruits; stay away from products made with fresh fruit, such as juices and extracts. If you eat fruits, then keep it in moderation.

Grains

Obviously, avoid all foods made with processed grains. Grains contain additives that can negatively affect your insulin levels. Such grains include bread, pasta, cakes, breadcrumbs, cookies, and pastries.

acids, protein, zinc, and niacin. If you include zucchini in your diet, it can lead to an optimal healthy lifestyle.

Bell Peppers
Bell peppers are nutritious and packed with fiber and vitamins. Bell peppers also contain anti-inflammatory properties that are useful on the ketogenic diet.

Proteins

Following a ketogenic diet requires you to find a source of protein. Proteins consist of amino acids, which are essential nutrients for your body and brain. You need to consume protein, as it is your primary fuel source on this diet. Here are some things you might consider adding to your plate:

Meat and Poultry
Any kind of meat can be used for the ketogenic diet, especially if they are high in fat. Always choose meat from grass-fed and wild animal sources. Avoid hot dogs and sausages, and meat covered with starch or processed sauces.

Fish
Fish is another great source of protein. As with meat and poultry, always choose organic and wild fish caught naturally. Examples of good fish include salmon, trout, tuna, shrimp, cod, lobster, and catfish.

Eggs
Eggs are an incredible source of protein and contain low carbs, especially the egg yolk.

Fats and Oils

Since you will need to burn fat for energy, include fats and oils in your diet. Instead of vegetable oil, go for olive oil, coconut oil, avocado oil, and ghee.
Also, buy oils that are rich in polyunsaturated fats and have a low smoke level; these oils will retain their fatty acids. Such oils include walnut oil, flax oil, hemp seed oil, and grape seed oil.

Dairy Products
For a ketogenic diet, consider consuming raw and organic dairy products. You can use cheeses and creams to prepare ketogenic meals. Examples of the best dairy products to include in your diet are mozzarella cheese, cheddar cheese, parmesan cheese, cottage cheese, sour cream, cream cheese, heavy whipping cream, and Greek yogurt.

Nuts and Seeds
Nuts contain healthy fats and nutrients such as vitamin E. When choosing nuts, purchase roasted nuts because they already have their anti-nutrients discarded.

magnesium, calcium, phosphorus, sodium, niacin, folate, vitamin B6, vitamin A, and vitamin K. Lettuce can also be a healthy ketogenic alternative for hamburger buns and taco shells.

Broccoli

Broccoli is healthy and delicious and rich in nutrients, fiber, calcium, protein, and potassium.

Spinach

Spinach is one of the best vegetables rich in potassium, proteins, and iron. Spinach is also delicious and can be used for salads, stuffing, side dishes, and much more.

Cauliflower

Cauliflower is an excellent source of choline, dietary fiber, omega-3 fatty acids, phosphorus, biotin, vitamins B1, B2, and B3. You can use cauliflower to prepare rice, pizza crusts, hummus, and breadsticks.

Tomatoes

Tomatoes carry many positive health benefits and are a great source of vitamin A, C, and K. Including these vitamins, tomatoes are high in potassium, which can reduce blood pressure levels and decrease stroke risks. When you roast tomatoes with olive oil, you can enhance the lycopene content, boosting its effects. It can also protect heart health and reduce the risk of cancer.

Avocados

Avocados are rich in omega oils. Avocados can be consumed in salads or mixed with other ingredients such as yogurt and nuts. They are high in potassium and fiber and are great for your metabolism and heart. Most grocery stores will sell them in a semi-ripened condition, so you can keep them for up to a week as they ripen. Avocados also have high oil content and minerals, which reduce your appetite and provide nutrients all around for your body.

Asparagus

Asparagus is a great source of minerals and vitamins, including vitamin A, C, and K. Studies have shown that asparagus can help cope with anxiety and protect mental health. Consider eating roasted asparagus for dinner or add raw asparagus in your salads.

Mushrooms

Mushrooms contain strong anti-inflammatory properties, which can improve inflammation for those who have metabolic problems. Mushrooms are also packed with copper, potassium, protein, and selenium. It is also a great source of phosphorus, niacin, pantothenic acid, and zinc, especially if you cook them until brown.

Zucchini

Zucchini is low-carb vegetable and a great source of vitamin A, magnesium, potassium, copper, phosphorus, and folate. Zucchini is also high in omega-3 fatty a scale, instead be patient and trust that the ketogenic diet will help you lose weight.

8. Use vitamins and mineral salts

Foods high in carbohydrates contain many micronutrients, such as vitamins and minerals. When you stop eating carbohydrates, it can cause nutritional deficiency to your body. To help fight through this, you should use proper vitamins that can provide your body with nutrients.

9. Restock your fridge and pantry

If you are preparing to follow the ketogenic diet, the best way to begin is to rid the keto-unfriendly ingredients from your kitchen and restock with keto-friendly ones. This will make you more attentive and help you resist the urge to eat keto-unfriendly recipes.
Get everything you need to prepare your meals and plan ahead to avoid any inconveniences that may make you lose track of your diet.

<u>What Foods Should Be on Your Plate?</u>
There are specific guidelines for you to follow on the ketogenic diet. It was designed to help people with various diseases and for those looking to shed extra weight. It is best to take note of all the healthy and essential foods that are allowed on this diet.
Below is a list you should include on your menu:

Vegetables

You will eat tons of vegetables on the keto diet. However, you should be more attentive about the kinds of vegetables you consume. Eat vegetables high in nutrients and low in carbohydrates. Organic vegetables are the best, as they contain fewer chemicals and pesticides. The greatest advantage for eating non-starchy vegetables is that they do not raise your blood glucose levels, which would throw your ketosis off balance. Non-starchy vegetables can also help you lose weight by reducing your appetite because they are loaded with fiber.
Here is a short list of some of the best vegetables to eat on the ketogenic diet:
Lettuce
Lettuce is the best vegetable for a ketogenic lifestyle. Lettuce contains few carbohydrates and is a great source of potassium, protein, fiber, and energy. Lettuce also contains many beneficial minerals and vitamins including iron,

3. Turn your favorite foods into ketogenic foods

Thinking of the foods you are not permitted to eat can become quite discouraging. Instead, learn keto-friendly versions of your favorite dishes. There are plenty of ketogenic cookbooks and internet recipes for tips and ideas on how to turn your favorite dishes into tasty ketogenic-friendly versions.

Following the ketogenic diet does not mean depriving yourself from your favorite meals, but about improving your diet and making it healthier. As the keto diet is high in fat, you will maintain all the flavors and texture from your favorite recipes. In many cases, the ketogenic diet has enhanced the flavor of many recipes.

4. Don't be afraid to ask for advice

If you have questions or confusions about the ketogenic diet, don't be afraid to ask for help. Ask professionals, ketogenic dieters, and maybe even certified nutritionists for advice, recipes, and experiences. You will be surprised by the experiences of others, and the information they share.

5. Be alert of alcohol consumption

You can still drink alcohol while on the keto diet without ruining the process. This is one of the great aspects of this diet. However, don't go overboard and drink all the time. It is preferred to go for unsweetened liquors, like scotch, tequila, vodka, whiskey, rum, and reduced-carb beer.

6. Be mindful of condiments and sauces

Not all condiments and sauces are healthy or ketogenic friendly. If you must use sauce and condiments, choose ones that are low in carbs, like soy sauce, lemon, salad dressings, mayonnaise, mustard, olive oil, and coconut oil (just to name a few).

In cases in which you can't tell if something is keto-friendly or not, you can always ask the server or chef. If they are not sure, it would be best to not use the sauce.

7. Be patient

Even though the ketogenic lifestyle is known for rapid weight loss, losing weight will take some time. Do not quit the diet when you are not experiencing quick results. Getting rid of fat will change throughout the day. Try not to get too worked up with

6. Do be patient

It is common nature for us to seek immediate gratification. When you start a diet, you may be discouraged to continue if you are not experiencing the benefits immediately. Losing weight and being healthy takes time. In order to do this, allow your body some time to start burning fat instead of glucose. It may take a few days or a couple of weeks, but be patient and don't bail on the diet.

Important Tips for Successful Ketogenic Journey
If you are just beginning the ketogenic journey, it may be hard for you to stick to this new eating regime, even if you know it's good for you. We are always influenced by unhealthy foods around us, and the accessibility to these foods make them difficult to pass up. Changing your diet is a long-term process; not something you do right off the bat. Here are some valuable tips for a successful ketogenic journey:

1. Gradually follow the ketogenic diet

A common mistake of many when starting the ketogenic diet is immediately eliminating carbohydrates. Doing this is not healthy for your body. While this may work in the short term, doing this can cause serious health problems over the long-term.
Give yourself time to maneuver into the keto lifestyle by making small but essential changes, like giving up one carb source every week or so. It's critical to give your body time to adjust to changes. An excellent way to overcome transition discomfort is to replace a healthy nutrient source to your diet for every unhealthy one. For example, if you use all-purpose flour, start substituting it with almond flour or coconut flour.

2. Drink plenty of water

When you start the ketogenic diet, your body will have a difficult time keeping the proper amount of water you need, so staying perfectly hydrated is the best way to go about it. Drink eight, 8-ounce glasses, which is equivalent to 2 liters every day. To know if you are well hydrated is to determine the color of your urine. Whenever your urine is light yellow or clear, you are properly hydrated.

people follow a diet where they consume 100 to 150 grams of carbs a day. To achieve ketosis, be sure that your carbohydrate intake is low.

Most keto dieters manage the state of ketosis by consuming between 20 to 100 grams of carbs a day.

2. Don't fear fat

If you are on a ketogenic diet, don't be scared of fat. Especially if you consume healthy fats like Omega-3s, monounsaturated fats, and saturated fats. This is encouraged in the ketogenic diet plan; a limit of 60 to 70% fat intake is best. To achieve these levels of fat, you must consume meat and healthy fats, such as olive oil, lard, butter, and coconut or alternatives on a daily basis.

3. Don't eat fast food

If you don't have time to cook, you may turn to fast foods. However, don't even think about it. Fast foods are incredibly unhealthy and can deter you from your keto journey. Fast foods contain too many harmful chemicals and preservatives, and some fast foods don't use real cheese, and meats that contain hidden sugars among other ingredients.

4. Do increase your protein intake

Protein is an essential and important nutrient that is needed for your body. It can soothe your appetite and burn fat more than any other nutrient. Generally, protein is said to be very effective in weight loss, increase muscle mass, and improve your body composition.

5. Do increase your sodium intake

By reducing carbohydrate consumption, your insulin levels fall, which in turn gets rid of extra sodium stored in your body, causing problems such as sodium deficiency. If your body experiences sodium deficiency, you might experience exhaustion, headaches, constipations, etc.

To relieve this problem, increase your sodium intake on a keto diet. Add a teaspoon of salt to daily meals or drink a glass of water with a ¼ teaspoon of salt mixed with it.

5. Headaches

As with many changes in your diet, headaches can occur for no reason. It is possibly you may become light-headed and start to have flu-like symptoms, which could occur over a few days. These headaches normally come about because of a mineral imbalance due to a change in diet. One way to resolve this is to add one-quarter teaspoon of salt to a glass of water and drink it. If you are just beginning the keto lifestyle, you should increase both your salt and water intake for the first couple of days to combat this effectively.

6. Difficulty Sleeping

Another symptom of embarking on the ketogenic diet is trouble sleeping. After cutting down on carbs, many novices to this diet often find themselves staying up later than usual, or frequently waking up at night. Remember, this is temporary. Over time, you will not have trouble sleeping. In fact, many people who remain on the ketogenic diet had their quality of sleep significantly improved.

7. Constipation

In your first week of the ketogenic diet, you may experience constipation because your body may need time to adjust to this new eating regime. To help you cope with this symptom, you can eat more vegetables loaded with fiber. This will keep your intestines moving and increase bowel movements. You can also drink more water to help fight dehydration, which is the contributing factor for constipation. These are the most common signs of what your body could go through when embarking on the ketogenic diet. Not everyone experiences the same symptoms or may even encounter different symptoms. Do not feel discouraged or unmotivated about the diet. Remember, the symptoms will pass within a few weeks and you can reap the positive benefits from ketogenic lifestyle.

Dos and Don'ts of Ketogenic Diet
If you are not familiar with the Keto, mistakes can be made to to keep you from having good health and the benefits of this diet. To enhance the success with the ketogenic diet, here are some dos and don'ts about following the diet:

1. Don't increase your carb intake

The ketogenic diet is a low-carb diet, which means you should lower your carb intake. A specific number of carbs you should have in a diet is not there. Many

- Dizziness.
- Insomnia.

To help cope with the ketogenic flu, you should increase your water and salt intake, as this can prevent you from feeling lousy and tired.

2. Temporary Fatigue

For most dieters feeling fatigued and weak is one of the most common side effects in entering ketosis. This is mostly because your body is being deprived of carbohydrates, which is the only fuel source that your body has been used to. After a week or two, when your body has successfully adapted to burning fats, you will feel more energized and sense an improvement in mental clarity.

In the meantime, how can you cope with temporary fatigue? One thing you can do is take vitamin supplements. One essential nutrient your body always needs is Vitamin B5. If you do not have Vitamin B5, you will start to feel more fatigued or lethargic.

Vitamin B5 helps the adrenaline by boosting metabolism with more energy. Visit your local health store and purchase Vitamin B5, as it can help with temporary fatigue during your ketogenic journey.

3. Bad Breath

Something you should expect from your body under the ketogenic diet is stinky breath. It's not because the foods you eat cause bad breath. Bad breath is a common sign of ketosis because of the elevated levels of ketones in your blood. Notably, it's caused by a specific ketone known as acetone. This type of ketone usually leaves your body through your breath and urine, thus creating stinky breath. Luckily, this symptom will last a short time. As with fatigue, bad breath will go away once your body is fully adapted to the ketogenic diet. Moreover, while waiting for your body to adjust to this diet, you can brush your teeth more frequently and use mouthwash more often.

4. Leg Cramps

Under the ketogenic diet, you may experience muscle cramps. They are common due to hyponatremia, which occurs when your level of sodium in the blood is low. To cope with muscle cramps, you can add an extra teaspoon of salt in your meals and stay well hydrated.

converts to glycogen and gets stored in your liver for later use. When your glycogen levels are full, the excess is stored as fat, thus leading to weight gain. This means that the main cause of weight gain is not eating fats, but the excessive consumption of carbs. Once you eliminate or reduce your carb intake and raise your fat intake, your body changes from burning carbs for energy to burning fats for energy. This means that the excess fats stored in your body will be burned for your energy source, consequently leading to weight loss.

Alongside, the ketogenic lifestyle also helps suppressing your appetite. This is largely because the foods you eat under the ketogenic diet, like fats and protein are quite filling; thus, you will stay full longer and don't feel the urge to eat often.

What Happens to Your Body Under the Ketogenic Diet?

When it comes to improving your health, losing weight, lowering health risks, gaining more energy, and mental clarity, t the ketogenic diet is so efficient because of ketosis, which is a status when your body produces ketones to provide energy for your brain and body. Usually, your body will break down carbohydrates and turn them into glucose for a source of fuel. However, when you adjust to a ketogenic diet, your body will go from storing carbohydrates to burning fat.

Over time, when you have successfully entered ketosis, your body will adapt to this new eating regime. During this short period of transitioning to ketogenic lifestyle, you may experience side effects.

Here is what may happen when your body enters the ketogenic diet:

1. Ketogenic Flu

In the first week of starting the ketogenic diet, it might be challenging for some. Your body may be used to relying mainly on glucose for energy, so it needs to evolve to using ketones for fuel. You may feel tired, unmotivated, and lethargic; this is generally caused by salt deficiency and dehydration that is promoted by the transitory increase in urinating. It also implies that your body will need to take more time to adjust to the different and new ingredients being digested and consumed.

Some of symptoms you may experience with Keto flu:
- Brain fogginess.
- Nausea.
- Cravings.
- Irritability.
- Sniffles.
- Coughing.
- Heart palpitations.

5. Improve Digestion

The ketogenic diet contains low carbs, low grains, and low sugars, which can significantly improve your digestion. When you consume carbs and sugars on a regular basis, it can result in gas, bloating, stomach pains, and constipation. Reducing sugars and carbohydrates in your diet can restore your digestive system.

6. Reduce Triglycerides

Triglycerides are also known as fat molecules. Increased levels of triglycerides are connected to heart health. Thus, it is important to lower triglyceride levels, which can be achieved with the ketogenic diet. The more carbohydrates you consume, the more triglycerides you will have in your blood, which can provoke heart disease. When you cut down carbohydrate consumption, the number of triglycerides in the body is dramatically reduced.

7. Increase Energy

A ketogenic diet can increase energy levels in multiple ways. It increases the mitochondrial function, and at the same time decreases the harmful radicals inside your body, thus making you feel more energetic and revitalized.

8. Improve Mental Health

The ketone bodies released when following ketogenic diet are directly connected to mental health. Research has shown that increased ketone levels can lead to stabilization of neurotransmitters, like dopamine and serotonin. This stabilization helps fight mood swings, depression, and other psychological issues.

Lose Weight Faster with the Ketogenic Diet than Other Diets

Obesity has become one of the largest health epidemics in the world. Many have tried multiple methods to fight obesity and excess weight, but their methods were not successful. To overcome obesity and lose weight, you must change your diet. The ketogenic diet has worked for many to preserve muscle mass and shed excess fat, without putting much effort.

The sole purpose of the ketogenic diet is to make your body enter a state of glycogen deprivation and maintain a state of ketosis, which is great for weight loss. Usually, in carb-based diets, carbohydrates are transformed into glucose, which is then used as the main fuel source for the body and brain. The remaining glucose

1. Weight Loss

The ketogenic diet focuses on keeping carbs to a minimum. Studies have proven that ketogenic practitioners lose weight easier and faster, compared to other people. Why? Because on a ketogenic diet, you drastically reduce the number of carbohydrates in every meal.

When you begin to consume fewer carbohydrates, the excess water in your body will shed. Thereby, reducing the levels of insulin, which directly affect your sodium levels, cultivating weight loss.

2. Diminish Your Appetite

Following a low-carb diet can alleviate your hunger. The worst side effect of this diet is feeling hungry. Hunger is the main reason why many people bail. However, when you follow the low-carb diet, your appetite is reduced. The more carbs you cut from your diet, the more protein and healthy fats is added. Thus, the fewer calories you consume. In other words, once you eliminate carbohydrates from your diet, your appetite will decrease and you end up consuming fewer calories, without even trying to eat less.

3. Decrease Blood Pressure

When your blood pressure is high or if you suffer from hypertension, you become prone to developing several health issues, like heart disease, kidney failure, or strokes. One of the most efficient ways to reduce your blood pressure is to maintain a low-carb diet. Successfully following a low-carb diet, your exposure to diseases is reduced. Research has also shown that by decreasing the consumption of carbohydrates leads to a significant reduction in blood pressure, thus reducing the risk of developing various diseases.

4. Improve Your HDL Cholesterol

HDL cholesterol is a special kind of protein that runs by transferring the "bad cholesterol" from your body and into your liver, where the cholesterol is either exerted or reused. When your HDL cholesterol level is high, your cholesterol deposits within your blood vessel walls, and this helps to prevent blockage that can provoke heart disease or heart pain. High-fat diets like the ketogenic diet are known for raising your blood vessels with HDL, which means you can reduce the risk of developing cardiovascular disease.

Chapter 2: Everything About the Ketogenic Diet

There are many low-carb diets available. One of the most popular is the "ketogenic diet". More and more people are turning to the ketogenic diet because of the various advantages this diet carries. The ketogenic diet is a powerful way to lose weight and offers multiple benefits leading to a healthy lifestyle that fad diets do not. In this chapter, you will learn everything you need to know about the ketogenic diet.

What is the Ketogenic Diet?

The ketogenic diet is a high-fat, moderate protein, low-carbohydrate diet. This diet concentrates on decreasing your carbohydrate intake and replacing it with healthy fats and proteins. Normally, your body burns carbohydrates to convert into glucose, which is then carried around your body and is essential for brain fuel. However, when your body has low amounts of carbohydrates, the liver will convert fat into fatty acids and ketone bodies. The ketone bodies then move into the brain and replace glucose as the primary energy source.

The ketogenic diet was created to reach a state of ketosis. Ketosis is a metabolic state where your body produces ketones. Ketones are produced by your liver and used as fuel toward your body and brain instead of glucose. To make ketones, you must consume a substantial number of carbs and a bare minimum amount of proteins. The traditional ketogenic diet contains a 4:1 ratio by weight of fat to combined protein and carbohydrate. This is accomplished by eliminating high-carbohydrate foods, such as starchy fruits, vegetables, breads, grains, pasta, and sugar while boosting the consumption of foods high in fats, such as nuts, cream, and butter. The bottom line is the ketogenic diet is a low-carb diet useful in burning body fat.

Benefits of the Ketogenic Diet.

The ketogenic diet comes with many positive benefits. For beginners, it has been used to treat epileptic seizures and various other diseases, including cancer and Alzheimer's. Overall, the ketogenic diet can be used to improve and enhance your health by preventing and controlling the substances in your body. Here are some of the benefits of the ketogenic diet:

It is not necessary that you preheat your pot, if you do, you will get better results. Just let the appliance pre-heat for 5 minutes before cooking.

Is it possible to open the lid while cooking?

As long as you are using any of the convection methods such as Air Crisp, Bake/Roast, you are allowed to open the lid at any time you want. Once you open up the lid, the cooking will pause and will only resume once you have securely placed the lid.

However, while Pressure Cooking/Steaming, you should never open the lid until the whole cook cycle and pressure release cycle is complete!

Are the different parts of the Foodi Dishwasher safe?

Yes, all the accessories of the Ninja Foodi are dishwasher safe, alongside the inner pot as well. However, keep in mind that the base, Crisping Lid, and Pressure Lid are NOT dishwasher safe and should be cleaned by using a sponge or wet cloth.

How to get rid of the unpleasant smell from the Sealing Ring?

The most basic step to do is to remove the sealing ring after every cook session and washing/drying I before putting it back. You can do this either by hand or by using your dishwasher. If that doesn't do the trick, try to leave it under the sun for a while.

- This is something that many people don't know, once the cooking timer of your appliance hits '0', the pot will automatically go into "Natural Pressure Release" mode where it will start to release the pressure on its own. You can use a quick release anytime to release all the steam at once, or you can wait for 10-15 minutes until the steam vents off.
- It is important that you place the lid properly while closing the appliance as it greatly affects the cooking. Therefore, make sure that your lid is tightly close by ensuring that the silicone ring inside the lid is placed all the way around the groove.
- If you are in a rush and want to release the pressure quickly, turn the pressure valve to "Open Position," which will quick release all the pressure. But this can be a little risky as a lot of steam comes out at once, so be sure to stay careful.
- Once your start using the appliance for cooking, make sure to check if the Pressure Valve is in the "Locked Position." If it is not, your appliance won't be able to build up pressure inside for cooking.
- If you are dealing with a recipe that calls for unfrozen meat, make sure to use the same amount of cooking time and liquid that you would use if you were to use frozen meat of the same type.
- Make sure to keep in mind that the "Timer" button isn't a button to set time! Rather it acts as a Delay Timer. Using this button, you will be able to set a specific time, after which the Ninja Foodi will automatically wake up and start cooking the food.

FAQ's

Below are the answers to some of the most commonly asked questions that should help you clear up some confusion (if you have any).

Why do some foods such as rice, or veggies call for different cooking times in different recipes?

The cooking time does not only depend on the type of ingredient that you are using but on various other factors as well.

When considering vegetables, you have to consider how the veggies are cut. If using a whole cauliflower head, it might be cubed, cut into florets, alternatively, you can have cubed potatoes and whole potatoes.

Cubed variations will always take less time than the whole veggie itself.

The same goes for meat as well, the thickness and the cut largely vary the time taken to cooking the meal properly.

If you are cooking rice, you might be interested to know that pressure cooking rice directly into the pot will cook much faster than pressure cooking the rice in a bowl that is set on the rack.

Is it possible to adjust the temperature of Sautéing or Searing?

Yes, all you have to do is press the Temperature Up and Down arrows twice, and the appliance will change the heat setting and allow you to Saute/Sear at your selected mode.

Is Pre-heating necessary when using the Crisping or Roasting feature?

At its heart, the Ninja Foodi is an electric pressure cooker, and making foods utilizing this single aspect will yield you extremely juicy and tender meals in no time!

But why should you limit yourself to only that?

Asides from being able to prepare mouthwatering pressure cooked and fried air meals, the Ninja Foodi comes with a plethora of advantages that will make your cooking experience even more delightful.

Below are just some of the many!

Allows you to cook frozen food: With the awesome power of the Ninja Foodi, you will be able to save a huge amount of time by skipping the "defrosting" phase and adding your meat right out of the freezer! The advanced cooking technologies allow the Foodi to defrost the meat and cook them to perfection in no time!

Let's you cook healthier meals: The precise cooking mechanism of the Ninja Foodi allows the appliance to preserve most of the nutrition of your meal while ensuring that your meals are undeniably delicious.

Acts as a one-stop shop: This single appliance acts as a one-stop shop for all of your meals! You can cook, roast, steam in the single pot itself and have everything ready by the end!

Allows cooking in a single pot: Just using a single pot, you will be able to convert a simple and regular looking soup into an amazing casserole dish or something exquisite. The versatility of the Ninja Foodi means that you won't have to use multiple pots for your cooking, the single pot provided with the Foodi is more than enough to prepare your meal from scratch to finish.

Frees up a lot of kitchen space: Regardless o the size of your kitchen, the ergonomic design of the Ninja Foodi means that you will always be able to make up space for this nifty appliance! And since this pot can perform the job of a Slow Cooker, Air Fryer, Pressure Cooker, etc. all alone, you won't even have to keep any other appliances around!

Easy Cleaning: Cleaning is a nightmare for every chef and homemaker! Since all the cooking is done in a ceramic coated non-stick pot in the Ninja Foodi, cleaning the appliance is a breeze! All it takes is a little bit of soapy water, and you are good to go!

Kills Any And All Harmful Micro-Organism: Sophisticated Electric Pressure Cookers such as the Ninja Foodi allows the internal temperature inside the pot to reach extremely high levels! This allows the pot to destroy most viruses and bacteria that might otherwise be harmful to your body. Some of the more resistant ones found in raw maize or corns can also be destroyed as well.

Useful Tips for Success

As time goes on, you will learn how to utilize the power of your Ninja Foodi to its full extent. However, the following tips will help you during the early days of your life with the Foodi and ensure that your experience is as pleasant and smooth as possible.

- It is crucial that you don't just press the function buttons randomly! Try to read through the function of each button and use them according to the requirement of your recipe.

The different parts of the Ninja Foodi are as follows:

- **Pressure Release Valve:** These valves are used to control the entrapment or release of the pressure inside the pot.
- **Pressure Lid:** The pressure lid is used when pressure is cooking your meals.
- **Crisping Lid:** The crisping lid is used when trying to Air Fryer your meals using the TenderCrisp technology.
- **Cooking Pot:** The cooking pot is the actual inner pot where you dump the ingredients and let it cook.

Asides from the above-mentioned core parts, there are some others that you should know about as well.

The Reversible Rack: This particular rack can be used both ways for your desired effect. The reversible rack is primarily used for broiling (when placed in the upper position), while it can also be used for steaming, cooking, baking, and roasting, should you choose to place it in the lower position.

Cook And Crisp Basket: The crisping basket is an easily removable basket that is specially designed for Air Crisping.

Various other accessories are also available for the Ninja Foodi. Some of the more useful ones are as follows:

Extra Reversible Rack/ 8 Inch Round Wire Cooling Rack: Some recipes might ask you to use a rack twice, once for steaming and once for broiling for example. Instead of using the same rack over and over again, it's a pretty good idea to have an extra rack around, and it makes life a whole lot easier.

And as a bonus, you will also be able to use it as a cooling rack as well.

Extra Sealing Ring: Overtime and despite your best efforts, the Silicone ring might pick up dirt and unpleasant odor. Despite its pretty long-lasting durability, they tend to become nicked or stretched after prolonged usage!

Having a damaged or compromised Sealing Ring is never a good idea as it will render your pot useless in the future. Therefore, keeping an extra ring always helps in the long run. You When buying an extra ring, make sure to check that you are buying a ring that is specifically designed for the Foodi. Otherwise, it won't fit properly.

Multi-Purpose Pan/Metal/Ceramic Bowl: If you do a lot of Pot-In-Pot cooking, then having a ceramic or metal bowl would be a Godsend! These are excellent for when you are making dishes such as quiches, casseroles or even cake. Just make sure to buy a one that it no more than about 8 and ½ inches across. The official Multi-Purpose Pan sold by Ninja is excellent for this purpose.

Roasting Rack Insert: This rack is specifically designed to work with the Cook and Crisp Basket, and comes in real handy if you want to roast or glaze meat/ribs.

Cook and Crisp Layered Insert: This layout helps to increase the capacity of the Cook and Crisp Basket by allowing you to create layers of meals and crisp them all at once.

Amazing advantages of the Ninja Foodi

this function is to suck out the moisture and dehydrate your ingredient into a hearty edible snack.

The different parts and accessories of the Ninja Foodi

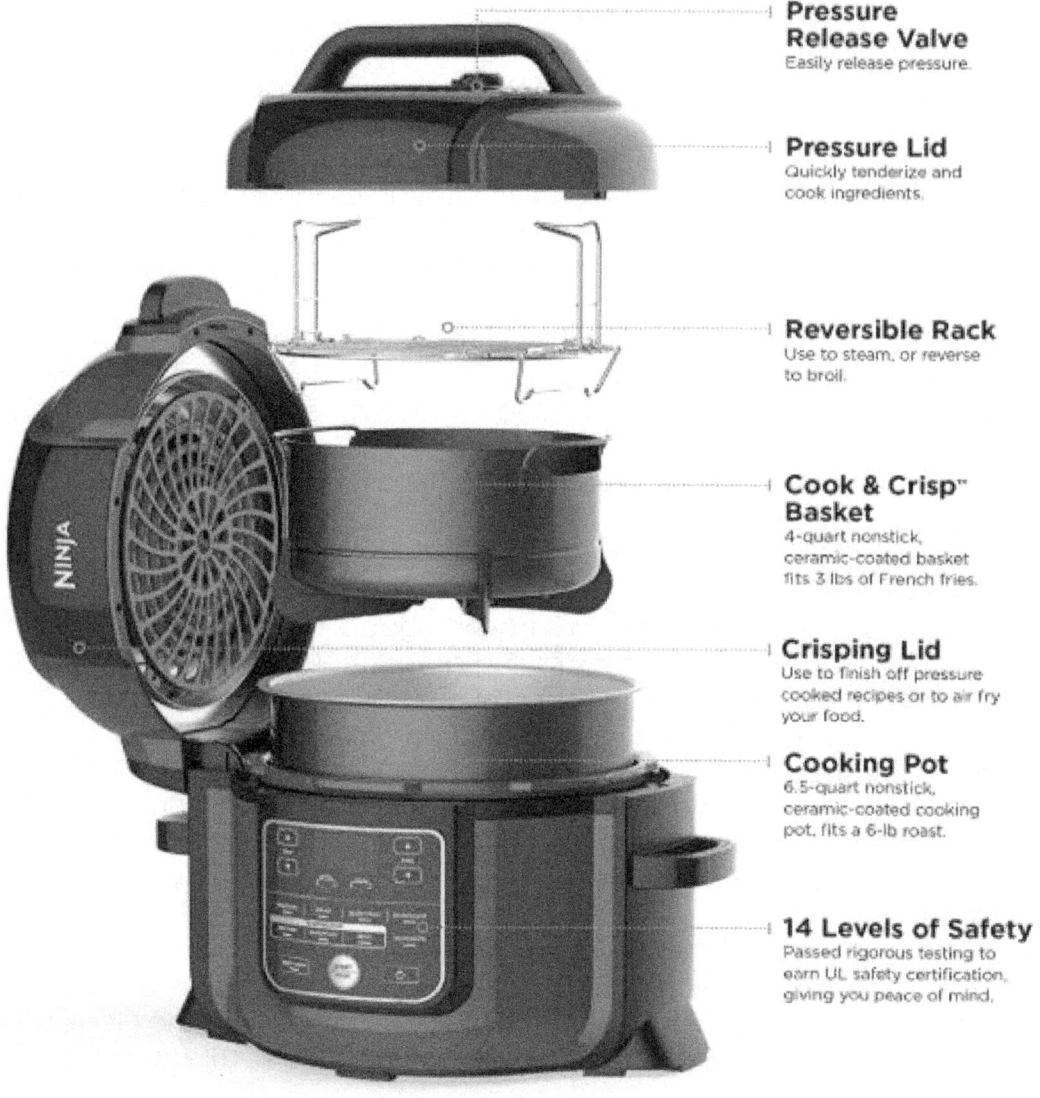

THE NINJA FOODI

Pressure Release Valve
Easily release pressure.

Pressure Lid
Quickly tenderize and cook ingredients.

Reversible Rack
Use to steam, or reverse to broil.

Cook & Crisp Basket
4-quart nonstick, ceramic-coated basket fits 3 lbs of French fries.

Crisping Lid
Use to finish off pressure cooked recipes or to air fry your food.

Cooking Pot
6.5-quart nonstick, ceramic-coated cooking pot, fits a 6-lb roast.

14 Levels of Safety
Passed rigorous testing to earn UL safety certification, giving you peace of mind.

Sear/Saute

The Browning/Saute or Sear/Saute mode of the Ninja Foodi provides you with the means to brown your meat before cooking it using a just a little bit of oil. This is similar to when you are browning meat on a stovetop frying pan. And keeping that in mind, the Ninja Foodie's browning mode comes with five different Stove Top temperature settings that allow you to set your desired settings with ease.

Asides from browning meat, the different Stove Top temperatures also allows you to gently simmer your foods, cook or even sear them at very high temperatures.

Searing is yet another way to infuse the delicious flavors of your meat inside and give an extremely satisfying result.

This particular model is also excellent if you are in the mode for a quick Sautéed vegetable snack to go along with your main course.

Air Crisp

This is probably the feature that makes the Ninja Foodi so revolutionary and awesome to use! The Tendercrisp lid that comes as a part of the Ninja Foodi allows you to use the appliance as the perfect Air Fryer device.

Using the Tendercrisp lid and Air Crisp mode, the appliance will let you bake, roast, broil meals to perfection using just the power of superheated air! In the end, you will get perfectly caramelized, heartwarming dishes.

The Foodi comes with a dedicated crisping basket that is specifically designed for this purpose, which optimizes the way meals are air fried in the Foodi.

But the best part in all of these is probably the fact that the using the Air Crisp feature, you will be able to cook your meals using almost none to minimal amount of oil!

It is also possible to combine both the pressure cooking mechanism and Air Crisp function to create unique and flavorful dishes.

The Pressure cooking phase will help you to seal the delicious juices of the meal inside the meat, while the crisping lid and Air Crisp mechanism will provide you to cook/roast your meal to perfection, giving a nice heartfelt crispy finish.

This combined method is also amazing when roasting whole chicken meat or roasts, as all the moisture remains intact and the final result turns out to be a dramatic crispy finish.

Bake/Roast

For anyone who loves to bake, this function is a dream come true! The Bake/Roast function allows the Foodi to be used as a traditional convection oven. This means you will be do anything that you might do with a general everyday oven! If you are in the mode to bake amazing cakes or casseroles, the Foodi has got you covered!

Broil

The main purpose of the Broil function is to allow you to use your appliance like an oven broiler and slightly brown the top of your dish if required. If you are in the mood for roasting a fine piece of pork loin to perfection or broiling your dish until the cheese melts and oozes, this mode is the perfect one to go with!

Dehydrate

In some more premium models of the Ninja Foodi appliance, you will notice a function labeled as "Dehydrate." This particular function is best suited for simple dried snacks such as dried apple slices, banana chips, jerky, etc. As you can probably guess, the core idea of

To make things easier for you and ensure that you don't have to face any troubles in the future, I have tried to outline the basic functions of all of the buttons present in most models of the Ninja Foodi.

Pressure

Let's first talk about the single feature that you will be using most of the time. The Pressure function will allow you to use your Ninja Foodi as a Pressure Cooker appliance and cook your meals as you would in an electric pressure cooker such as the Instant Pot.

In this feature, foods are cooked at high temperature under pressure.

Just make sure to be careful when releasing the pressure! Otherwise, you might harm yourself.

There are essentially two ways through which you can release the pressure, which is discussed later on in the chapter.

Steam

Asides from Air Crisp, the Steam Function is probably one of the healthiest cooking option available in the Foodi!

The basic principle is as follows- Water is boiled inside the Ninja Foodi that generates a good amount of steam. This hot steam is then used to cook your ingredients kept in a steaming rack situated at the top of the inner chamber of your Pot.

Steaming is perfect for vegetables and other tender foods as it allows to preserve the nutrients while maintaining a nice crispy perfectly.

Asides from vegetables, however, the Steam function can also be used for cooking various fish and seafood, which are much more delicate than other red meats and chicken.

The process of steaming fish are the same, all you have to do is place them on the steaming rack.

Steaming the fish helps to preserve the flavor and moisture as well perfectly.

Slow Cooker

Despite popular belief, some foods tend to taste a whole lot better when Slowly Cooked over extremely low temperature for hours on end. This is why Slow Cookers such as the CrockPot are so popular amongst chefs and house makers!

The Slow Cooker feature of the Ninja Foodi allows you to achieve the same result, but without the need for a different appliance.

Ideal scenarios to use the Slow Cooker function would be when you want to cook your foods for longer to bring out the intense flavor of spices and herbs in stews, soups, and casseroles.

Since it takes a lot of time to Slow Cook, you should prepare and toss the ingredients early on before your feeding time.

For example. If you want to have your Slow Cooker meal for breakfast, prepare ingredients the night before and add them to your Foodi. The Foodi will do its magic and have the meal prepared by morning.

The Slow Cooker feature also comes with a HIGH or LOW setting that allows you to decide how long you want your meal to simmer.

Start/Stop Button

The function of this particular button is pretty straightforward; it allows you to initiate or stop the cooking process.

However, general Slow Cookers are only designed to do just one thing, that is to cook your meals for an extended period at extremely low temperatures. (There are multifunctional Slow Cookers, but we are not considering them here).

Instant Pots, on the other hand, are multifunctional Electric Pressure Cookers, which were pretty much the king of the game until the arrival of the Ninja Foodi, which might dethrone them. Similar to the Ninja Foodi, Instant Pot's also come packed with a large number of different features that allows users to bake, roast, simmer, boil, steam and pressure cook their meals.

However, the crucial point where the Ninja Foodi stands out is that alongside most of the features of the Instant Pot and Slow Cooker, the Ninja Foodi is capable of Air Frying meals using the Crisping Lid and TenderCrisp technology.

So in short, the Ninja Foodi is essentially the combination of all three appliances in on nifty package.

Understanding the Revolutionary Tendercrisp Technology

The Tendercrisp Technology stands at the heart of the Ninja Foodi cooking appliance that seemingly differentiates itself from the rest of the world. So, I strongly believe that it is really important that you have a good understanding of what this unique technology does.

So when you are pressure cooking tough ingredients such as meats, you end up with meals that are extremely juicy and satisfying to eat, but tender as well. Just pressure cooking alone won't be able to provide you with any crispy finish! This is where Air Frying comes in.

Air Frying utilizes the power of air to make foods crispier by giving it a nice tasty crust.

The revolutionary technology used in the Ninja Foodi allows a user to infuse both the effects of Pressure Cooking and Air Frying using just the single device! This basic cooking principle of combining both cooking methods is known as Ninja Foodi's proprietary TenderCrisp Technology.

In short, it allows you to create meals that are extremely tender and juicy on the side while having a satisfying crust on the surface.

The basic cooking procedure will ask you first to cook you a meal using pressure cooking, then use the Crisping Lid and Crisping Basket accompanied by the Air Crisp function to achieve your desired level of crispiness.

To better understand the mechanism at work here, the TenderCrisp technology utilizes superheated steam to infuse both flavors and moisture into your pressure cooked food. Afterward, the crisping lid blows extremely hot air to every side of your meal that gives it a fine golden color and crisp finish.

This unique combination is so far unachievable by any other appliance to date!

Looking at the different function buttons of the Ninja Foodi

Given the versatility of the Ninja Foodi, it is very easy to understand why some individuals might get confused when dealing with the plethora of amazing functions available in the appliance.

Chapter 1: Understanding the Fundamentals Of Ninja Foodi

What is Ninja Foodi?

The Ninja Foodie is probably the most versatile, and undoubtedly revolutionary kitchen appliance out there in the market.

This is the only appliance of its kind that can work as Slow Cooker, Saute pan, Electric Pressure Cooker, Rice Cooker, and even an Air Fryer! All under one hood.

The unique technology that allows it's designers to blend the functionalities of Air Fryer and Pressure Cooker means that chefs can cook their food more efficiently and faster than any other kitchen appliance to date.

And just in case you are wondering, with this amazing device, you won't only be limited to simple pressure cooker dishes! The versatility of this appliance will allow you to create anything from soups, stews, chili's to breakfast and desserts! Your imagination is the only limitation here.

For new beginners though, the barrage of functionalities might seem a little bit confusing at first, but rest assured, the appliance is very easy to use.

All you need is a little understanding of what each function button does, and you are good to go!

The differences between Ninja Foodi and Instant Pot/Slow Cooker/Air Fryer

At its heart, the core difference between all three of the above-mentioned appliances and the Ninja Foodi is that the Ninja Foodi is the combination of all three. Meaning, with this revolutionary appliance, you will be able to Pressure Cook, Slow Cook, and even Air Fryer your meals with ease.

Asides from that, there are some fundamental differences that you should about as well.

Considering the Ninja Foodi and Air Fryer: The Air Fryer is essentially an appliance that is strictly designed for just the purpose of Air Frying various and preparing various meals, using the minimum amount of oil. This appliance is excellent at what it does and using an Air Fryer; you can prepare a plethora of different types of meals. However, it is not an all in one.

Comparing the Ninja Foodi with an Air Fryer, you would immediately notice that they both sport a very distinctive shape. The Ninja Foodi is like a round pot, similar to the Instant Pot while the Air Fryer extrudes a little a bit on the top side.

The Crisping Lid alongside the TenderCrisp technology that allows the Ninja Foodi to Air Fry meals, while working as an advanced and versatile is what sets it apart from the Air Fryer.

Considering the Ninja Foodi and Instant Pot and Slow Cooker: The Slow Cooker and Instant Pot are probably the two appliances can be considered as being the closest sibling to the Ninja Foodi Electric Pressure cooker!

All three of the appliances sport a similar shape, which is like a pot.

Improves blood profile indicators.
Reduces or eliminates the need for diabetic medications.
Regulates blood pressure without medication.
Eliminates insulin resistance.
Be wiser by increasing mental focus and clearing mental fog.

And once you are done with the intro's, feel free to explore the amazing Keto-Friendly Ninja Foodi recipes found in this booklet and let your creativity go wild! You will find: *Breakfast, Vegetarian and Vegan, Chicken and Poultry, Beef, Pork and Lamb, Seafood and Fish, Dessert and Snacks, etc. Everything you will find to make you feel happy every meal.*

Welcome, to the world of Ketogenic Diet with the revolutionary Ninja Foodi!

Introduction

Are you looking for a way to lose your weight fast and permanently?
Do you want to save your precious time and money while have your favorite dishes everyday?
Do you want to cook all your meals just by using one kitchen appliance, which can be used as Instant Pot pressure cooker, slow cooker and air fryer, etc.?
If yes of any questions above, then you are absolutely reading your right book already!
Come on, friends! Let's dive into this amazing but effective book now!

Even though the Instant Pot could replace most of the everyday kitchen appliances such as **Saute Pan, Steamer, Slow Cooker**, etc., the one thing that it wasn't able to do, was replicate the effects of an Air Fryer. And this is exactly where the revolutionary Ninja Foodi came in and completely flipped the paradigm with its revolutionary new "**TenderCrisp**" technology!

At its heart, the amazing Ninja Foodi is an all-in-one kitchen appliance like that no other, that is designed to replace not only an Instant Pot and CrockPot but also an Air Fryer! The meticulously crafted design of this single appliance allows you to *Saute, Broil, Bake, Roast, Pressure Cook, Steam, Slow Cook and even Air Fry!* All under the same hood.

This Ninja Foodi can accomplish this feat, thanks to the crisping lid that comes attached with the Foodi itself. When needed, this particular lid alongside the Air Crisp Function and Crisping Basket allows the users to seamless Air Fry their dishes and give them a satisfying crispy finish!

Throughout the first chapter, you will find that I have discussed the core concepts of the Ninja Foodi in greater details, so if this is your first time diving into the world of Ninja Foodi, this is the perfect opportunity to get the hang of this amazing device!

And don't worry, I haven't forgotten about the Ketogenic part either! Since this particular book focuses on the awesome Ketogenic Diet cooking, another chapter is also provided that will cover up all essentials of the Keto diet itself. Nowadays, Keto Diet is the most popular and easy-to-follow diet, which has been written in many websites and books. You may have already known much information about it. This book will give you a complete guide of Ketogenic Diet for weight loss and overall health in a very easy-to-understand way!

By following a ketogenic diet, you will get many benefits, below are some of them:
No undernourishment.
Lose weight faster.
A stable energy level.
Increases endurance.

Tasty Brussels...128

Visible Citrus And Cauli Salad...128

Faithful Roasted Garlic...129

Feisty Chicken Thighs...129

Garlic And Tomato "Herbed" Chicken Thighs..............................129

The Kool Poblano Cheese Frittata...130

The Divine Fudge Meal...130

The Original Braised Kale And Carrot Salad.................................130

Delicious Bacon- Wrapped Drumsticks...131

Stuffed Chicken Mushrooms...131

A Hot Buffalo Wing Platter...131

Garlic And Mushroom Crunchies..132

Delicious Cocoa Almond Bites...132

Keto Chicken Crescent Wraps..132

Diced And Spiced Up Paprika Eggs...133

Faux Daikon Noodles...133

Simple Vegetable Stock..134

Conclusion...135
Appendix: Measurement Conversion Table.................136

Just A Simple Egg Frittata...115

Ultimate Cheese Dredged Cauliflower Snack...116

Chapter 10: Snacks Recipes..117

Ultimate Creamy Zucchini Fries..117

The Onion And Smoky Mushroom Medley..117

Cool Beet Chips..117

Lovely Cauliflower Soup...118

Elegant Broccoli Pops..118

Great Brussels Bite..118

Simple Mushroom Saute...119

Delicious Assorted Nuts..119

Garlic And Sage Spaghetti Squash..119

Spicy Cauliflower Steak...120

Subtle Buffalo Chicken Meatballs..120

The Original Steamed Artichoke..121

Crispy Avocado Chips..121

The Crazy Egg-Stuffed Avocado Dish..121

The Great Mediterranean Spinach...123

Quick Turkey Cutlets..123

Veggies Dredged In Cheese...123

Egg Dredged Casserole...124

Excellent Bacon And Cheddar Frittata...124

Pork Packed Jalapeno...124

Juicy Garlic Chicken Livers...125

The Original Zucchini Gratin...125

Quick Bite Zucchini Fries..125

Pickled Up Green Chili...126

Spaghetti Squash And Chicken Parmesan..126

Spice Lover's Jar Of Chili...126

Easy To Swallow Beet Chips...127

Bacon Samba Bok Choy..127

Sour Cream Mushroom Appetizer..127

Heart-Throb Buttery Scallops..103

Sensational Coconut Fish Curry...104

Warm Cajun Bass Stew...104

The Great Lobster Bisque..105

Elegant Fish Curry...105

Almond Cod Fillets..106

Simple Sweet And Sour Fish Magnifico...106

Cod With Broccoli, Lemon And Dill Mismash..106

Butter Dredged "Rich" Lobster...106

The Extremely Wild Alaskan Cod...107

Magical Shrimp Platter...107

Gentle Salmon Stew..108

Chapter 9: Dessert Recipes.................................. 109

The Divine Fudge Delight...109

Keto-Friendly Nut Porridge...109

Heartfelt Vanilla Yogurt..109

Delicious Lemon Mousse..110

The Generous Strawberry Shortcake..110

Sensational Lemon Custard...110

Hearty Carrot Pumpkin Pudding..111

Creative Crème Brulee...111

The Original Pot-De-Crème..111

Inspiring Cauliflower Hash Browns...112

Everybody's Favorite Cauliflower Patties..112

Kale And Almonds Mix..113

Simple Treat Of Garlic...113

Buttered Up Garlic And Fennel..113

Obvious Paprika And Cabbage...114

Authentic Western Omelet..114

Bowl Full Of Broccoli Salad..114

Rise And Shine Breakfast Casserole..115

Cauliflower And Egg Dish..115

Decisive Kalua Pork...91

Easy-Going Kid Friendly Pork Chops..92

Amazing Mexican Pulled Pork Lettuce...92

Cuban And Garlic Pork Meal..93

Mean Cream Mushroom Garlic Chicken...93

Chapter 8: Seafood And Fish Recipes...................... 94

Hearty Swordfish Meal..94

Gentle And Simple Fish Stew...94

Cool Shrimp Zoodles...94

Heartfelt Sesame Fish...95

Awesome Sock-Eye Salmon..95

Buttered Up Scallops..95

Awesome Cherry Tomato Mackerel..96

Lovely Air Fried Scallops...96

Packets Of Lemon And Dill Cod...96

Adventurous Sweet And Sour Fish...97

Garlic And Lemon Prawn Delight..97

Lovely Carb Soup...97

The Rich Guy Lobster And Butter...98

Lovely Panko Cod..98

Salmon Paprika..99

Heartfelt Air Fried Scampi...99

Ranch Warm Fillets...99

Alaskan Cod Divine..100

Kale And Salmon Delight..100

Breathtaking Cod Fillets..101

Lemon And Pepper Salmon Delight..101

Fresh Steamed Salmon...101

Small-Time Herby Cods..102

Tomato And Shrimp Medley..102

The Smoked White Fish...103

Cool Lemon And Dill Fish Packages..103

Quick Picadillo Dish...78

Simple/Aromatic Meatballs...79

Generous Shepherd's Pie..79

Hybrid Beef Prime Roast...80

The Epic Carne Guisada..80

No-Noodle Pure Lasagna..80

The Wisdom Worthy Corned Beef...81

Hearty Korean Ribs...81

Traditional Beef Sirloin Steak...82

Beef And Broccoli Platter..82

Chapter 7: Pork Recipes...**83**

Spicy "Faux" Pork Belly...83

Spiced Up Chipotle Pork Roast...83

Happy Burrito Bowl Pork...83

Awesome Sauerkraut Pork..84

Spice Lover's Jalapeno Hash...84

The Premium Red Pork..84

Cool Spicy Pork Salad Bowl..85

Dill And Butter Pork Chops..85

Cranberry Pork BBQ Dish...86

Definitive Pork Carnita..86

Technical Keto Pork Belly...87

Jamaican Pork Pot..87

The Mexican Pulled Pork Ala Lettuce......................................87

Pork With Cranberries And Pecan...88

Mesmerizing Pork Carnitas...88

Mustard Dredged Pork Chops..89

Authentic Beginner Friendly Pork Belly.....................................89

Deliciously Spicy Pork Salad Bowl...90

Special "Swiss" Pork chops..90

Perfect Sichuan Pork Soup..90

Healthy Cranberry Keto-Friendly BBQ Pork.............................91

Taiwanese Chicken Delight..66

Cabbage And Chicken Meatballs...66

Poached Chicken With Coconut Lime Cream Sauce............................66

Hot And Spicy Paprika Chicken...67

Inspiring Turkey Cutlets..67

Lemongrass And Tamarind Chicken..68

Fluffy Whole Chicken Dish...68

Sensible Chettinad Chicken..68

Hawaiian Pinna Colada Chicken Meal...69

Garlic And Butter Chicken Dish...69

Creamy Chicken Curry...70

Lemon And Artichoke Medley..70

Awesome Sesame Ginger Chicken...70

Chicken Korma...71

Turkey With Garlic Sauce..71

Awesome Ligurian Chicken..72

Chapter 6: Beef and Lamb Recipes....................................... 73

Warm And Beefy Meat Loaf...73

Wise Corned Beef...73

Elegant Beef Curry..73

Mesmerizing Beef Sirloin Steak...74

Epic Beef Sausage Soup..74

The Indian Beef Delight..74

Fresh Korean Braised Ribs..75

The Classical Corned Beef And Cabbage...75

Crazy Greek Lamb Gyros...76

The Ultimate One-Pot Beef Roast..76

Easy To Swallow Beef Ribs..76

Everyday Lamb Roast...77

The Gentle Beef And Broccoli Dish..77

The Juicy Beef Chili...78

Generous Ground Beef Stew..78

Chives And Radishes Platter...52

Garlic And Swiss Chard Garlic..53

Healthy Rosemary And Celery Dish..53

Awesome Veggie Hash...53

Thyme And Carrot Dish With Dill..54

Creative Coconut Cabbage..54

Complete Cauliflower Zoodles...55

Simple Mushroom Hats And Eggs..55

Ginger And Butternut Bisque Yum..55

Hearty Cheesy Cauliflower...57

Mesmerizing Spinach Quiche..57

Running Away Broccoli Casserole...58

Spaghetti Squash Fancy Noodles...58

Dill And Garlic Fiesta Platter..59

Quick Red Cabbage...59

Simple Rice Cauliflower...59

Very Spicy Cauliflower Steak..60

Authentic Indian Palak Paneer...60

Chapter 5: Chicken And Poultry Recipes........................61

Juicy Sesame Garlic Chicken Wings..61

Perfectly Braised Chicken Thigh With Chokeful Of Mushrooms.................................61

Lemon And Butter Chicken Extravagant...62

Creative Cabbage And Chicken Meatball..62

Spicy Hot Paprika Chicken...62

Elegant Chicken Stock..63

Hot Turkey Cutlets..63

Pulled Up Keto Friendly Chicken Tortilla's...64

Fully-Stuffed Whole Chicken..64

Ham-Stuffed Generous Turkey Rolls...64

Sensational Lime And Chicken Chili..65

Funky-Garlic And turkey Breasts...65

Mexico's Favorite Chicken Soup..65

The Early Morning Ballet Of Ham And Spinach...41

The Coolest New York Strip Steak...42

French Onion Pork Chops...42

Hearty Apple Infused Water...42

Simple And Easy Chicken Breast...42

Italian Dark Kale Crisps...43

Quick Ginger And Sesame Chicken...43

Butter Melted Broccoli Florets...43

The Epic Fried Eggs...44

Gentle Keto Butter Fish...44

Sensational Carrot Puree...44

Simple Broccoli Florets...45

Awesome Magical 5 Ingredient Shrimp...45

Romantic Mustard Pork...45

Creative And Easy Lamb Roast...46

Crispy Tofu And Mushrooms...46

Chapter 4: Vegetarian And Vegan Recipes..................................47

Cheese Dredged Cauliflower Delight...47

Garlic And Dill Carrot Fiesta...47

Cool Indian Palak Paneer...47

Astounding Caramelized Onions...48

Special Lunch-Worthy Green Beans...48

Healthy Cauliflower Mash...48

Beets And Greens With Cool Horseradish Sauce...49

Summertime Veggie Soup...49

Delicious Mushroom Stroganoff...50

Everyday Use Veggie-Stock...50

Groovy Broccoli Florets...50

Offbeat Cauliflower And Cheddar Soup...51

Powerful Medi-Cheese Spinach...51

Awesome Butternut Squash Soup...52

Comfortable Mushroom Soup...52

2. Don't fear fat..30
3. Don't eat fast food..30
4. Do increase your protein intake..30
5. Do increase your sodium intake..30
6. Do be patient...31

Important Tips for Successful Ketogenic Journey..31

1. Gradually follow the ketogenic diet..31
2. Drink plenty of water...31
3. Turn your favorite foods into ketogenic foods..32
4. Don't be afraid to ask for advice...32
5. Be alert of alcohol consumption...32
6. Be mindful of condiments and sauces...32
7. Be patient..32
8. Use vitamins and mineral salts...33
9. Restock your fridge and pantry...33

What Foods Should Be on Your Plate?..33

Vegetables..33
Proteins...35
Fats and Oils...35
Fruits...36

What Foods Should not be on Your Plate?...36

Root Vegetables...36
Sweet Fruits..36
Grains...36
Diet Soda...37
Alcohol..37
Processed Foods...37

Chapter 3: Breakfast Recipes...38

The Early Morning Veggie Hash Brown..38

Sicilian Cauliflower Roast Crunch..38

Heartfelt Spinach Quiche...38

Breakfast Broccoli Casserole...39

Creamy Early Morning Asparagus Soup...39

Good-Day Pumpkin Puree..40

Amazing Bacon And Veggie Delight...40

Hearty Broccoli And Scrambled Cheese Breakfast..40

Original Onion And Scrambled Tofu..41

Contents

Introduction..13

Chapter 1: Understanding the Fundamentals Of Ninja Foodi..15

What is Ninja Foodi?...15

The differences between Ninja Foodi and Instant Pot/Slow Cooker/Air Fryer.....15

Understanding the Revolutionary Tendercrisp Technology............................16

Looking at the different function buttons of the Ninja Foodi........................16

The different parts and accessories of the Ninja Foodi..................................19

Amazing advantages of the Ninja Foodi...20

Useful Tips for Success..21

FAQ's..22

Chapter 2: Everything About the Ketogenic Diet........................24

What is the Ketogenic Diet?...24

Benefits of the Ketogenic Diet..24

    1. Weight Loss...25
    2. Diminish Your Appetite..25
    3. Decrease Blood Pressure..25
    4. Improve Your HDL Cholesterol...25
    5. Improve Digestion...26
    6. Reduce Triglycerides...26
    7. Increase Energy..26
    8. Improve Mental Health...26

Lose Weight Faster with the Ketogenic Diet than Other Diets......................26

What Happens to Your Body Under the Ketogenic Diet?..............................27

    1. Ketogenic Flu..27
    2. Temporary Fatigue...28
    3. Bad Breath...28
    4. Leg Cramps..28
    5. Headaches..29
    6. Difficulty Sleeping..29
    7. Constipation...29

Dos and Don'ts of Ketogenic Diet..29

    1. Don't increase your carb intake...29

© Copyright 2020 -All rights reserved.

Legal Notice: This book is copyright protected. This is only for personal use. You cannot amend, distribute, sell, use, quote or paraphrase any part or the content within this book without the consent of the author or copyright owner. Legal action will be pursued if this is breached.

The information provided herein is stated to be truthful and consistent, in that any liability, regarding inattention or otherwise, by any usage or abuse of any policies, processes, or directions contained within is the solitary and complete responsibility of the recipient reader. Under no circumstances will any legal liability or blame be held against the publisher for any reparation, damages, or monetary loss due to the information herein, either directly or indirectly.

MW01568535

700 Ninja Foodi Keto Diet Cookbook 2020

The Complete Guide to Keto Ninja Foodi Diet Cooking Book, Have 700 Simple Quick Ninja Foodi Recipes, Lose Your Weight Fast and Never Let It Back

Laurel Andrews